EMT-B
National Standards
Self-Test

Third Edition

MS. CHARLY D. MILLER, Paramedic

Emergency Medical Services
Educator/Author/Consultant

Based on the
The 1994 Emergency Medical Technician-Basic
National Standard Curriculum
as set forth by the
U.S. Department of Transportation,
National Highway Traffic Safety Administration

and

The 2010 American Heart Association
Guidelines for Cardiopulmonary Resuscitation
and Emergency Cardiovascular Care Science
(*Circulation*, Volume 122, Issue 18 Supplement:
November 2, 2010

PEARSON

Prentice
Hall

Upper Saddle River, New Jersey 07458

Library of Congress Cataloging-in-Publication Data

Miller, C. D. (Charly D.)
  EMT-B national standards self-test / Charly D. Miller.-- 3rd ed.
     p. ; cm.
  "Based on the the 1994 Emergency Medical Technician-Basic National Standard
Curriculum as set forth by the U.S. Department of Transportation, National Highway
Traffic Safety Administration."
  "Answer-key reference-pages provided for: Brady's Emergency Care, 10th Edition, (c)
2005; Brady's Prehospital Emergency Care, 7th Edition, (c) 2004."
  ISBN 0-13-170787-6
  1. Emergency medicine--Examinations, questions, etc. 2. Emergency medical
technicians--Examinations, questions, etc.
  [DNLM: 1. Emergencies--Examination Questions. 2. Emergency Medical Services--
Examination Questions. 3. Emergency Medical Technicians--education--Examination
Questions. WB 18.2 M647e 2006] I. Mistovich, Joseph J. Prehospital emergency care.
7th ed. II. United States. National Highway Traffic Safety Administration. III.
Emergency care. 10th ed. IV. Title.
  RC86.9.M54 2006
  616.02'5'076--dc22   2005017474

Publisher: Julie Levin Alexander
Publisher's Assistant: Regino Bruno
Executive Editor: Marlene McHugh Pratt
Senior Managing Editor for Development: Lois Berlowitz
Editorial Assistant: Matthew Sirinides
Director of Marketing: Karen Allman
Executive Marketing Manager: Katrin Beacom
Senior Channel Marketing Manager: Rachele Strober
Marketing Coordinator: Michael Sirinides
Director of Production and Manufacturing: Bruce Johnson
Managing Editor for Production: Patrick Walsh
Production Liaison: Faye Gemmellaro
Production Editor: Mark Corsey, nSight, Inc.
Manufacturing Manager: Ilene Sanford
Manufacturing Buyer: Pat Brown
Senior Design Coordinator: Christopher Weigand
Cover Design: Kevin Kall
Composition: Laserwords
Printing and Binding: Command Web
Cover Printer: Phoenix Color

Pearson Education Ltd.
Pearson Education Singapore, Pte. Ltd.
Pearson Education Canada, Ltd.
Pearson Education—Japan
Pearson Education Australia Pty., Limited
Pearson Education North Asia Ltd.
Pearson Educación de Mexico, S.A. de C.V.
Pearson Education Malaysia, Pte. Ltd.
Pearson Education Upper Saddle River, NJ

Notice: The author and the publisher of this book have taken care to make certain that the information given is correct and compatible with the standards generally accepted at the time of publication. Nevertheless, as new information becomes available, changes in treatment and in the use of equipment and procedures become necessary. The reader is advised to carefully consult the instruction and information material included in each piece of equipment or device before administration. Students are warned that the use of any techniques must be authorized by their medical advisor, where appropriate, in accordance with local laws and regulations. The author and the publisher disclaim any liability, loss, injury, or damage incurred as a consequence, directly or indirectly, of the use and application of any of the contents of this book.

Studentaid.ed.gov the U.S. Department of Education's website on college planning assistance, is a valuable tool for anyone intending to pursue higher education. Designed to help students at all stages of schooling, including international students, returning students, and parents, it is a guide to the financial aid process. The website presents information on applying to and attending college as well as on funding your education and repaying loans. It also provides links to useful resources, such as state education agency contact information, assistance in filling out financial aid forms, and an introduction to various forms of student aid.

16 15 14 13 12 11 10

0-13-170787-6

Contents

Drug and Alcohol Abuse

Dual Lumen Airways

Eye Injuries

Glasgow Coma Scale, Revised Trauma Score, Apgar Score

Head and Spine Injuries

Inhaled and Injected Poisonings

Medical Terminology

TEST SECTION TEN (AN *ELECTIVE SECTION*)   **289**

ADVANCED AIRWAY MANAGEMENT

(75 questions; 1 hour and 15 minutes allotted for completion.)

Airway Anatomy Review (repeated per DOT emphasis)

Adult Orotracheal Intubation

Pediatric Orotracheal Intubation

Endotracheal Tube Suctioning

Nasogastric Tube Insertion

TEST SECTION ELEVEN (AN *ELECTIVE SECTION*)   **307**

ALS-ASSIST SKILLS

(40 questions; 40 minutes allotted for completion.)

Assisting with Endotracheal Intubation

Assisting with ECG Application and Use

Assisting with IV Therapy

APPENDIX:

Acknowledgments

I continue to be extremely grateful for, and deeply appreciative of, the extraordinary Brady editors I have worked with throughout the years: Natalie Anderson, Susan B. Katz, Judy Streger, and Marlene Pratt. Most importantly, Brady's remarkable staff of sales reps and marketing folks are the "best evah"!

I gratefully acknowledge the efforts expended and the valuable feedback provided by the following reviewers of my manuscript:

Liza Burrill, Education Coordinator, NH DOS Bureau of EMS, Berlin, NH

Bruce L. Gadol, NREMT, CCT EMS, I/C NRMA, Director of Education, Emergency Medical Training Institute, School of EMS and Allied Health Medicine, Miami, Florida

Bill Locke, EMS Instructor/Coordinator, Moraine Park Technical College, Fond du Lac, Wisconsin

Estevan Pacheco, NREMT-B, EMT-T, B.S., Program Director for EMS Programs, Education, and Training, US Naval Hospital, Okinawa, Japan

Terry Taylor II, Blockport, NY

Donald L. Whitely, Jr., B.A., NREMT-P, Manager, Training & Certification, SC DHEC Division of EMS, Columbia, SC

Next: James J. Wohlers is an incredibly talented and well-educated paramedic firefighter in Grand Island, Nebraska. I met JJ back in the '90s when we both were working as "Denver General" paramedics. JJ has been helping me in many aspects of the educational and Expert Witness work I've done since I "left the streets" in 1998. And, now he's helping me with my Brady self-test textbooks. **BLESS YOU, JJ!**

Lastly, to my parents, Ray and Carol Miller (and all my "sibling-units"), I extend a resounding, "Thank you for all you've done for me!!!"

Ms. Charly D. Miller

About the Author

Charly D. Miller is a nationally known Emergency Medical Services author, instructor, and consultant who lives in Lincoln, Nebraska. A paramedic since 1985 (including nine years as a Denver General paramedic, in Denver, Colorado), Charly is a seasoned prehospital emergency care provider. With her additional experience as a psychiatric medical technician (in the '70s) and an Army National Guard combat helicopter medic, Charly is one of the United States' most exciting and entertaining EMS educators.

Charly specializes in the following educational and consultation topics:

"All Tied Up & No Place To Go": Patient Restraint Issues, Safe & Effective Techniques

"Restraint Asphyxia—Silent Killer": Understanding & Avoiding Restraint-Related Positional Asphyxia

"Because I Said So!": Patient Communication Techniques

"Need The Info!": Patient Interview Techniques

In addition to this text, Charly's other Brady-published texts include the *Paramedic National Standards Self-Test*, 5th Edition, and (as lead co-author) *Taigman's Advanced Cardiology (In Plain English)*.

Charly has been a contributing author for several EMS magazines, including the *Journal of Emergency Medicine (JEMS)*, and the Internet EMS Webzine, *MERGInet.com*.

To learn more about Charly or to contact her, visit her Website at: ***www.charlydmiller.com***.

About This Text

Dear EMT,

This text was written *by* an EMT (and EMS Educator), specifically *for* EMTs. It was designed to assist you in your preparation for, and execution of, *any* EMT-Basic written examination. Specifically written to challenge you and to help you identify subjects requiring additional study, this text will also significantly improve your skill at reading and responding to "tricky" test questions.

Many new "Case-Based Scenario questions" have been added to this 3rd Edition. Also, many of the questions in the previous edition have been replaced or rewritten.

The majority of questions and answers presented in this text remain based upon the 1994 EMT-Basic National Standard Curriculum as set forth by the National Highway Traffic Safety Administration's Department of Transportation (DOT). Many of the original 3rd edition's questions and answers were affected by the changes recommended within the "Guidelines for Cardiopulmonary Resuscitation and Emergency Cardiovascular Care," published in the December 2010 edition of the American Heart Association's journal, *Circulation*. This updated 3rd edition has corrected those questions and answers.

Every test section's Answer Key identifies each question's subject, in addition to providing reference page numbers that correspond to the following Brady texts:

- *Emergency Care*, 10th Edition Update, © 2007
- *Prehospital Emergency Care*, 8th Edition, © 2008
- EMT Complete: A Basic Worktext, © 2007

If you don't have access to these Brady textbooks, simply use the question's subject to search the index of the texts you *do* have access to, in order to obtain information on the subjects you have difficulty with. PDF files of *Circulation*'s special 2010 AHA Guidelines supplement are freely available on the World Wide Web. If you wish to obtain them, go to: http://circ.ahajournals.org/ Click on the "Circulation Supplements" link. Then, click on the link to Circulation, Volume 122, Issue 18 Supplement: November 2, 2010

The questions in this text are designed to be more demanding than average test questions. If you can pass each of these eleven self-test sections with a score of 90% or better, you will easily achieve a significantly higher score on your actual written exam.

Be sure to read the "**How To Use This Text**" section. These directions will help you use this text to your greatest advantage. All too frequently, EMTs fail written tests only because they haven't developed good test-taking skills, because they haven't learned how to carefully read test questions, or because they haven't reviewed critical information. Used as suggested, this text will enable you to avoid failure for any of those reasons.

Also, be sure to read my "**Suggestions for Written Examination Preparation and Execution**." This section provides important tips for mental and physical preparation before taking any actual written exam. Again, all too frequently, EMTs fail written tests even when they know the material, because they haven't developed good test-taking skills.

Lastly, I strongly suggest that you read my "**Suggestions for Practical Examination Preparation and Execution**." EMTs who operate with exceptional competency in the "real world" often fail practical (situational) examinations, because they were ill-prepared to successfully perform in the simulated-emergency testing environment. This text will help you excel during the written exam. However, your performance during practical exams is also vitally important to your successful certification or recertification.

I sincerely hope that this text assists you to excel in your examination.

I *do not* wish you "Good Luck!" Luck is simply not a consideration when it comes to successful test-taking, either written or practical. Your dedicated preparation and review are the only factors that will help you to achieve the high scores you seek.

Sincerely yours,

Ms. Charly D. Miller

www.charlydmiller.com

How to Use This Book

This "self-test" book was developed to help you determine the strengths and weaknesses of your knowledge base, to help you determine the subjects you have difficulty with (the subjects you should especially study), and to help you practice your written test-taking skills. Here are some important suggestions for using this book, so that you do better when taking your practice (and actual) exams:

Read each question carefully. Knowledgeable and experienced EMTs often fail written exams simply because they don't read the questions thoroughly.

- *Pay very close attention to the kind of answer the question requires.* Is the question asking you to identify a correct or "true" answer, an incorrect or "false" answer? Is the phrase "except for" contained in the question?
- *Do not read more into the question or the answers than what is presented.* Do not ask, "Well, what if . . .?" Each question and its answer options (whether it's a basic-information question or a scenario-based question) clearly present all the "clues" you need to select the correct answer—if you know the subject.

Read all the answer options carefully.

- *Does there seem to be more than one correct answer?* If so, you must consider all the answer options against each other, and use the answer option that is "most correct." For instance, is there a multiple-answer option; such as "(d) Answers (a) and (c)"?

  After selecting the answer you think is "most correct," go back and reread the question, inserting that answer (or each of the multiple-answer option selections).

- *Does the answer option you selected still seem correct?* If not, or if you're not sure, you should review this question's subject. Circle this question's answer sheet number lightly, in pencil, so you'll be reminded to review it later.

Do not guess when you don't know the answer! When taking an actual written exam, a guess is always better than an unanswered question (unanswered questions are always an "error"). However, when practicing with Self-Tests, do not guess! If you guess on a Self-Test, you may correctly answer the question purely by accident, and thus you'll not be reminded to review that subject. Without review, when answering a similar question on an actual exam, there is no guarantee that you'll make the same, accidentally correct, guess. When practicing with Self-Tests, if you cannot answer a question with confidence, circle that question's answer sheet number, skip it, and move on. Later, your circled question number will cue you to review the subject identified by the Answer Key.

The Self-Test Answer Key is your "structured review guide."
When you have completed each Self-Test section, compare your answers to the Answer Key provided in the Appendix of this text. Note the reference page numbers or subjects for each question you skipped or answered incorrectly. Go to the referenced texts or the EMT text you have and review that subject's material. Then, retake the Self-Test. If you again encounter difficulty with one or more subjects, repeat your review. The more often you repeat this process, the better you will fare on the actual examination.

Time yourself as you take the Self-Tests.   Most examinations allow one minute per question. For instance: 60 questions = a one-hour time limit; 120 questions = a two-hour time limit; 180 questions = a three-hour time limit; and so on.

- Timed practice sessions help you learn to improve your test-taking speed.
- This 3rd Edition consists of 11 Test Sections, containing a total of 1,285 questions. If you use each Test Section even only once, you will have accomplished over 21 hours of test-taking practice!

Use group study sessions.   During the weeks before the test, get together with coworkers or friends who are taking the same exam and study as a group, especially in preparation for practical examinations. "Teaching" is a great way to "learn."

Suggestions for Written Examination Preparation and Execution

Most of us consider written examinations about as delightful as a tooth extraction accomplished without the use of anesthetic! However, when taking a written examination, anesthesia is entirely inappropriate and unhelpful. As long as you've prepared well, you'll do well!

Test preparation should start long before exam day. First, read the "**How To Use This Text**" section, if you haven't already. Then, using this Self-Test text, determine your strengths and weaknesses, study the subjects you have difficulty with, and practice your test-taking skills.

TEST-DAY PREPARATION TIPS

Get a good night's sleep before taking the actual test. Losing sleep by furiously studying the night before an exam is sure to cause you more harm than good. Even if you've delayed your review and can't avoid last-minute studying, you still need to get plenty of sleep before the exam!

Go to bed earlier than usual on the night before, and then get up early enough to study on the morning of the test. Or, if you are one of those "night shift" people who cannot think efficiently in the early morning hours, take a good, long nap the previous afternoon or evening. Then study into the wee hours of the morning, and take another nap before the test.

Eat a good breakfast on Test Day. Contrary to popular EMT behavior (of all certification levels), a good breakfast does not consist of coffee and donuts. The donut's sugar-energy burst will quickly peak, thereafter resulting in a rebound lethargy, perhaps during the time of the test. The coffee's caffeine provides artificial stimulation but does not improve your concentration or mental acuity.

Whether or not you adopt good nutritional habits in your normal day-to-day living, it will be a great advantage for you to do so just prior to an event as stressful and demanding as a written or practical examination. A good meal (breakfast or lunch), high in complex carbohydrates and protein, eaten before the exam is the key to fueling the sustained energy levels and mental acuity you'll need during the high-stress test situation. Complex carbohydrates are found in things like fresh fruits and juices, whole-grain breads, or rice products. Lean meats, eggs, and milk products (yogurt, cheeses, and low-fat milk) are good sources of protein.

Allow yourself at least one hour between a good meal and the test time.   An important point to remember is that immediately after a meal, a large proportion of your body's blood supply is diverted from your brain to your stomach, to aid in food digestion. If you follow this recommendation, during the test your brain will be fueled slowly and efficiently, helping you perform at your absolute best.

TIPS FOR TAKING THE ACTUAL WRITTEN EXAMINATION

Remember: Read each question carefully.   Is the question asking you to identify a correct or "true" answer, an incorrect or "false" answer, or the "best" answer? Don't read more into the question or answers that is stated. Avoid "what ifs" when considering your answer. Each question (or case scenario), and the answer options provided, should clearly present all the "clues" you need to select the correct answer.

Read each answer option carefully.   Then, after making your selection, go back and reread the question, inserting that answer. Does your answer still seem correct? If not, try another answer. If you're unsure, consider skipping the question (lightly circling the answer sheet's question number) and coming back to it later.

Budget your test-taking time.   Do not dwell upon any question that you can't confidently and quickly answer. Spending too much time on one difficult or confusing question gives you less time to answer questions you can confidently, correctly, and quickly complete. Skip any troublesome question and come back to it later. By doing so, even if you run out of time before completing the entire test, you've confidently answered the maximum number of questions you possibly can.

When you skip a question, LIGHTLY circle (in pencil) its question number on your answer sheet.   Test proctors will strongly warn you against making any "unnecessary stray marks or erasures" on your answer sheet. This is because, on answer forms designed to be scored by computers, "unnecessary stray marks" or print damage caused by heavy "erasures" can cause interpretation errors that might result in correct answers being counted as wrong answers!

However, when you skip a question, you *must* be sure to *also skip that question's answer sheet selection.* It is far better to lightly circle the number of a skipped question's answer set than to cause all subsequent questions to be incorrectly answered because you accidentally lost your place on the answer sheet. So, when circling a skipped question number, do it lightly and avoid crossing over any of the form's print.

Make sure that you gently, but completely, erase all "stray" marks or circles before submitting your completed answer sheet. When erasing pencil marks, erase them completely but GENTLY, so that you avoid dimming or blurring any of the answer sheet's print. Again, any stray marks or computerized answer form print damage may cause computer interpretation errors that might count correct answers as wrong answers.

As a last resort, GUESS—but only after you've "come back" to a skipped question. An unanswered question is always counted as an incorrect answer. If you can't confidently (and quickly) answer a question, lightly circle its answer sheet number and come back to it later. Sometimes, subsequent questions or answer options will help you recognize the correct answer to a skipped question! Even if that is not the case, it is best not to "dwell" upon a question you can't confidently and quickly answer. Move on.

Once you've been through the entire test and have answered all the questions you are confident of, go back to your skipped questions. If you're still in doubt, make your best guess; a guess is always better than no answer!

What about case-based questions? Sometimes, medics with little "field" experience approach case-based "scenario" questions with extreme self-doubt and trepidation. Such worry is completely unnecessary! "Field" experience has very little to do with correctly answering written test questions, whether they are "straight" informational questions, or case-based "scenario" questions.

Case-based "scenario" questions simply test your ability to integrate your training and knowledge when considering situational information, as provided to you by the test questions. They test how well you are able to solve mysteries, given a limited amount of information. Approach case-based "scenario" questions with confidence, and play "EMS Detective." You have the knowledge that is being tested, but you are not "running a call." You're simply figuring out a mystery, based only upon the information provided by the test questions.

SUMMARY

Structured review, adequate rest, and efficient nutrition will give you an undeniable advantage and vastly improve your performance in any testing situation. Following the tips I've provided will help you confidently answer the greatest number of questions possible, in the shortest amount of time. After that, return to the questions that require more thought (or a guess). Once you get to the "return" point, simply relax and have faith in yourself! You've already done well!

Suggestions for Practical Examination Preparation and Execution

Throughout your entire EMS career, you will periodically be subjected to the dreaded "practical skills," "assessment," or "situational" examination stations. Practical examinations accompany all levels of EMS training courses, local and state certification and recertification tests, and all National Registry examinations. More and more often, practical examinations also accompany continuing education workshops or courses (such as Advanced Cardiac Life Support or Pre-Hospital Trauma Life Support).

However, sometimes even the most "veteran" EMS providers tremble in their boots when faced with the ordeal of performing in the practical examination environment. There may be a number of reasons for this trepidation, including the following:

- A written test evaluates only your medical knowledge and test-question/answer-reading skills. A practical examination places your medical knowledge, your equipment-use skills, and your physical performance under the strictest scrutiny. It's unnerving to be so closely observed and evaluated, especially when failure to "pass" and obtain certification threatens your livelihood!
- Even the most elaborately recreated practical examination simulations contain situational components that you must recognize and remember, without actually seeing, feeling, hearing, or smelling them.
- You may be facing the practical exam station alone, or you may be teamed with people you have never worked with before.
- The equipment you are given is rarely, if ever, presented in a manner you are accustomed to dealing with. Consequently, you may fumble around, hunting for instruments that, in a "real-life" situation, your hands would normally find on their own.

Often, the equipment is of a different brand, make, or model than what you're familiar with using.

- In addition to all of the above problems, in their effort to remain unbiased and objective, even the friendliest practical examination evaluators often appear cold, or even hostile.

Throughout my years of EMS service, I've participated in practical examinations as a test-taker, a "patient," and an evaluator. From these experiences, I've developed several suggestions for how to dramatically diminish your trepidation and significantly improve your performance on practical examinations.

PREPARING FOR A PRACTICAL EXAMINATION

Periodic practice and review are essential. Regardless of the volume or variety of calls you've experienced, it is imperative that you remain skilled at operating all EMS equipment, that you frequently refresh your knowledge of patient assessment and treatment protocols, and that you especially refresh your knowledge of skills performance prior to performing in a practical examination situation.

We all know that "real-life" situations often require us to deviate from, alter, or augment any "established" order of skills performance. But, in the practical examination situation, following a precise order of assessment or skills performance has a significant effect upon how you're scored. Even though you complete every individual step, if the order in which you complete the steps deviates from the established order of skills performance, your score will be diminished. Thus, to prepare for a practical examination, you must memorize the precise order of assessment and skills performance steps required for each station. Any testing authority's performance-order requirements should be available to you for study purposes. (In the Appendix of this text, you will find copies of the skills station score sheets used by the National Registry of EMTs.) Get them. Memorize them. Practice following them!

Prior to the practical examination, get together with a small group of your peers and practice the skills, using the performance-order guidelines you are provided. Take turns being an examination evaluator, a "patient," and a skills performer. Experience in all three of these roles is enormously helpful in developing your awareness of common performance mistakes, and in training yourself to avoid these common mistakes.

APPROACHING THE PRACTICAL EXAMINATION

Remember the notes about sleep and nutrition from my "**Suggestions for Written Examination Preparation and Execution**." Get a lot of rest before the exam. Also, whether or not you adopt good nutrition in your normal day-to-day living, it will be a great advantage for you to do so just prior to an event as stressful as a practical examination. A breakfast or lunch high in complex carbohydrates and protein is key to fueling the sustained energy levels you'll need during such high-stress situations.

Also remember to time your pretest meal so that you have at least an hour to "digest" it before the time of the practical examination. By doing so, your body will be sending energy and nutrients to your brain (rather than to your stomach) during the time of your practical examination performance.

PERFORMING IN THE PRACTICAL EXAMINATION

"Dress for Success!"   Your goal should be to clothe and equip yourself in a manner that makes you feel as "normal" and comfortable as possible, a manner that will help make your surroundings as familiar as possible.

Actually changing into your uniform before performing in the practical examination is ideal. This may appear "gung-ho" to others, but those others are not grading your performance. (They may laugh right up until the moment when they discover how far you out-performed them in the practical examination! Then, who'll have the "last laugh"?!)

At the very least, wear your own equipment holster and pants with "cargo pockets." That way, vital and frequently used items such as scissors, penlight, pens, etc., will be found precisely where you are used to finding them. Your own stethoscope ought to be draped, strapped, or tucked-into wherever it is usually draped, strapped, or tucked-into.

Indeed, if you have a personal emergency care equipment kit that you routinely use, bring it and request permission to use it!

Again, your goal is to clothe and equip yourself in a manner that makes you feel as "normal" and comfortable as possible, making your surroundings as familiar as possible. This will enormously improve your performance in any practical examination.

SPECIFIC PERFORMANCE RULES FOR "ASSESSMENT" OR "SITUATIONAL" PRACTICAL EXAMINATIONS

Practical examinations involving the utilization or application of a single piece of emergency care equipment are relatively easy to prepare for and perform in. The greatest challenge to any EMS provider is the "Assessment" or "Scenario" practical examination station. To improve your performance in these exams, the most vital "secret for success" is to train yourself in some specific ways of approaching and performing in them. Based upon my experience as an "Assessment" or "Scenario" practical examination EVALUATOR, here are my suggestions for SUCCESS:

- **As you begin the practical examination, fix your EYES and your ATTENTION *only* upon the evaluator.** When you first enter the station and the evaluator is giving you an "introduction," do not preoccupy yourself with "eyeballing" the patient or scene, thinking you'll get "a head start" on the situation. Good listening requires complete concentration. Eyeballing the patient or scene will significantly distract you from hearing (and processing) the evaluator's introductory information, causing you to miss important details! Upon entering the station, fix your eyes and your attention on the evaluator, and concentrate entirely upon the instructions and information she/he is providing you.

- **When the evaluator describes the situation and scene, be especially alert for indications of the mechanism of injury, or the nature of illness, or descriptions of the scene itself—things that *cannot be simulated*.** If you are told that the steering wheel is bent, that the windshield fractured, or that items of furniture are broken, this information is given to you for a reason. Take time to consider these important clues.

- **If this type of information is not offered, ask for it.** Scene size-up is important to every call, and important to every practical examination station. Ask the evaluator questions like: "What is the condition of the apartment? Is it tidy? Messy? What does it smell like? What does the car look like? Where was the point of impact, and where was the patient sitting? Is there compartmental intrusion involving the patient's space? What does the patient look like on my approach?" and so on.

- **If you are offered time to examine the available equipment before your evaluation begins, *DO IT!*** Even if you don't think you need to, carefully look at all the equipment provided, especially if anything differs from equipment you are accustomed to using. Arrange the equipment in a manner that is familiar to you. Certainly, do not leave it in a messy pile at the corner of the room or beside the patient! Use the entire time offered to become as familiar as possible with the equipment provided, and to rearrange it so that you know where everything is. (Remember the old rule of "take your pulse first!" when responding to an emergency call? Anyone who discounts this rule is a fool. Whenever you're offered time to do something, take the entire amount of time offered and do it. At the very least, this will give you time to let your anxiety-driven adrenalin burst wear off, so that you can function at your best.)

- **As you are directed to actually begin your performance, no matter what the situation is, the first question you should voice is, "*Is the scene safe?*"** In real life, you can usually sense potential dangers on approach. You can see smoke, smell a gas leak, hear a domestic altercation, or observe that the police have not yet arrived. Practical examinations are rarely able to simulate such normally apparent indications of danger. So, when beginning the practical examination, the very first words out of your mouth should be, "Is the scene safe?" It is important to verbalize this consideration, to let the evaluator know that you are considering it.

- **FROM THIS MOMENT ON, THERE IS NO LONGER ANY REASON FOR YOU TO LOOK AT THE EVALUATOR!** This is very, very important. Continually glancing at the evaluator and then back at the patient is extremely distracting. It interrupts both your concentration and the continuity of your performance. After the introductory and scene information has been provided by the evaluator, and you've begun your patient assessment and care, your eyes and hands should never leave the patient and the simulated environment, except to obtain equipment. The evaluator does not need to see your face to answer your questions! She/he can listen to what you say, respond to your questions, and watch your skills performance without ever having eye contact with you.

- **Never stop talking.** Whether you are questioning the evaluator, addressing or questioning the patient, or describing your thoughts and actions, you should never stop talking. Frequently, even the best evaluators fail to observe the SILENT performance of skills because they are busy making notes on a performance score sheet. If you aren't verbalizing your every single thought or activity while the evaluator is making notes, she/he may miss things such as your initial pulse check, or your sweep of the patient's clothing to detect gross bleeding. Thus, even though you performed something, if you did it SILENTLY, you might not be credited for doing so. However, if you verbalize every single thing you do, verbalize everything you are thinking, you will be credited with all the activities and skills you are performing, whether or not the evaluator actually "observes" your performance.

- **Continuously talk to your patient.** This may sound difficult (or weird), but it is easily combined with the previous suggestion. Focus your attention on the patient, and tell the patient about everything you are thinking and doing. Not only will this help to alert the evaluator to what you are doing and thinking (preventing the evaluator from "missing" anything), it will help to keep YOU calm, and increase the effectiveness of your performance in the practical examination. (Oddly enough, this works to keep YOU calm in "real-life" situations, too!) Address ALL your questions, explanations, and descriptions to the patient. The evaluator should provide you with any information that the patient is unable to verbalize in response to your direct questions; thus you'll not need to disrupt your concentration by looking at the evaluator to receive this information!

- **Ask for information.** If the patient doesn't exhibit or give you the answers you need, the evaluator should provide the information. If the evaluator doesn't volunteer the information, it's because she/he is waiting for you to ask for it. Again, you should not break your eye contact with the patient to ask for information! The evaluator is in the same room. She/he can respond to your questions without you having to look at her/him.

The following is a written example of what a successful practical examination performance should *sound like*. Except for the first couple of cues, only the medic being tested (the performer) can be "heard."

Evaluator: You may begin.

Performer: Is the scene safe?

Evaluator: The scene is safe.

Performer: I am observing the scene as I approach. Is the mechanism of injury apparent?

I can see that my patient has some blood on his left thigh. Is the blood spurting as though it is an arterial bleed? It's not? Good.

First, I place my hand on his head and assess his level of consciousness.

Sir? Sir? Can you hear me?

Hi. My name is Mork. I'm a medic and I'm here to help you. I need you to stay very still and not move your head, please. Thank you!

What's your name?

Great, Endor, thank you. Any pain in your neck as I run my fingers down it, Endor?

My invisible partner, Mindy, is going to hold your head to help you keep it absolutely still while I examine you. She will not stop holding your head until we have secured you to a long backboard.

First, I'd like to check your airway. I'm going to look inside your mouth and make sure everything's cool there. Anything loose or bothering you in there, Endor?

Good. How does your breathing feel?

When I listen to Endor's chest with this stethoscope, what do I hear?

How does your chest feel, Endor? How about when I compress it, like this?

It feels even in excursion, and I don't feel any crepitus. I don't see any wounds or deformities.

Endor, my invisible partner, Mindy, will observe your airway and respiratory effort as she continues to maintain immobilization of your c-spine—that's your neck—and she'll alert me to any changes while I examine you further.

I'm going to check your pulses now, Endor. Do I feel Endor's radial pulse?

What quality and rate do I feel?

Is Endor sweaty?

What's Endor's skin color?

Temperature?

Endor, I'm going to give you some oxygen to help you feel better. This mask may seem a little confining, but I'm going to run oxygen into it at fifteen liters per minute, and it will help you feel much, much better.

YES: An evaluator could be scoring this medic's performance over the TELEPHONE!

A continuous narration of your thoughts and activities, whether delivered to your patient or to the evaluator (while still focusing on the patient), assists your score in a number of ways. It keeps you focused on the situation and your task performance, improves your mental concentration, and ensures that you proceed without forgetting things. It also helps to calm you and improve your physical performance. Most importantly, though, verbalizing everything you do and think will make it almost impossible for the evaluator to miss the things you have done, even if she/he doesn't actually see your performance of something.

PARTNERED OR GROUP APPROACHES TO A PRACTICAL EXAMINATION

All of the previous suggestions apply here as well. However, now you are teamed with one or more other participants—people who may have been total strangers only moments before the practical examination. The old adage, "Too many cooks spoil the broth," applies here in quadruplicate. Few things are as debilitating and disastrous as having two, three, or four EMTs crawling all over each other, each trying to treat the patient and "run the call" at the same time.

The secret to group success is organization and assignment of tasks. Each group member must have an assigned role, with one group leader assigned to be in charge of directing the entire group's performance. Obviously, these assignments must be made and agreed upon before the group enters the practical examination station. And, as each new station is approached, the roles should be clearly reassigned, allowing each participant an opportunity to rotate through each different role.

Groups of Two are Easy. For trauma practical examinations, one partner is the group leader, and the other is the c-spine/airway monitor. The group leader introduces self and partner, directing the partner to maintain immobilization of the c-spine continuously and to monitor for changes in airway status after the initial airway/ breathing examination. The group leader continues examination of the patient and performs all other necessary treatments. The group leader is also the team member in charge of verbalizing all the activities.

The c-spine/airway monitor maintains spinal immobilization and observes airway/respiratory status, no matter how tempted she/he is to help with other treatment. While doing so, (unless prohibited from "cuing" the group leader by the evaluator), she/he should provide verbal cues whenever the group leader appears to have forgotten something.

For medical practical examinations, one partner is the group leader, and the other is the airway monitor/equipment operator. The airway monitor/equipment operator's primary task is to manage oxygen equipment and delivery. If the patient does not require active airway maintenance and ventilation, this person is free to take vital signs, apply the ECG monitor (if available), start IVs, position the wheeled stretcher, and so on.

The group leader is still responsible for patient examination and assessment. However, when the airway monitor is free to also be an equipment operator, the group leader should direct the application of treatments, periodically participating in equipment operation.

Groups of three responders can be broken down into assignments of group leader, c-spine/airway monitor, and equipment operator.

Groups of four responders can be broken down into assignments of group leader, c-spine immobilizer, airway monitor, and equipment operator. If continued airway maintenance is not required, the airway monitor may also act as a secondary equipment operator (yet never forgetting to watch the airway).

If you have the misfortune of operating in a team consisting of five or more members, send all but four team members to direct traffic, boil water, anything to get them out of the way!

The most important key to group performance, no matter how you designate the tasks or roles, is that the assignments (responsibilities) are clearly understood by each member before you begin the practical examination.

IN SUMMARY

A brief recap of the essential points to remember for the practical examination:

- **Wear your uniform, and bring your own equipment holster, stethoscope, and jump-kit if you have them and regularly work with them!** Make the practical examination's environment as comfortable and familiar as you possibly can.
- **As you first enter the station, fix your eyes and attention only upon the evaluator.** Carefully listen to the clues provided by the evaluator. Take all of the time you are offered to consider the clues. Ask for any and all scene or situation information if it

is not offered. If you're offered time to check the available equipment before starting the exam, do it.

- **Ask, out loud, "Is the scene safe?"**
- **After beginning your performance, after the scene size-up, never let your eyes or hands leave the patient.** There is no need to look at the evaluator again.
- **Never stop talking.** Talk to the patient, and ask the patient ALL your questions. Verbalize everything you are doing and everything you are thinking. When asking questions of the evaluator, do not look away from the patient; the evaluator does not need your eye contact to answer you.
- **Clearly assign specific tasks to group members before beginning a group exam, and take turns with roles and task performance.**
- **When you are not the group leader, do not deviate from your assigned task.** However, if allowed, provide reminders of business that should be performed (or questions that should be asked) when the group leader seems to have forgotten something.
- **Above all, enjoy yourself!** Really. Why not? When examination day arrives, set aside your fears. Take pride in the performance level you have worked so hard to achieve. Have confidence in your abilities.

DOT Module One:
Preparatory

Subjects:

- Introduction to Emergency Medical Care
- Well-being of the EMT-Basic
- Medical/Legal and Ethical Issues
- The Human Body
- Baseline Vital signs and SAMPLE History
- Lifting and Moving Patients

Test Section One consists of 225 questions and is allotted 3 hours and 45 minutes for completion.

1.   Roles and responsibilities of an EMT include patient assessment, patient care based on assessment findings, lifting and moving, patient transportation or transfer of patient care, patient advocacy, and
     (a) personal safety.
     (b) safety of the crew and patient.
     (c) safety of bystanders.
     (d) Answers (a) and (b).
     (e) Answers (a), (b), and (c).

2.   Professional attributes of an EMT include a neat and clean appearance; knowledge of local, state, and national EMS issues; and
     (a) a pleasant personality and a positive attitude.
     (b) the ability to place the patient's needs ahead of personal safety.
     (c) attending continuing education and refresher courses.
     (d) Answers (a) and (c).
     (e) Answers (b) and (c).

3.   The definition of _____ is: A system of internal/external reviews and audits of all aspects of an EMS system so as to identify those aspects that need improvement to assure that the public receives the highest quality of prehospital care.
     (a) Quality Improvement
     (b) Medical Direction
     (c) Patient Advocacy
     (d) Any of the above.
     (e) None of the above.

4.   The definition of _____ is: A physician responsible for the clinical and patient care aspects of an EMS system. This is a requirement for every ambulance service or rescue squad.
     (a) Quality Improvement Officer
     (b) Medical Director
     (c) Patient Advocate
     (d) Any of the above.
     (e) None of the above.

5.   Quality improvement requires that an EMT attends continuing education and skills-maintenance refresher courses, gathers feedback from patients and hospital staff, attends run reviews and audits, and
     (a) documents patient contacts completely and legibly.
     (b) conducts basic maintenance on equipment to assure proper functioning.

    (c) performs patient care without deviating from care protocols without permission.

    (d) Answers (a) and (c).

    (e) Answers (a), (b), and (c).

6.   "On-line" medical direction is when care is performed according to

    (a) telephone contact instructions from the Medical Director or receiving facility during a specific call.

    (b) radio contact instructions from the Medical Director or receiving facility during a specific call.

    (c) "Standing Orders" or care protocols previously written by the Medical Director.

    (d) Answers (a) and (b).

    (e) Answers (a), (b), and (c).

7.   "Off-line" medical direction is when care is performed according to

    (a) telephone contact instructions from the Medical Director or receiving facility during a specific call.

    (b) radio contact instructions from the Medical Director or receiving facility during a specific call.

    (c) "Standing Orders" or care protocols previously written by the Medical Director.

    (d) Answers (a) and (b).

    (e) None of the above.

8.   Which of the following statements regarding EMS stress is false?

    (a) Multiple-casualty incidents (MCIs) are the only stressful events any EMT may ever have to face.

    (b) Incidents of pediatric or elderly abuse/neglect are often causes of great stress to the EMT.

    (c) Severe injuries (distortion of the human face from crushing, limb amputations, hangings, and the like) are very stressful for any prehospital provider.

    (d) Any single event may affect any EMT with profound stress, depending upon his private history or personal responses.

    (e) Personal life problems combined with stressful EMS incidents may result in a serious stress level for any EMT.

9.   Signs and symptoms of stress include irritability, inability to concentrate, indecisiveness, difficulty sleeping, and

    (a) feelings of guilt.

    (b) loss of appetite.

    (c) loss of interest in sexual activities.

    (d) Answers (a) and (b).

    (e) Answers (a), (b), and (c).

10.   All of the following lifestyle or work environment changes can be helpful in dealing
      with EMS stress, except

      (a) dietary changes: reducing intake of sugar, caffeine, alcohol, and fatty
          foods.
      (b) avoiding the embarrassment of seeking "professional" help.
      (c) requesting a duty assignment to a less busy area.
      (d) requesting work shift changes to allow extra relaxation time with family or
          friends.
      (e) safely increasing physical exercise and also learning relaxation techniques.

11.   Which of the following statements regarding Critical Incident Stress Debriefing
      (CISD) is true?

      (a) A CISD team is composed only of mental health professionals.
      (b) CISD is designed to accelerate the normal recovery process after experiencing
          a critically stressful incident.
      (c) CISD team activation is reserved for MCIs of 20 or more casualties.
      (d) CISD is only helpful if it occurs within 12 to 24 hours of the incident.
      (e) As all information shared during a CISD meeting is considered "public
          record," CISD is also a helpful method of incident investigation.

12.   Dealing with death and dying produces specific stages of reactions that are
      experienced by terminally ill or injured patients. Which of the following statements
      regarding death and dying stages is false?

      (a) These stages may occur in any order.
      (b) Some stages may be experienced simultaneously.
      (c) Some people display emotions or attitudes that don't seem to fit any of the
          "stages" of death and dying.
      (d) The dying individual's family members will experience these stages.
      (e) All patients with foreknowledge of their death experience each stage at least
          once.

13.   Death and dying response stages include all of the following, except the

      (a) bargaining stage ("If I can live, I'll never do such-and-such again."); an
          attempt to postpone death.
      (b) healing stage ("I'm feeling much better! Really!"); a sudden remission of all
          signs and symptoms of the patient's illness, often occurring immediately
          before death.
      (c) anger stage ("Why me?!"); the patient focuses anger about his impending
          death upon those around him.
      (d) denial stage ("Not me!"); a defense mechanism creating a buffer between the
          shock of dying and dealing with the illness/injury.
      (e) acceptance stage ("Well, I need to get everything in order now"); when the
          patient accepts the fact of impending death.

14. When dealing with the death of a patient, the EMT
    (a) may go through the same grief stages as the family.
    (b) may need to express feelings of guilt or helplessness.
    (c) should recognize that it is inappropriate for a professional to express personal emotions felt for the death of a stranger.
    (d) Answers (a) and (b).
    (e) Answers (a), (b), and (c).

15. Diseases are caused by _____, such as viruses and bacteria.
    (a) halogens
    (b) carcinogens
    (c) pathogens
    (d) biogens
    (e) chromogens

16. Infectious diseases may be spread by
    (a) direct contact with infected blood or other body fluids.
    (b) droplet infection from airborne organisms (coughing, sneezing, or breathing).
    (c) indirect contact via handling objects or materials contaminated with infectious secretions.
    (d) Answers (a) and (c).
    (e) Answers (a), (b), and (c).

17. Which of the following statements regarding personal protective equipment is false?
    (a) Hand washing before and after every patient contact is required only if protective gloves are not worn throughout the entire patient contact.
    (b) Protective gloves must be worn for every patient contact, and a separate pair used for each patient.
    (c) Eye protection should be worn whenever airborne droplet (or fluid splashing) contact is anticipated.
    (d) Masks should be worn whenever airborne droplet (or fluid splashing) contact is anticipated.
    (e) A gown should be worn whenever spilling or splashing of infectious fluid is anticipated.

18. Immunizations are available for EMS personnel against all the following diseases except
    (a) tetanus.
    (b) hepatitis-C.
    (c) hepatitis-B.
    (d) chickenpox.
    (e) measles.

19. Which of the following statements regarding hazardous material incidents is false?
    (a) Every ambulance should be equipped with a pair of binoculars and *The North American Emergency Response Handbook (RSPA P 5800.7)*, published by the U.S. Department of Transportation, so that hazardous material may be identified from a safe distance.
    (b) If a patient is in immediate life threat, untrained EMTs may borrow hazardous-material suits and enter the contaminated area to provide emergency patient care.
    (c) A self-contained breathing apparatus (SCBA) is required for entering any scene where poisonous gases, dust, or fumes are present or are suspected to be present.
    (d) EMTs should provide emergency care only after the patient is decontaminated.
    (e) Placards with symbols, colors, and identification numbers of hazardous materials must be displayed on all vehicles (or containers) carrying hazardous materials.

20. Rescue operations often involve potential life threats from hazards such as electricity, fire, explosion, hazardous materials, cave-ins and the like. Which of the following statements regarding hazardous rescue operations is true?
    (a) Appropriate protective clothing (such as turnout gear, puncture-proof gloves, or helmets) must be worn by any responder before engaging in a rescue operation.
    (b) An EMT's first responsibilities are to ensure personal and public safety, identify potential dangers or rescue needs, and to call for appropriate rescue teams to be dispatched.
    (c) Untrained persons must *never* attempt rescues.
    (d) Answers (a) and (b) are true.
    (e) Answers (a), (b), and (c) are true.

21. Scenes involving violence are not uncommon. Crime perpetrators, bystanders, family members, and even patients may present a personal threat to the responding EMT. Which of the following statements regarding violent scenes is true?
    (a) A potentially violent scene should be controlled by law enforcement before an EMT provides care.
    (b) EMS crews should have preplanned procedures for dealing with violence that erupts after entering the scene and should never be without radio contact.
    (c) When wearing body armor (such as a bulletproof vest) the EMT is safe, and his first responsibility is to shield the patient from further harm.
    (d) Answers (a) and (b) are true.
    (e) Answers (a), (b), and (c) are true.

22. The EMT has legal, medical, and ethical duties to his patient, public, and Medical Director. Which of the following statements regarding the EMT's *scope of practice* is false?
    (a) The *scope of practice* defines the extent and limits of an EMT's job responsibilities.
    (b) The medical skills and the interventions that an EMT is allowed to perform are defined by state legislation.

    (c) Within the limits set by state legislation, the medical skills and the interventions that an EMT is allowed to perform are defined by local protocols (as set forth by the EMT's Medical Director) and may vary from region to region within a state.

    (d) All regions within a state must share the same definition of an EMT's scope of practice, as set forth by state legislation.

    (e) Legislation about an EMT's scope of practice, skills, and intervention may vary from state to state.

23. When considered in the context of EMS, the term *battery* may be defined as

    (a) unlawfully touching a competent patient without his consent.

    (b) providing emergency care to a competent patient who does not consent to the treatment.

    (c) providing emergency care to an unconscious patient.

    (d) Answers (a) and (b).

    (e) Answers (a), (b), and (c).

24. Which of the following requirements for *expressed consent* is false?

    (a) To be effective, the patient expressing consent must be of legal age and be able to make a rational decision.

    (b) The patient must be informed of the steps of any procedure and all related risks before expressed consent will be effective.

    (c) Expressed consent must be obtained from every conscious, mentally competent adult before rendering treatment or transportation.

    (d) Explanations of treatment must be provided in terms the patient can understand before expressed consent will be effective.

    (e) Expressed consent is only required when someone other than the patient is the person who called for help.

25. Which of the following statements regarding *implied consent* is false?

    (a) If a parent or legal guardian is not present, any injured child may be treated on the basis of implied consent.

    (b) Any unconscious adult patient may be treated on the basis of implied consent.

    (c) Treatment may be provided to an unconscious patient on the basis of implied consent, even if the patient was competent and refusing treatment before becoming unconscious.

    (d) Any disoriented or confused adult who is refusing care may be treated against his will on the basis of implied consent.

    (e) To be effective, implied consent must be *informed* consent.

26. Which of the following statements regarding minors (children) and mentally incompetent adults is true?

    (a) If the patient's parent or legal guardian is present, consent for treatment must be obtained from him prior to beginning care.

    (b) Some states consider a married minor to be "emancipated," and to have the same rights of consent or refusal of treatment as adults.

    (c) Some states consider a minor who is also a parent to be "emancipated," and to have the same rights of consent or refusal of treatment as adults.

    (d) All of the above are true.

    (e) None of the above is true.

27. Which of the following statements regarding refusal of care is false?

    (a) In the United States, every patient has a right to refuse treatment or transport, regardless of age, color, sex, or mental capacity.

    (b) Treatment and transport refusals are honored only when made by mentally competent adults following the rules of expressed consent.

    (c) Every patient refusing treatment or transport must be informed of all the risks and consequences associated with such refusal, and should be able to demonstrate understanding of those risks and consequences.

    (d) Any unconscious patient who regains consciousness and demonstrates mental competency has a right to refuse further treatment or transportation.

    (e) Even if the patient signs a "release from liability" form, the EMT is *not* guaranteed freedom from liability for failing to provide treatment and transportation.

28. An EMT's best protection from liability when a patient refuses treatment or transportation is

    (a) a good EMS lawyer.

    (b) an accurate, detailed written report, describing all attempts made to obtain the patient's consent to treatment and transportation.

    (c) a more experienced partner (the most experienced provider will be blamed).

    (d) to have the police arrest the patient so that he can be treated against his will.

    (e) a "release from liability" form, signed by the patient and witnesses.

29. Which of the following statements regarding Do Not Resuscitate (DNR) orders is false?

    (a) Every mentally competent patient has the right to refuse resuscitative efforts in advance of his actual need.

    (b) Some forms of DNR orders do not require a physician's signature to be effective; the notarized or witnessed signature of the patient, or the patient's legal guardian, is sufficient.

    (c) Some forms of DNR orders stipulate only that intubation, CPR, and chemical resuscitation be withheld.

    (d) When in doubt, or when written orders are not present, the EMT should perform all possible resuscitation efforts.

    (e) If the patient is unconscious and no written orders are present, any competent immediate family member (a parent, spouse, or adult child) has the legal right to act as the patient's "health care proxy" and refuse treatment for the patient.

30. Another term for a DNR order is
  (a) a Death Wish Directive (DWD).
  (b) a dying will.
  (c) an advanced directive.
  (d) a Hold Treatment Directive (HTD).
  (e) a hospice directive.

31. For an EMT to be convicted of *negligence*, which of the following must be proven to have occurred?
  (a) The EMT had to act and provide care for the patient, but failed to do so.
  (b) The EMT performed care in a manner that deviated from his allowed scope of practice, *or* failed to perform care in a manner stipulated by his scope of practice.
  (c) The EMT's actions or inactions caused the patient to suffer physical or psychological injury.
  (d) Answers (a) and (b).
  (e) Answers (a), (b), and (c).

32. You have transferred a nursing-home resident to the emergency department (ED) for evaluation and treatment of a urinary problem. As you arrive, your dispatcher notifies you that a 911 emergency call is waiting for you. All of the ED nurses are busy, but the ED clerk (who is not a medical professional) listens to your report and assures you that she will inform the nurse. You leave the patient in the care of the clerk. Which of the following statements regarding this situation is true?
  (a) In every state of the United States, this action is viewed as abandonment.
  (b) Only some states view this action as abandonment.
  (c) Emergency calls take precedence over simple patient transfers; therefore, this is not abandonment.
  (d) Because the patient was received by the ED clerk, your transfer to the ED was legally completed; therefore, this is not abandonment.
  (e) None of the above statements is true.

33. Many states have "Good Samaritan Laws." These laws grant immunity from medical negligence prosecution to
  (a) all EMTs who are licensed or certified within that state.
  (b) all EMTs who are licensed or certified within any U.S. state.
  (c) all individuals who, in good faith, volunteer to help an injured person at the scene of an accident, even if untrained to provide medical care.
  (d) All of the above.
  (e) None of the above.

34.   Patient confidentiality rules stipulate that information obtained through the
       interview or examination of a patient may be shared with other persons
       (a) only when a written release is signed by the patient or an established legal
            guardian.
       (b) only when a verbal release is made by the patient or an established legal
            guardian.
       (c) under no circumstances.
       (d) when the patient (or established legal guardian) gives permission either in
            writing or over the telephone.
       (e) only after the patient's physician signs a Release of Information form.

35.   Exceptions to patient confidentiality rules regarding information disclosure include
       provision of information
       (a) to the health care providers who receive the patient from you and need the
            information to continue patient care.
       (b) regarding incidents that the state requires reporting of, such as sexual
            assault, child or elderly abuse or neglect.
       (c) after receiving a legal subpoena, and the court orders you to disclose the
            information.
       (d) Answers (a) and (b).
       (e) Answers (a), (b), and (c).

36.   A medical identification device is designed to provide emergency medical
       information about a patient. It may list allergies, diabetic conditions, epilepsy,
       or other pertinent medical information about the patient. Types of medical
       identification devices include information tubes kept in the refrigerator, or
       (a) a bracelet on the patient.
       (b) a necklace on the patient.
       (c) a card in the patient's wallet, pocket, or purse.
       (d) Answers (a) and (b).
       (e) Answers (a), (b), and (c).

37.   Which of the following statements regarding crime scenes and preservation of
       evidence is false?
       (a) If a crime has been committed, the EMT has a duty to preserve evidence, even
            if that means a delay in providing care to a seriously injured or ill patient.
       (b) An EMT should not touch or disturb any item at the scene unless emergency
            care requires it.
       (c) When cutting off clothing, the EMT should avoid cutting through holes made
            by gunshot wounds or stabbings.
       (d) If the police order the EMT to leave the patient in place until after photos are
            taken or evidence is collected, but the patient appears to be seriously injured
            or ill, the EMT has a duty to act against the wishes of the police by providing
            the patient with rapid treatment and transport.
       (e) An EMT should never enter a potential crime scene until after the police have
            secured it.

38. State legislation requires the reporting of special situations, which may vary from state to state. Situations that commonly require reporting include medical emergencies suspected to have resulted from all of the following except
    (a) child or elderly abuse.
    (b) acts of prostitution.
    (c) sexual assault.
    (d) gunshot or stabbing wounds.
    (e) spousal (domestic) abuse.

39. In addition to giving the body shape, the musculoskeletal system functions to
    (a) provide for body movement.
    (b) protect vital internal organs.
    (c) produce red blood cells (within bone marrow).
    (d) Answers (a) and (b).
    (e) Answers (a), (b), and (c).

40. The skull consists of
    (a) the cranium (which contains the brain).
    (b) the cranium (which contains the brain) and the face.
    (c) the cranium (which contains the brain), the face, and the first vertebra of the spine.
    (d) the cranium (which contains the brain), the face, and the first two vertebrae of the spine.
    (e) None of the above.

41. The bony facial structure that surrounds each eye is called the
    (a) mandible.
    (b) orbit.
    (c) nasal bone.
    (d) maxillae (maxilla).
    (e) zygoma (zygomatic bone).

42. The bony facial structure that provides shape to the nose is called the
    (a) mandible.
    (b) orbit.
    (c) nasal bone.
    (d) maxillae (maxilla).
    (e) zygoma (zygomatic bone).

43. The bony facial structure that is the upper jaw is called the
    (a) mandible.
    (b) orbit.
    (c) nasal bone.
    (d) maxillae (maxilla).
    (e) zygoma (zygomatic bone).

44.   The bony facial structure that is also called the cheekbone is the
        (a) mandible.
        (b) orbit.
        (c) nasal bone.
        (d) maxillae (maxilla).
        (e) zygoma (zygomatic bone).

45.   The bony facial structure that is the lower jaw is called the
        (a) mandible.
        (b) orbit.
        (c) nasal bone.
        (d) maxillae (maxilla).
        (e) zygoma (zygomatic bone).

46.   Which of the following statements regarding the spinal column is false?
        (a) The spinal column encloses the spinal cord.
        (b) The spinal cord connects with the brain through an opening at the base of the
             skull.
        (c) The spinal column consists of 33 bones known as *vertebrae*.
        (d) The spine is divided into five sections.
        (e) The coccyx does not enclose any portion of the spinal cord, and therefore is
             not considered a part of the spine.

47.   The sacral section of the spine (the sacrum) is located
        (a) in the upper back, having ribs attached to it.
        (b) immediately inferior to the lower back, forming the posterior wall of the pelvis.
        (c) in the lower back and does not have attached ribs.
        (d) in the neck.
        (e) at the very end of the spine.

48.   The thoracic section of the spine is located
        (a) in the upper back, having ribs attached to it.
        (b) immediately inferior to the lower back, forming the back wall of the pelvis.
        (c) in the lower back and does not have attached ribs.
        (d) in the neck.
        (e) at the very end of the spine.

49.   The cervical section of the spine is located
        (a) in the upper back, having ribs attached to it.
        (b) immediately inferior to the lower back, forming the back wall of the pelvis.
        (c) in the lower back and does not have attached ribs.
        (d) in the neck.
        (e) at the very end of the spine.

50. The lumbar section of the spine is located
   (a) in the upper back, having ribs attached to it.
   (b) immediately inferior to the lower back, forming the back wall of the pelvis.
   (c) in the lower back and does not have attached ribs.
   (d) in the neck.
   (e) at the very end of the spine.

51. The coccyx is located
   (a) in the upper back, having ribs attached to it.
   (b) immediately inferior to the lower back, forming the back wall of the pelvis.
   (c) in the lower back and does not have attached ribs.
   (d) in the neck.
   (e) at the very end of the spine.

52. The chest is also sometimes called the
   (a) cervical cavity (cervix).
   (b) lumbar cavity.
   (c) thoracic cavity (thorax).
   (d) sacral cavity (sacrum).
   (e) coccygeal cavity (coccyx).

53. The cervical spine consists of _____ vertebrae.
   (a) 12
   (b) 10
   (c) 7
   (d) 5
   (e) 4

54. The thoracic spine consists of _____ vertebrae.
   (a) 12
   (b) 10
   (c) 7
   (d) 5
   (e) 4

55. The lumbar spine consists of _____ vertebrae.
   (a) 12
   (b) 10
   (c) 7
   (d) 5
   (e) 4

56. The sacral spine (sacrum) consists of _____ fused vertebrae.
  (a) 12
  (b) 10
  (c) 7
  (d) 5
  (e) 4

57. The coccyx consists of _____ fused vertebrae.
  (a) 12
  (b) 10
  (c) 7
  (d) 5
  (e) 4

58. The chest consists of ___ pairs of ribs.
  (a) 11
  (b) 12
  (c) 8
  (d) 7
  (e) 14

59. Almost all of the pairs of ribs are attached posteriorly to vertebrae and anteriorly to the breast bone. ___ pair(s) is/are attached only to the vertebrae and are called "floating" ribs.
  (a) One
  (b) Two
  (c) Three
  (d) Four
  (e) Five

60. Another term for the breast bone is the
  (a) xiphoid process.
  (b) ilium.
  (c) sternum.
  (d) manubrium.
  (e) acetabular process.

61. Another term for the superior section of the breast bone is the
  (a) xiphoid process.
  (b) ilium.
  (c) sternum.
  (d) manubrium.
  (e) acetabular process.

62. Another term for the inferior tip of the breast bone (lying over a portion of the liver) is the
    (a) xiphoid process.
    (b) ilium.
    (c) sternum.
    (d) manubrium.
    (e) acetabular process.

63. The *hip* is defined as
    (a) the pelvis.
    (b) the joint between the pelvis and the thighbone.
    (c) the thighbone.
    (d) the joint between the spine and the thighbone.
    (e) the joint between the spine and the pelvis.

64. The pelvis consists of several bones fused together. Two large, wide bones that form each lateral (and superior) portion of the pelvis are often called the "wings" of the pelvis. Each of these bones is called the _____, and its top is called the _____.
    (a) ilium / iliac crest
    (b) ischium / ischiac crest
    (c) pubis / pubic crest
    (d) Any of the above.
    (e) None of the above.

65. The anterior pelvis is formed by the joining of bones that are collectively called the
    (a) ilium.
    (b) ischium.
    (c) pubis.
    (d) Any of the above.
    (e) None of the above.

66. The socket portion of the hip is the
    (a) tibia.
    (b) fibula.
    (c) femur.
    (d) acetabulum.
    (e) patella.

67. The anatomical term for the thighbone is the
    (a) tibia.
    (b) fibula.
    (c) femur.
    (d) acetabulum.
    (e) patella.

68.   The anatomical term for the knee cap is the
   (a) tibia.
   (b) fibula.
   (c) femur.
   (d) acetabulum.
   (e) patella.

69.   The anatomical term for the anterior bone in the lower leg is the
   (a) tibia.
   (b) fibula.
   (c) femur.
   (d) acetabulum.
   (e) patella.

70.   The anatomical term for the posterior bone in the lower leg is the
   (a) tibia.
   (b) fibula.
   (c) femur.
   (d) acetabulum.
   (e) patella.

71.   The anatomical term for the ankle bone on the great-toe side of the foot is the
   (a) medial malleolus.
   (b) lateral malleolus.
   (c) medial tuberosity.
   (d) lateral tuberosity.
   (e) dorsal tuberosity.

72.   The anatomical term for the ankle bone on the small-toe side of the foot is the
   (a) medial malleolus.
   (b) lateral malleolus.
   (c) medial tuberosity.
   (d) lateral tuberosity.
   (e) dorsal tuberosity.

73.   The anatomical term(s) for the bones of the toes is (are) the
   (a) tarsals and metatarsals.
   (b) carpals and metacarpals.
   (c) phalanges.
   (d) calcaneus.
   (e) sacrals and metasacrals.

74.   The anatomical term(s) for the bones of the foot is (are) the
       (a)   tarsals and metatarsals.
       (b)   carpals and metacarpals.
       (c)   phalanges.
       (d)   calcaneus.
       (e)   sacrals and metasacrals.

75.   The anatomical term for the heel bone is the
       (a)   megatarsal.
       (b)   megacarpal.
       (c)   phalanx.
       (d)   calcaneus.
       (e)   posterior tuberosity.

76.   The anatomical term(s) for the bones of the fingers is (are) the
       (a)   tarsals and metatarsals.
       (b)   carpals and metacarpals.
       (c)   phalanges.
       (d)   calcaneus.
       (e)   sacrals and metasacrals.

77.   The anatomical term(s) for the bones of the hands is (are) the
       (a)   tarsals and metatarsals.
       (b)   carpals and metacarpals.
       (c)   phalanges.
       (d)   calcaneus.
       (e)   sacrals and metasacrals.

78.   The shoulder is composed of several bones. The anatomical term for the collarbone
       is the
       (a)   ulna.
       (b)   acromion.
       (c)   scapula.
       (d)   clavicle.
       (e)   olecranon.

79.   The anatomical term for the shoulder blade (in the back) is the
       (a)   ulna.
       (b)   acromion.
       (c)   scapula.
       (d)   clavicle.
       (e)   olecranon.

80.   The very end of the collarbone, at the shoulder joint, is called the
   (a)   ulna.
   (b)   acromion.
   (c)   scapula.
   (d)   clavicle.
   (e)   olecranon.

81.   The bone of the upper arm is the
   (a)   ulna.
   (b)   humerus.
   (c)   radius.
   (d)   carpalus.
   (e)   olecranon.

82.   The lateral bone of the lower arm is the
   (a)   ulna.
   (b)   humerus.
   (c)   radius.
   (d)   carpalus.
   (e)   olecranon.

83.   The medial bone of the lower arm is the
   (a)   ulna.
   (b)   humerus.
   (c)   radius.
   (d)   carpalus.
   (e)   olecranon.

84.   The _____ is an example of a ball-and-socket joint.
   (a)   elbow
   (b)   hip
   (c)   neck
   (d)   Answers (a) and (c).
   (e)   Answers (a) and (b).

85.   The _____ is an example of a hinge joint.
   (a)   elbow
   (b)   hip
   (c)   neck
   (d)   Answers (a) and (c).
   (e)   Answers (a) and (b).

86. Muscles come in three different types. Voluntary muscle is best described as the type of muscle that
      (a) requires no conscious control.
      (b) is consciously controlled.
      (c) has properties of automaticity (is able to generate and conduct its own electrical impulses).
      (d) Answers (a) and (c).
      (e) Answers (b) and (c).

87. Involuntary muscle is best described as the type of muscle that
      (a) requires no conscious control.
      (b) is consciously controlled.
      (c) has properties of automaticity (is able to generate and conduct its own electrical impulses).
      (d) Answers (a) and (c).
      (e) Answers (b) and (c).

88. Cardiac muscle is best described as the type of muscle that
      (a) requires no conscious control.
      (b) is consciously controlled.
      (c) has properties of automaticity (is able to generate and conduct its own electrical impulses).
      (d) Answers (a) and (c).
      (e) Answers (b) and (c).

89. _____ attaches to the bones of the skeleton, forms the major muscle mass of the body, and is controlled by the nervous system and the brain. It also can be contracted and relaxed by the individual's will and is responsible for body movement.
      (a) Involuntary muscle
      (b) Cardiac muscle
      (c) Voluntary muscle
      (d) Any of the above.
      (e) None of the above.

90. _____ is found in the walls of the gastrointestinal tract and urinary system as well as the blood vessels and bronchi. It controls the flow of materials through these structures, carries out the automatic muscular functions of the body, is under no direct control by the individual, and responds to stimuli such as stretching, heat, and cold.
      (a) Involuntary muscle
      (b) Cardiac muscle
      (c) Voluntary muscle
      (d) Any of the above.
      (e) None of the above.

91. _____ is found only in the heart and has its own rich supply of blood. It can tolerate only a very short interruption of blood supply.
  (a) Involuntary muscle
  (b) Cardiac muscle
  (c) Voluntary muscle
  (d) Any of the above.
  (e) None of the above.

92. The respiratory system is responsible for the
  (a) provision of carbon dioxide to the blood stream and excretion of oxygen.
  (b) provision of oxygen to the blood stream and excretion of carbon dioxide.
  (c) muscular function of inhalation and exhalation.
  (d) Answers (a) and (c).
  (e) Answers (b) and (c).

93. When breathing through the mouth, the first area that air enters is the
  (a) pharynx.
  (b) oropharynx.
  (c) larynx.
  (d) endopharynx.
  (e) nasopharynx.

94. When breathing through the nose, the first area that air enters is the
  (a) pharynx.
  (b) oropharynx.
  (c) larynx.
  (d) endopharynx.
  (e) nasopharynx.

95. A leaf-shaped valve that prevents food and liquid from entering the wind pipe is called the
  (a) cricoid cartilage.
  (b) larynx.
  (c) valecula.
  (d) epiglottis.
  (e) trachea.

96. The medical term for the "wind pipe" is the
  (a) cricoid cartilage.
  (b) larynx.
  (c) valecula.
  (d) epiglottis.
  (e) trachea.

97. The firm ring that forms the lower portion of the voice box is the
    (a) cricoid cartilage.
    (b) larynx.
    (c) valecula.
    (d) epiglottis.
    (e) trachea.

98. The medical term for the "voice box" is the
    (a) cricoid cartilage.
    (b) larynx.
    (c) valecula.
    (d) epiglottis.
    (e) trachea.

99. The windpipe divides into two large air tubes at a junction commonly called "the cough center." The medical term for these two large air tubes is the
    (a) right and left rhonchi.
    (b) right and left bronchi.
    (c) right and left alveoli.
    (d) anterior and posterior rhonchi.
    (e) anterior and posterior bronchi.

100. At the end of the respiratory "tree" are groups of tiny sacs. These sacs are called the
    (a) rhonchi.
    (b) bronchi.
    (c) alveoli.
    (d) petechia.
    (e) cilia.

101. The respiratory rate considered normal for an adult at rest is _____ breaths per minute.
    (a) 10 to 12
    (b) 12 to 20
    (c) 15 to 30
    (d) 25 to 35
    (e) 25 to 50

102. The respiratory rate considered normal for an infant (not a newborn) at rest is _____ breaths per minute.
    (a) 10 to 12
    (b) 12 to 20
    (c) 15 to 30
    (d) 20 to 30
    (e) 25 to 40

103. The respiratory rate considered normal for a child at rest is _____ breaths per minute.

    (a) 10 to 12

    (b) 12 to 20

    (c) 15 to 30

    (d) 20 to 30

    (e) 25 to 40

104. The complete assessment of respiration includes assessing the rate of breathing, the rhythm of breathing (is it regular or irregular?), and the

    (a) clarity and equality of breath sounds.

    (b) equality and fullness of chest expansion.

    (c) the use of accessory muscles.

    (d) Answers (a) and (b).

    (e) Answers (a), (b), and (c).

105. Which of the following statements regarding pediatric airway anatomy considerations is false?

    (a) In general, all pediatric airway structures are smaller and more easily obstructed than adult airway structures.

    (b) A child's trachea is harder and less flexible than an adult's, providing greater protection from direct injury.

    (c) Children's tongues take up proportionally more space in the mouth than adults'.

    (d) All of the above are false.

    (e) None of the above is false.

106. Which of the following statements regarding pediatric airway anatomy considerations is true?

    (a) Children have narrower tracheas that can be obstructed more easily by swelling.

    (b) Like other cartilage in the child, the cricoid cartilage is less developed and less rigid than that in the adult.

    (c) The pediatric chest wall is softer, and children tend to depend more heavily on the diaphragm for breathing.

    (d) All of the above are true.

    (e) None of the above is true.

107. The heart is the circulatory pump of the body. The right side of the heart pumps _____ blood through the _____ circulation.

    (a) oxygen-rich / systemic

    (b) oxygen-poor / systemic

    (c) oxygen-rich / pulmonary

    (d) oxygen-poor / pulmonary

    (e) either oxygenated or deoxygenated / systemic or pulmonary

108. The _____ receives blood from the veins of the body and the heart.
    (a) left ventricle
    (b) right ventricle
    (c) ventricular septum
    (d) right atrium
    (e) left atrium

109. The _____ receives blood from the lungs.
    (a) left ventricle
    (b) right ventricle
    (c) ventricular septum
    (d) right atrium
    (e) left atrium

110. The _____ pumps blood to the lungs.
    (a) left ventricle
    (b) right ventricle
    (c) ventricular septum
    (d) right atrium
    (e) left atrium

111. The _____ pumps blood to the body.
    (a) left ventricle
    (b) right ventricle
    (c) ventricular septum
    (d) right atrium
    (e) left atrium

112. The cardiac valves
    (a) propel blood from one chamber of the heart to another.
    (b) propel blood from the heart chambers into the blood vessels.
    (c) prevent back flow of blood.
    (d) Answers (a) and (c).
    (e) Answers (b) and (c).

113. All arteries
    (a) carry blood away from the heart.
    (b) carry blood back to the heart.
    (c) carry only oxygenated blood.
    (d) Answers (a) and (c).
    (e) Answers (b) and (c).

114. All veins
  (a) carry blood away from the heart.
  (b) carry blood back to the heart.
  (c) carry only deoxygenated blood.
  (d) Answers (a) and (c).
  (e) Answers (b) and (c).

115. Pulmonary arteries
  (a) carry blood away from the heart.
  (b) carry blood back to the heart.
  (c) carry only deoxygenated blood.
  (d) Answers (a) and (c).
  (e) Answers (b) and (c).

116. Pulmonary veins
  (a) carry blood away from the heart.
  (b) carry blood back to the heart.
  (c) carry only oxygenated blood.
  (d) Answers (a) and (c).
  (e) Answers (b) and (c).

117. A major blood vessel that originates from the heart, then descends through the thoracic and abdominal cavities, is the
  (a) superior vena cava.
  (b) inferior vena cava.
  (c) aorta.
  (d) Answers (a) or (b).
  (e) Answers (b) or (c).

118. A major blood vessel that returns blood to the heart is the
  (a) superior vena cava.
  (b) inferior vena cava.
  (c) aorta.
  (d) Answers (a) or (b).
  (e) Answers (b) or (c).

119. The heart muscle is supplied with blood by the _____, which branch off from the aorta.
  (a) femoral arteries
  (b) radial arteries
  (c) carotid arteries
  (d) coronary arteries
  (e) brachial arteries

120.   The head is supplied with blood by the _____, which have a pulse that can be palpated on either side of the neck.
   (a)   femoral arteries
   (b)   radial arteries
   (c)   carotid arteries
   (d)   coronary arteries
   (e)   brachial arteries

121.   As the major arteries in each thigh, the _____ supply the groin and both lower extremities with blood and can be palpated in the groin area.
   (a)   femoral arteries
   (b)   radial arteries
   (c)   carotid arteries
   (d)   coronary arteries
   (e)   brachial arteries

122.   The _____ produce a pulse that can be palpated between the elbow and the shoulder on the inside of the arm.
   (a)   femoral arteries
   (b)   radial arteries
   (c)   carotid arteries
   (d)   coronary arteries
   (e)   brachial arteries

123.   The _____ produce a pulse that can be palpated on the _____ side of either wrist.
   (a)   radial arteries / small finger (medial)
   (b)   radial arteries / thumb (lateral)
   (c)   pulsitile arteries / small finger (lateral)
   (d)   brachial arteries / thumb (lateral)
   (e)   brachial arteries / small finger (medial)

124.   The pulse produced by the _____ is auscultated when using a sphygmomanometer and stethoscope to determine the blood pressure.
   (a)   femoral artery
   (b)   radial artery
   (c)   carotid artery
   (d)   coronary artery
   (e)   brachial artery

125. An artery on the posterior surface of the medial malleolus that can be palpated for a pulse is the
    (a) anterior tibial artery.
    (b) posterior tibial artery.
    (c) dorsalis pedis artery.
    (d) superior pedal artery.
    (e) posterior pedal artery.

126. An artery on the top of the foot that can be palpated for a pulse is the
    (a) anterior tibial artery.
    (b) posterior tibial artery.
    (c) dorsalis pedis artery.
    (d) superior pedal artery.
    (e) posterior pedal artery.

127. Capillaries are found in all parts of the body. They are tiny blood vessels that
    (a) receive blood from the smallest arteries and send it to the smallest veins.
    (b) receive blood from the smallest veins and send it to the smallest arteries.
    (c) are responsible for the exchange of nutrients and waste, oxygen and carbon dioxide, at the cellular level of the body.
    (d) Answers (a) and (c).
    (e) Answers (b) and (c).

128. The smallest branch of an artery is called
    (a) a capillary.
    (b) an arteriette.
    (c) an arteriole.
    (d) Answers (b) or (c).
    (e) None of the above.

129. The smallest branch of a vein is called
    (a) a capillary.
    (b) a veinette.
    (c) a venule.
    (d) Answers (b) or (c).
    (e) None of the above.

130. Blood is made up of several components. Red blood cells (RBCs or red corpuscles) carry oxygen to the tissues and carbon dioxide away from the tissues. Another medical term for RBCs is
    (a) leukocytes.
    (b) platelets.
    (c) erythrocytes.
    (d) plasma.
    (e) packed cells.

131. White blood cells (WBCs or white corpuscles) are the body's immune defense against infections. Another medical term for WBCs is

    (a) leukocytes.

    (b) platelets.

    (c) erythrocytes.

    (d) plasma.

    (e) packed cells.

132. The formation of blood clots is largely dependent upon the _____ found in blood.

    (a) leukocytes

    (b) platelets

    (c) erythrocytes

    (d) plasma

    (e) packed cells

133. The fluid that carries blood cells and nutrients from place to place within the circulatory system is called

    (a) whole blood.

    (b) platelets.

    (c) erythroliquid.

    (d) plasma.

    (e) packed cells.

134. A palpable pulse is formed when the _____ contracts, sending a wave of blood through the arteries.

    (a) left atrium

    (b) right atrium

    (c) left ventricle

    (d) right ventricle

    (e) ventricular septum

135. A pulse can be palpated

    (a) only at the neck, inner arm, wrist, groin, and foot.

    (b) anywhere an artery simultaneously passes near the skin surface and over a bone.

    (c) anywhere a vein simultaneously passes near the skin surface and over a bone.

    (d) anywhere a vein or artery simultaneously passes near the skin surface and over a bone.

    (e) only at the neck, inner arm, wrist, groin, ankle, and foot.

136. *Peripheral* pulses include all of the following except the _____ pulse.
- (a) femoral
- (b) brachial
- (c) radial
- (d) dorsalis pedis
- (e) posterior tibial

137. *Central* pulses consist of the carotid pulse and the _____ pulse.
- (a) femoral
- (b) brachial
- (c) radial
- (d) dorsalis pedis
- (e) posterior tibial

138. When measuring the blood pressure, the pressure on the walls of the artery when the left ventricle contracts is called the _____ blood pressure.
- (a) diastolic
- (b) endostolic
- (c) systolic
- (d) Any of the above.
- (e) None of the above.

139. When measuring the blood pressure, the pressure on the walls of the artery when the left ventricle is at rest or relaxed is called the _____ blood pressure.
- (a) diastolic
- (b) endostolic
- (c) systolic
- (d) Any of the above.
- (e) None of the above.

140. Which of the following statements regarding the nervous system is false?
- (a) It controls voluntary activities of the body.
- (b) It controls involuntary activities of the body.
- (c) It governs sensation.
- (d) It governs movement.
- (e) It does not govern thought processes.

141. The components of the central nervous system include the brain and the
- (a) spinal cord.
- (b) sensory nerves.
- (c) motor nerves.
- (d) Answers (a) and (b).
- (e) Answers (a) and (c).

142. Peripheral nervous system components include the
      (a) spinal cord.
      (b) sensory nerves.
      (c) motor nerves.
      (d) Answers (a) and (b).
      (e) Answers (b) and (c).

143. The spinal cord is located within the spinal column. It begins at the brain and ends
      in the
      (a) cervical vertebrae.
      (b) thoracic vertebrae.
      (c) lumbar vertebrae.
      (d) sacrum.
      (e) coccyx.

144. The _____ nerves carry information from the body to the brain.
      (a) motor
      (b) sensory
      (c) antegrade
      (d) Answers (a) and (b).
      (e) Answers (b) and (c).

145. The _____ nerves carry information from the brain to the body.
      (a) motor
      (b) sensory
      (c) retrograde
      (d) Answers (a) and (b).
      (e) Answers (b) and (c).

146. Involuntary motor functions are controlled by a division of the peripheral nervous
      system called the
      (a) heterogenic nervous system.
      (b) independent nervous system.
      (c) autonomic nervous system.
      (d) Any of the above.
      (e) None of the above.

147. All of the following functions are performed by the skin, except
      (a) protection of the body from the environment and provision of a barrier to keep
          out bacteria and other organisms.
      (b) prevention of body water loss and provision of a barrier to keep out
          environmental water.
      (c) production of white blood cells within special skin tissues.
      (d) body temperature regulation.
      (e) reception and transmission of environmental information to the brain.

148.   The outermost layer of skin that is composed primarily of dead cells that are
        constantly rubbed or sloughed off and replaced is the
        (a) endodermis.
        (b) epidermis.
        (c) dermis.
        (d) subcutaneous layer.
        (e) sebaceous layer.

149.   The layer of skin containing sweat and sebaceous glands is the
        (a) endodermis.
        (b) epidermis.
        (c) dermis.
        (d) subcutaneous layer.
        (e) sebaceous layer.

150.   The layer of skin containing fat and soft tissue is largely responsible for
        temperature insulation and shock absorption (protection from impact injuries to
        the body organs). This layer is called the
        (a) endodermis.
        (b) epidermis.
        (c) dermis.
        (d) subcutaneous layer.
        (e) sebaceous layer.

151.   The layer of skin containing hair follicles, blood vessels, and nerve endings is the
        (a) endodermis.
        (b) epidermis.
        (c) dermis.
        (d) subcutaneous layer.
        (e) sebaceous layer.

152.   The endocrine system of the body is responsible for the secretion of chemicals that
        regulate body activities and functions (such as insulin and adrenaline). These
        chemicals are called
        (a) glycogens.
        (b) hormones.
        (c) immunosuppressants.
        (d) Answers (a) or (b).
        (e) Answers (b) or (c).

153.   The thoracic and abdominal cavities are separated by the
        (a) duodenum.
        (b) xiphoid process.

    (c) lower rib margin.

    (d) cerebellum.

    (e) diaphragm.

154. If a patient sustained an isolated blunt injury to the right upper quadrant of the anterior abdomen, what organ would you be most concerned about?

    (a) The heart.

    (b) The kidney.

    (c) The liver.

    (d) The spleen.

    (e) The appendix.

155. If a patient sustained an isolated penetrating injury to the left lower quadrant of the abdomen, what organ would you be most concerned about?

    (a) The heart.

    (b) The large intestine.

    (c) The liver.

    (d) The spleen.

    (e) The appendix.

156. If a patient sustained an isolated blunt injury to the lateral aspect of the left upper abdominal quadrant, what organ would you be most concerned about?

    (a) The heart.

    (b) The large intestine.

    (c) The liver.

    (d) The spleen.

    (e) The appendix.

157. If a patient complained of severe pain in the right lower quadrant of the anterior abdomen, what organ would you be most concerned about?

    (a) The heart.

    (b) The kidney.

    (c) The liver.

    (d) The spleen.

    (e) The appendix.

158. "Vital signs" include all of the following indicators of a patient's condition, except

    (a) mental status.

    (b) respirations.

    (c) pulse.

    (d) skin color, temperature, and condition.

    (e) pupil size and reactivity.

159. Which of the following statements regarding respiratory rate measurement is false?

    (a) Be sure to inform the patient when you are counting his respiratory rate so that the patient will cease talking or crying and breathe normally.

    (b) Respiratory rates are assessed by observing the patient's chest rise and fall.

    (c) Respiratory rates are assessed by observing the patient's abdomen rise and fall.

    (d) Age influences the normal range of respiratory rates.

    (e) When assessing the rate of respirations, the quality of respirations should simultaneously be determined.

160. To determine an official respiratory-rate-per-minute measurement, you should count the number of complete breaths (an inhalation and exhalation cycle) the patient takes within

    (a) a full 60 seconds.

    (b) 30 seconds, then multiply that number by 2.

    (c) 15 seconds, then multiply that number by 4.

    (d) 10 seconds, then multiply that number by 6.

    (e) 6 seconds, then multiply that number by 10.

161. Determining the *quality* of respiratory effort includes assessing all of the following, except

    (a) rate of chest movement.

    (b) equality of chest wall movement.

    (c) depth of chest excursion.

    (d) effort of chest excursion (use of accessory muscles).

    (e) presence or absence of noisy respirations (snoring, wheezing, gurgling, crowing, or the like).

162. In the adult patient, assessment of accessory muscle use includes observing for any or all of the following, except

    (a) pulling in of the shoulder or neck muscles when inhaling (suprasternal retractions).

    (b) excessive abdominal movement when inhaling.

    (c) pulling in of the skin between the ribs when inhaling (intercostal retractions).

    (d) grasping the neck with both hands while inhaling.

    (e) widening of the nostrils (nasal flaring) while inhaling.

163. To count a pulse rate, the EMT should place his

    (a) thumb on the pulse site, because the thumb is the most sensitive to touch.

    (b) small finger ("pinkie") on the pulse site, because the small finger is the most sensitive to touch.

    (c) first two or three fingers on the pulse site.

    (d) Answers (a) or (b), according to personal preference.

    (e) Answers (b) or (c), according to personal preference.

164. The carotid pulse is located in the patient's
     (a) wrist.
     (b) groin.
     (c) upper arm.
     (d) neck.
     (e) foot.

165. Which of the following statements regarding assessment of the carotid pulse is false?
     (a) It is important to check both carotid pulses at the same time, to assess for bilateral equality.
     (b) Placing excessive pressure upon the carotid pulse can slow the patient's heart rate.
     (c) Placing excessive pressure upon the carotid pulse can interfere with blood flow to the brain.
     (d) If the carotid pulse cannot be felt on one side, the other side should immediately be assessed for a carotid pulse.
     (e) Carotid pulse assessment may be dangerous to perform on elderly patients.

166. The radial pulse is located in the patient's
     (a) wrist.
     (b) groin.
     (c) upper arm.
     (d) neck.
     (e) foot.

167. In all patients over the age of 1 year, the radial pulse should be assessed first. Per the DOT EMT guidelines, the method of determining a patient's official pulse rate per minute consists of counting the number of pulse beats that can be felt within
     (a) 6 seconds, then multiplying that number by 10.
     (b) 10 seconds, then multiplying that number by 6.
     (c) 30 seconds, then multiplying that number by 2.
     (d) 15 seconds, then multiplying that number by 4.
     (e) a full 60 seconds.

168. While counting the pulse rate, the *quality* of the pulse also should be assessed. Pulse quality is characterized by whether the pulse is
     (a) strong (normal or "full"), or weak and thin (abnormal or "thready").
     (b) regular in rhythm (normal) or irregular in rhythm (abnormal).
     (c) fast or slow.
     (d) Answers (a) and (b).
     (e) Answers (a) and (c).

169. Per the DOT EMT guidelines, if the patient's pulse is noted to be irregular in rhythm, the pulse rate per minute should be obtained by counting the number of pulse beats that can be felt within

    (a) 10 seconds, then multiplying that number by 6.
    (b) 15 seconds, then multiplying that number by 4.
    (c) 30 seconds, then multiplying that number by 2.
    (d) a full 60 seconds.
    (e) a full five minutes.

170. Your patient is alert and well oriented, but when you first assess his pulse at his right wrist, you cannot find one. You should next assess the patient's

    (a) left radial pulse.
    (b) right dorsalis pedis pulse.
    (c) left popliteal pulse.
    (d) left femoral pulse.
    (e) right carotid pulse.

171. If a patient has no pulse in either arm, the EMT should immediately assess the patient's

    (a) brachial pulse.
    (b) dorsalis pedis pulse.
    (c) popliteal pulse.
    (d) femoral pulse.
    (e) carotid pulse.

172. In an average adult, the "normal" resting pulse rate is between

    (a) 20 and 40 beats per minute.
    (b) 40 and 60 beats per minute.
    (c) 60 and 100 beats per minute.
    (d) 80 and 120 beats per minute.
    (e) 100 and 150 beats per minute.

173. In the adult athlete, the "normal" resting pulse rate may be between

    (a) 20 and 40 beats per minute.
    (b) 40 and 60 beats per minute.
    (c) 60 and 100 beats per minute.
    (d) 80 and 120 beats per minute.
    (e) 100 and 150 beats per minute.

174. Emergency situations often cause the "normal" adult patient's pulse to be temporarily between _____. Thus, this finding should not be considered unusual, or a sign of serious injury, unless it is maintained throughout several pulse checks.

    (a) 20 and 40 beats per minute.
    (b) 60 and 80 beats per minute.

    (c) 80 and 100 beats per minute.

    (d) 100 and 150 beats per minute.

    (e) 150 and 200 beats per minute.

175. In the adult patient, any maintained pulse rate that is slower than ___ or faster than ___ beats per minute is a sign of serious injury or illness.

    (a) 20 / 80

    (b) 60 / 120

    (c) 80 / 150

    (d) 150 / 200

    (e) 80 / 100

176. The medical term for a fast heart rate is

    (a) normocardia.

    (b) cardiomyopathy.

    (c) tachycardia.

    (d) bradycardia.

    (e) endocardia.

177. The medical term for a slow heart rate is

    (a) normocardia.

    (b) cardiomyopathy.

    (c) tachycardia.

    (d) bradycardia.

    (e) endocardia.

178. The pulse rate considered normal for an infant (not a newborn) at rest is _____ beats per minute.

    (a) 120 to 150

    (b) 100 to 120

    (c) 60 to 105

    (d) 70 to 110

    (e) 80 to 140

179. The pulse rate considered normal for a 13-year-old adolescent at rest is _____ beats per minute.

    (a) 120 to 150

    (b) 100 to 120

    (c) 60 to 105

    (d) 70 to 110

    (e) 80 to 140

180. The pulse rate considered normal for a 6-year-old child at rest is _____ beats
      per minute.
      (a) 120 to 150
      (b) 100 to 120
      (c) 60 to 105
      (d) 70 to 110
      (e) 80 to 140

181. Skin assessment is most important in determining the adequacy of
      (a) hemodynamic perfusion.
      (b) pulse rate.
      (c) respiratory rate.
      (d) mental faculty.
      (e) blood pressure.

182. Pink skin color is normal in light-skinned patients. To determine the normal
      "pinkness" of dark-skinned patients, the EMT should assess pinkness of the
      (a) inner eyelids (conjunctiva).
      (b) inner lips or cheeks (oral mucosa).
      (c) nail beds.
      (d) Answers (a) and (b).
      (e) Answers (a), (b), or (c).

183. The color of cyanotic skin (cyanosis) is commonly described as being
      (a) red.
      (b) white.
      (c) normal.
      (d) blue-gray.
      (e) yellow.

184. Cyanosis usually indicates inadequate perfusion (lack of oxygen in the tissues)
      because of
      (a) poor ventilation.
      (b) poor circulation.
      (c) poor cardiac function.
      (d) Answers (a) or (b).
      (e) Answers (a), (b), or (c).

185. The color of jaundiced skin is commonly described as being
      (a) red.
      (b) white.

    (c) normal.

    (d) blue-gray.

    (e) yellow.

186. A patient's jaundiced skin color suggests the possibility of

    (a) liver disease.

    (b) shock.

    (c) high blood pressure.

    (d) Any of the above.

    (e) None of the above.

187. A patient's red, "flushed" skin color suggests the possibility of heat exposure, emotional excitement, or

    (a) high blood pressure.

    (b) spinal injury shock.

    (c) alcohol overdose.

    (d) Answers (a) or (b).

    (e) Answers (a), (b), or (c).

188. Pale skin or mucosal membranes may indicate poor perfusion from constriction of blood vessels because of

    (a) emotional distress.

    (b) blood loss or other types of shock.

    (c) heart attack.

    (d) Answers (b) or (c).

    (e) Answers (a), (b), or (c).

189. The best places for determining a pediatric patient's skin color include the inside of the lower eyelids and the

    (a) mucosa of the inner mouth.

    (b) palms of the hands.

    (c) soles of the feet.

    (d) Answers (a) or (b).

    (e) Answers (a), (b), or (c).

190. To determine skin temperature, place the back of your hand on the patient's skin, simultaneously noting skin moisture and other aspects of skin condition. Skin signs of moderate-to-high fever or brief exposure to heat commonly include

    (a) cool, moist ("clammy") skin.

    (b) cold, dry skin.

    (c) hot, dry skin.

    (d) hot, moist skin.

    (e) "goose pimples."

191. Skin signs of prolonged fever or extreme exposure to heat commonly include
    (a) cool, moist ("clammy") skin.
    (b) cold, dry skin.
    (c) hot, dry skin.
    (d) hot, moist skin.
    (e) "goose pimples."

192. Skin signs of poor cellular perfusion commonly include
    (a) cool, moist ("clammy") skin.
    (b) cold, dry skin.
    (c) hot, dry skin.
    (d) hot, moist skin.
    (e) "goose pimples."

193. Skin signs of extreme exposure to cold commonly include
    (a) cool, moist ("clammy") skin.
    (b) cold, dry skin.
    (c) hot, dry skin.
    (d) hot, moist skin.
    (e) "goose pimples."

194. Pediatric patients' capillary refill should be assessed by pressing on the patient's skin or nail beds and determining the amount of time for a return of the initial color. Normal capillary refill time in children is
    (a) less than one second.
    (b) less than two seconds.
    (c) two to three seconds.
    (d) three to four seconds.
    (e) four full seconds.

195. When bright light is shown into the pupils, they should react by
    (a) constricting, and becoming larger.
    (b) dilating, and becoming larger.
    (c) dilating, and becoming smaller.
    (d) constricting, and becoming smaller.
    (e) elongating, and becoming more oval in shape.

196. When introduced to a dark environment, the pupils should react by
    (a) constricting, and becoming larger.
    (b) dilating, and becoming larger.
    (c) dilating, and becoming smaller.
    (d) constricting, and becoming smaller.
    (e) elongating, and becoming more oval in shape.

197. Fright may cause pupils to become
   (a) constricted.
   (b) dilated.
   (c) elongated.
   (d) unequal in size or reactivity to light.
   (e) Answers (c) or (d).

198. Stroke or head injury may cause pupils to become
   (a) equally constricted.
   (b) equally dilated.
   (c) unequally elongated in shape.
   (d) unequal in size or reactivity to light.
   (e) Answers (c) or (d).

199. The term *auscultation* refers to the process of
   (a) listening to areas of the body with a stethoscope.
   (b) systematically gathering information from the patient.
   (c) touching and feeling the patient to detect injuries or pain.
   (d) watching the patient closely for changes in level of consciousness.
   (e) tapping on the chest or abdomen.

200. The term *palpation* refers to the process of
   (a) listening to areas of the body with a stethoscope.
   (b) systematically gathering information from the patient.
   (c) touching and feeling the patient to detect injuries or pain.
   (d) watching the patient closely for changes in level of consciousness.
   (e) tapping on the chest or abdomen.

201. The medical term for a blood pressure cuff is
   (a) spiromanometer.
   (b) hemomanometer.
   (c) stethomanometer.
   (d) sphygmomanometer.
   (e) None of the above.

202. To obtain the patient's blood pressure by listening with a stethoscope, you should place the diaphragm of the stethoscope over the
   (a) carotid artery.
   (b) brachial artery.
   (c) radial artery.
   (d) femoral artery.
   (e) coronary artery.

203. To obtain the patient's blood pressure by feeling for a return of the patient's pulse, you should find the pulse at the _____ pulse site prior to inflation, maintaining contact during inflation and deflation of the blood pressure cuff.

    (a) carotid
    (b) brachial
    (c) radial
    (d) femoral
    (e) coronary

204. To obtain the patient's blood pressure by listening with a stethoscope, you should place the diaphragm of the stethoscope on the

    (a) medial side of the antecubital area.
    (b) lateral side of the antecubital area.
    (c) side indicated by the blood pressure cuff arrow (either side works).
    (d) medial side of the anterior wrist.
    (e) lateral side of the anterior wrist.

205. To obtain the patient's blood pressure by feeling for a return of the patient's pulse, you should feel the pulse on the

    (a) medial side of the antecubital area (anterior to the elbow).
    (b) lateral side of the antecubital area (anterior to the elbow).
    (c) side indicated by the blood pressure cuff arrow (either side works).
    (d) medial side of the anterior wrist.
    (e) lateral side of the anterior wrist.

206. When listening to obtain a blood pressure, the gauge number where the pulse is first heard represents the patient's _____ blood pressure.

    (a) diastolic
    (b) hypostolic
    (c) systolic
    (d) superstolic
    (e) None of the above.

207. When listening to obtain a blood pressure, the gauge number where the pulse is last heard represents the patient's _____ blood pressure.

    (a) diastolic
    (b) hypostolic
    (c) systolic
    (d) superstolic
    (e) None of the above.

208. When feeling the patient's pulse to obtain a blood pressure, the gauge number where the return of a pulse is first felt represents the patient's _____ blood pressure.

    (a) diastolic

    (b) hypostolic

    (c) systolic

    (d) superstolic

    (e) None of the above.

209. When feeling the patient's pulse to obtain a blood pressure, the gauge number where the pulse is last felt represents the patient's _____ blood pressure.

    (a) diastolic

    (b) hypostolic

    (c) systolic

    (d) superstolic

    (e) None of the above.

210. When the patient is stable, vital signs should be assessed

    (a) after every medical intervention.

    (b) every 30 minutes.

    (c) every 15 minutes.

    (d) Answers (a) and (b).

    (e) Answers (a) and (c).

211. When the patient is unstable, vital signs should be assessed

    (a) after every medical intervention.

    (b) every 10 minutes.

    (c) every 5 minutes.

    (d) Answers (a) and (b).

    (e) Answers (a) and (c).

212. In the phrase "signs and symptoms," a sign is something

    (a) a bystander knows about the patient.

    (b) the patient refuses to explain.

    (c) the care provider is told about the scene.

    (d) the patient feels and describes to the care provider.

    (e) the care provider sees, hears, feels, or smells about the patient.

213. In the phrase "signs and symptoms," a symptom is something

    (a) a bystander knows about the patient.

    (b) the patient refuses to explain.

    (c) the care provider is told about the scene.

    (d) the patient feels and describes to the care provider.

    (e) the care provider sees, hears, feels, or smells about the patient.

214. To obtain a complete patient history, the EMT may use the mnemonic (memory aid) *SAMPLE* to remember what questions to ask. The "S" of a SAMPLE history stands for

    (a) Signs and Symptoms—What are the patient's complaints and vital signs?

    (b) Size—What is the weight and height of the patient?

    (c) Speech—How well does the patient speak?

    (d) Snoring—Does the patient have an airway?

    (e) Sleeping—Does the patient "pass out" often?

215. The "A" of a SAMPLE history stands for

    (a) Aftereffects—complaints following the incident.

    (b) Allergies—to medications, food, environmental substances.

    (c) Altered level of consciousness.

    (d) Affect—What does the patient look like?

    (e) Anxiety—Is the patient upset?

216. The "M" of a SAMPLE history stands for

    (a) Major—What are the patient's major complaints?

    (b) Minor—What are the patient's minor complaints?

    (c) Multiple—What is the number of the patient's complaints?

    (d) Married—Is the patient married, single, divorced, or widowed?

    (e) Medications—What are the patient's current prescription and nonprescription drugs? Have any recent additions, deletions, or dose changes been made?

217. The "P" of a SAMPLE history stands for

    (a) Plan—your planned course of treatment.

    (b) Potential—the suspected diagnosis.

    (c) Previous—the treatment already rendered.

    (d) Pertinent Past history—medical, surgical, or traumatic.

    (e) Pulse—Does the patient have a pulse?

218. The "L" of a SAMPLE history stands for

    (a) Likes and dislikes.

    (b) Last menstrual period.

    (c) Last meal or oral intake—time, quantity, substance(s).

    (d) Looks—What is the patient's appearance?

    (e) Late—late developing signs and symptoms.

219. The "E" of a SAMPLE history stands for

    (a) Equal—equality of grips, pupils, movement.

    (b) Energy—Is the patient fatigued?

    (c) Events leading to the injury or illness.

    (d) Extra—What extra things can you think of asking?

    (e) Evaluation—the suspected diagnosis.

220. Which of the following statements regarding EMT safety when lifting and moving patients is false?

    (a) Do not try to handle too heavy a load. When in doubt, call for help.

    (b) Avoid twisting when lifting, lowering, or pulling.

    (c) When lifting a heavy patient, keep your legs straight and rely on shoulder and arm muscles.

    (d) Avoid bending at the waist.

    (e) Communicate clearly and frequently with your partner.

221. Which of the following statements regarding EMT safety when pushing or pulling objects is false?

    (a) Whenever possible, push a heavy object, rather than pulling it.

    (b) Keep your back locked in, and bend your knees to keep the line of pull through the center of your body.

    (c) Keep the weight close to your body and your arms close to your side.

    (d) If the weight is below your waist level, bend over at the waist to access it, keeping your legs locked in.

    (e) Avoid pushing or pulling weight that is over your head.

222. An *emergency move* is when a patient is moved before thorough examination and without full spinal precautions. This type of move is indicated when there is a clearly apparent danger to the patient or others if the patient is not *immediately* moved. All of the following are situations that would require an emergency move, except

    (a) a fire or the clear danger of imminent fire exists near the patient.

    (b) the presence of explosives or other hazardous materials.

    (c) the inability to gain access to another patient who needs lifesaving care.

    (d) the patient is a "public spectacle" and must be moved before news cameras arrive so as to avoid patient's confidentiality from being breached.

    (e) the patient is in cardiac arrest and is sitting in a chair or lying on a bed.

223. An *urgent move* is when a patient is moved after only a brief examination but with full spinal precautions. This type of move is indicated when there are signs of serious life threat and the patient must be moved *quickly*. Which of the following is an example of such a situation?

    (a) Altered level of consciousness.

    (b) Inadequate breathing or ventilation.

    (c) Shock (hypoperfusion).

    (d) Answers (a) and (b).

    (e) Answers (a), (b), and (c).

224. Which of the following statements regarding emergency moves is false?

    (a) The greatest danger in moving a patient immediately is the possibility of aggravating a spine injury.

    (b) In an emergency, every effort should be made to push (rather than pull) the patient.

    (c) Move the patient in the direction of the long axis of the body to provide as much protection to the spine as possible.

    (d) Clothing at the patient's neck and shoulder area can be used to drag the patient to safety.

    (e) The patient's feet can be used to drag the patient to safety.

225. Which of the following statements regarding patient positioning is false?

    (a) A trauma patient in her third trimester of pregnancy (a very gravid abdomen) should be spinally immobilized supine, and then with the right side of the backboard should be elevated.

    (b) A medical patient with chest discomfort or difficulty in breathing should be allowed to sit in a position of comfort, as long as the position does not cause hypotension.

    (c) Every patient with a suspected spine injury must be immobilized to a long back board in the supine position.

    (d) An unresponsive patient with no suspected spine injury should be moved into the "recovery position" by rolling the patient onto his side (preferably the left).

    (e) A patient in shock must have his legs elevated 8 to 12 inches, especially if head or spine injury is suspected.

The answer key for Test Section One is on page 324.

DOT Module Two: Airway

2

Subjects:

- Respiration Anatomy
- Respiratory Assessment
- Techniques of Artificial Ventilation
- Airway Adjuncts
- Suctioning and Suction Devices
- Oxygen Therapy
- Special Airway Considerations
- Obstructed Airway Management
- Rescue Breathing

Test Section Two consists of 120 questions and is allotted 2 hours for completion.

1.   The respiratory system is responsible for the
        (a) provision of carbon dioxide to the blood stream and excretion of oxygen.
        (b) provision of oxygen to the blood stream and excretion of carbon dioxide.
        (c) muscular function of inhalation and exhalation.
        (d) Answers (a) and (c).
        (e) Answers (b) and (c).

2.   When breathing through the mouth, the first area that air enters is the
        (a) pharynx.
        (b) nasopharynx.
        (c) larynx.
        (d) endopharynx.
        (e) oropharynx.

3.   When breathing through the nose, the first area that air enters is the
        (a) pharynx.
        (b) nasopharynx.
        (c) larynx.
        (d) endopharynx.
        (e) oropharynx.

4.   A leaf-shaped valve that prevents food and liquid from entering the wind pipe is
        called the
        (a) carina.
        (b) larynx.
        (c) valecula.
        (d) epiglottis.
        (e) sphincter.

5.   The medical term for the main "wind pipe" is the
        (a) hyperpharynx.
        (b) larynx.
        (c) valecula.
        (d) epiglottis.
        (e) trachea.

6.   The firm ring that forms the lower portion of the voice box is the
        (a) cricoid cartilage.
        (b) larynx.
        (c) valecula.
        (d) epiglottis.
        (e) carina.

7. The medical term for the "voice box" is the
    (a) carina.
    (b) larynx.
    (c) valecula.
    (d) epiglottis.
    (e) trachea.

8. The windpipe divides into two large air tubes at a junction commonly called "the cough center." The medical term for this junction is the
    (a) carina.
    (b) larynx.
    (c) valecula.
    (d) epiglottis.
    (e) hyoid.

9. The medical terms for the two large air tubes that extend from the windpipe are the
    (a) anterior and posterior rhonchi.
    (b) anterior and posterior bronchi.
    (c) right and left bronchi.
    (d) right and left rhonchi.
    (e) right and left alveoli.

10. At the end of the respiratory "tree" are groups of tiny sacs. These sacs are called the
    (a) rhonchi.
    (b) bronchi.
    (c) alveoli.
    (d) petechia.
    (e) cilia.

11. When the diaphragm and the muscles between the ribs (intercostal) are activated,
    (a) the larynx opens and air flows in.
    (b) lung size decreases and air flows out when the airway is open.
    (c) the larynx opens and air flows out.
    (d) lung size increases and air flows in when the airway is open.
    (e) None of the above.

12. When the diaphragm and intercostal muscles relax,
    (a) the larynx opens and air flows in.
    (b) lung size decreases and air flows out when the airway is open.
    (c) the larynx opens and air flows out.
    (d) lung size increases and air flows in when the airway is open.
    (e) None of the above.

13. Because it requires energy to accomplish, inhalation is considered the _____ phase of respiration.
   (a) active
   (b) passive
   (c) primary
   (d) formal
   (e) informal

14. Because it does not normally require energy to accomplish, exhalation is considered the _____ phase of respiration.
   (a) active
   (b) passive
   (c) secondary
   (d) formal
   (e) informal

15. The respiratory gas exchange of oxygen and carbon dioxide occurs
   (a) only in the alveoli.
   (b) only in the rhonchi and bronchi.
   (c) only in the cells of the body (via capillaries).
   (d) in the alveoli and the cells of the body (via capillaries).
   (e) in the alveoli, rhonchi, bronchi, and the cells of the body.

16. For an adult, an adequate (normal) rate of respiration at rest is considered to be _____ breaths per minute.
   (a) 10 to 12
   (b) 12 to 20
   (c) 15 to 30
   (d) 25 to 35
   (e) 25 to 50

17. For an infant, an adequate (normal) rate of respiration at rest is considered to be _____ breaths per minute.
   (a) 10 to 12
   (b) 12 to 20
   (c) 15 to 30
   (d) 25 to 35
   (e) 25 to 50

18. For a child, an adequate (normal) rate of respiration at rest is considered to be _____ breaths per minute.
   (a) 10 to 12
   (b) 12 to 20

    (c) 15 to 30

    (d) 25 to 35

    (e) 25 to 50

19. The complete assessment of respiration includes assessing the rate of breathing, the rhythm of breathing (is it regular or irregular?), and the

    (a) clarity and equality of breath sounds.

    (b) equality and fullness of chest expansion.

    (c) use of accessory muscles.

    (d) Answers (a) and (b).

    (e) Answers (a), (b), and (c).

20. Which of the following statements regarding pediatric airway anatomy considerations is true?

    (a) In general, all pediatric airway structures are smaller and more easily obstructed than are adult airway structures.

    (b) The trachea is harder and less flexible in children, providing greater protection from direct injury than an adult's trachea does.

    (c) Children's tongues take up proportionally more space in the mouth than adults' tongues do.

    (d) Answers (a) and (c) are true.

    (e) Answers (a), (b), and (c) are true.

21. Which of the following statements regarding pediatric airway anatomy considerations is true?

    (a) Children have narrower tracheas that can be obstructed more easily by swelling.

    (b) Like other cartilage in the child, the cricoid cartilage is less developed and less rigid than in the adult.

    (c) The pediatric chest wall is softer and children tend to depend more heavily on the diaphragm for breathing.

    (d) All of the above are true.

    (e) None of the above are true.

22. The medical term for a faster-than-normal respiratory rate is

    (a) rapidnea.

    (b) apnea.

    (c) tachypnea.

    (d) bradypnea.

    (e) dyspnea.

23. The medical term for a slower-than-normal respiratory rate is

    (a) retardnea.

    (b) apnea.

    (c) tachypnea.

    (d) bradypnea.

    (e) dyspnea.

24.   The medical term for difficulty in breathing is
    (a) diffopnea.
    (b) apnea.
    (c) tachypnea.
    (d) bradypnea.
    (e) dyspnea.

25.   The medical term for the absence of breathing is
    (a) antiopnea.
    (b) apnea.
    (c) tachypnea.
    (d) bradypnea.
    (e) dyspnea.

26.   The slow and gasping, entirely ineffective respiration efforts that sometimes immediately follow cardiac arrest are called _____ respirations.
    (a) agonal
    (b) basilar
    (c) Cushing's
    (d) Kendrick
    (e) impugned

27.   In the adult patient, the assessment of accessory muscle use includes observing any or all of the following, except
    (a) pulling in of the shoulder or neck muscles when inhaling (suprasternal retractions).
    (b) excessive abdominal movement when inhaling.
    (c) pulling in of the skin between the ribs when inhaling (intercostal retractions).
    (d) grasping of the neck with both hands while inhaling.
    (e) widening of the nostrils (nasal flaring) while inhaling.

28.   Noises produced during breathing may indicate a respiratory obstruction. Snoring respirations generally indicate
    (a) the presence of fluid in the upper airway, indicating a need for suction.
    (b) a partial upper airway inhalation obstruction, usually relieved with airway-opening maneuvers.
    (c) difficulty exhaling past clogged lower airways, a condition that may respond to inhaled medications.
    (d) a partial upper airway inhalation obstruction that probably will not respond to airway-opening maneuvers, inhaled medications, or other treatments rendered by EMTs.
    (e) an anxiety-related form of noisy breathing that should not cause any concern to prehospital care providers.

29. Wheezing respirations generally indicate
    (a) the presence of fluid in the upper airway, indicating a need for suction.
    (b) a partial upper airway inhalation obstruction, usually relieved with airway-opening maneuvers.
    (c) difficulty exhaling past clogged lower airways, a condition that may respond to inhaled medications.
    (d) a partial upper airway inhalation obstruction that probably will not respond to airway-opening maneuvers, inhaled medications, or other treatments rendered by EMTs.
    (e) an anxiety-related form of noisy breathing that should not cause any concern to prehospital care providers.

30. Gurgling respirations generally indicate
    (a) the presence of fluid in the upper airway, indicating a need for suction.
    (b) a partial upper airway inhalation obstruction, usually relieved with airway-opening maneuvers.
    (c) difficulty exhaling past clogged lower airways, a condition that may respond to inhaled medications.
    (d) a partial upper airway inhalation obstruction that probably will not respond to airway-opening maneuvers, inhaled medications, or other treatments rendered by EMTs.
    (e) an anxiety-related form of noisy breathing that should not cause any concern to prehospital care providers.

31. When listening to the patient's lungs with your stethoscope, you hear a loud and harsh rattling noise. The medical term for this respiratory noise is
    (a) rhonchi.
    (b) crowing.
    (c) rales.
    (d) wheezing.
    (e) stridor.

32. When listening to the patient's lungs with your stethoscope, you hear fine crackling noises similar to the sound of hair strands being rubbed together next to your ear. The medical term for this respiratory noise is
    (a) rhonchi.
    (b) crowing.
    (c) rales.
    (d) wheezing.
    (e) stridor.

33.   The medical term for the harsh, high-pitched "windy" type of sound characteristic
      of an upper airway obstruction caused by swelling in the larynx is
      (a) rhonchi.
      (b) crowing.
      (c) rales.
      (d) wheezing.   _____
      (e) stridor.

34.   The medical term for the high- or low-pitched, musical noise characteristic of air
      being forced past swollen or mucous-filled lower airway structures (especially on
      expiration) is
      (a) rhonchi.
      (b) crowing.
      (c) rales.
      (d) wheezing.
      (e) stridor.

35.   The medical term for the harsh, low-pitched, musical noise characteristic of air
      being forced through a partially obstructed larynx (due to spasming or swelling) is
      (a) rhonchi.
      (b) crowing.
      (c) rales.
      (d) wheezing.
      (e) stridor.

36.   The medical term for the loud and harsh rattling noise that is commonly caused by
      lower airway obstruction from thick mucus (or infection-filled fluid) is
      (a) rhonchi.
      (b) crowing.
      (c) rales.
      (d) wheezing.
      (e) stridor.

37.   Hearing rales in a patient's lungs commonly indicates that the patient's
      (a) alveoli or smallest bronchioles have been filled or surrounded by fluid.
      (b) upper airway needs to be suctioned.
      (c) bronchioles are clogged with thick mucus.
      (d) bronchioles are spasming closed.
      (e) lungs are clear of mucus.

38.   "Crowing" respirations commonly indicate that
      (a) the alveoli or smallest bronchioles have been filled or surrounded by fluid.
      (b) a partial upper airway inhalation obstruction exists, that ought to be relieved
           with airway-opening maneuvers.

    (c) difficulty exhaling or inhaling past clogged lower airways exists—a condition that may respond to inhaled medications.

    (d) a partial upper airway inhalation obstruction exists, that probably will not respond to airway-opening maneuvers, inhaled medications, or other treatments rendered by EMTs.

    (e) respiratory arrest is about to occur.

39. Which of the following statements regarding respiratory rhythm is true?

    (a) Even and regular respirations are the only respirations considered "normal."

    (b) In an unconscious patient, irregular respirations are a cause for concern.

    (c) Irregular respirations are not a cause for concern when the patient is conscious, because things such as speech, mood, and physical activity normally cause irregular respiratory patterns.

    (d) Both answers (a) and (b) are true.

    (e) Both answers (b) and (c) are true.

40. The definition of *cyanosis* is

    (a) the absence of respiratory effort.

    (b) the absence of oxygen in the blood.

    (c) pale nail beds, palms, and skin.

    (d) a grayish-blue discoloration of the skin.

    (e) a lack of oxygen in the lungs.

41. Cyanosis usually indicates inadequate perfusion (lack of oxygen in the tissues) because of

    (a) poor ventilation.

    (b) poor circulation.

    (c) poor cardiac function.

    (d) Answers (a) or (b).

    (e) Answers (a), (b), or (c).

42. To open the airway when no spine injury is suspected, the EMT should use the

    (a) head-tilt, neck-lift technique.

    (b) head-tilt, chin-lift technique.

    (c) jaw-thrust maneuver.

    (d) Any of the above.

    (e) None of the above.

43. To open the airway when a spine injury is suspected, the EMT should use the

    (a) head-tilt, neck-lift technique.

    (b) head-tilt, chin-lift technique.

    (c) jaw-thrust maneuver.

    (d) Any of the above.

    (e) None of the above.

44.   When administering mouth-to-mask ventilations, if the pocket face mask has an oxygen inlet, oxygen tubing should be attached and oxygen should be run at _____ liters per minute (lpm).

  (a) 2 to 6
  (b) 6 to 8
  (c) 8 to 10
  (d) 12
  (e) 15

45.   The pocket face mask should be positioned on the adult patient with the apex of the mask

  (a) over the bridge of the nose.
  (b) under the chin.
  (c) between the lower lip and the chin.
  (d) Any of the above.
  (e) None of the above.

46.   When exhaling into the pocket face mask to ventilate the adult patient, the duration of each ventilation (exhalation) should last

  (a) $\frac{1}{2}$ second (use of a mask allows faster ventilation delivery).
  (b) 1 full second.
  (c) $1\frac{1}{2}$ to 2 seconds.
  (d) 2 to $2\frac{1}{2}$ seconds.
  (e) $2\frac{1}{2}$ to 3 seconds.

47.   When exhaling into the pocket face mask to ventilate the pediatric patient, the duration of each ventilation (exhalation) should last

  (a) $\frac{1}{2}$ second (children require faster ventilation delivery).
  (b) 1 full second.
  (c) $1\frac{1}{2}$ to 2 seconds.
  (d) 2 to $2\frac{1}{2}$ seconds.
  (e) $2\frac{1}{2}$ to 3 seconds.

48.   The bag-valve-mask (BVM) device should be equipped with all of the following except

  (a) a nonjam valve that allows an oxygen flow of 15 lpm.
  (b) a pop-off valve to prevent overinflation.
  (c) standardized 15/22 mm fittings (to fit face masks or endotracheal tubes).
  (d) a nonrebreathing valve that prevents the patient from breathing in his exhaled air.
  (e) a self-refilling bag or another form of oxygen reservoir.

49. The BVM device must be

    (a) equipped with a reservoir (a bag or tube) to deliver the highest possible concentration of oxygen. Without a reservoir, a less than optimal oxygen concentration will be delivered.

    (b) easy to clean and sterilize, or disposable after a single-patient use.

    (c) available in adult, pediatric, and infant sizes.

    (d) Answers (b) and (c).

    (e) Answers (a), (b), and (c).

50. Which of the following statements regarding the BVM device is false?

    (a) The BVM delivers smaller volumes of air than mouth-to-mask ventilation.

    (b) The volume of the BVM bag is approximately 1,600 mL of air.

    (c) Observation of chest rise and fall is vital to operating the BVM.

    (d) Use of adjunct airways (oropharyngeal or nasopharyngeal) is unnecessary when using the BVM correctly.

    (e) Obtaining an effective seal with the patient's face, while still maintaining an open airway, is the most difficult aspect of delivering effective BVM ventilations.

51. When supplemental oxygen is not available, the BVM device will deliver approximately _____ percent oxygen.

    (a) 51

    (b) 31

    (c) 21

    (d) 11

    (e) None of the above. A BVM should not be used until supplemental oxygen is available.

52. When supplemented with 15 lpm of oxygen, but without an oxygen reservoir, a BVM device will deliver approximately _____ percent oxygen.

    (a) 100

    (b) 90

    (c) 70

    (d) 50

    (e) 30

53. When supplemented with 15 lpm of oxygen, a BVM device with an oxygen reservoir will deliver approximately _____ percent oxygen.

    (a) 100

    (b) 90

    (c) 70

    (d) 50

    (e) 30

54. When delivering BVM ventilations to an adult, ventilate the patient every _____ seconds.
   (a) 10
   (b) 8
   (c) 5
   (d) 3
   (e) 2

55. When delivering BVM ventilations to children and infants, ventilate the patient every _____ seconds.
   (a) 10
   (b) 8
   (c) 5
   (d) 3
   (e) 2

56. Some ventilation techniques and devices provide better oxygenation and ventilation than others. Place the following in the order of their ventilation effectiveness, from the most effective to the least effective.
   (1) Single-person-operated BVM with supplemental oxygen
   (2) Two-person-operated BVM with supplemental oxygen
   (3) A flow-restricted oxygen-powered ventilation device
   (4) Mouth-to-mask ventilation with supplemental oxygen

   (a) 1, 3, 2, 4.
   (b) 4, 2, 3, 1.
   (c) 2, 1, 3, 4.
   (d) 2, 1, 4, 3.
   (e) 1, 2, 3, 4.

57. When a spinal injury is not suspected, and the patient's chest does not rise and fall with each BVM ventilation,
   (a) reposition the patient's head, gently hyperextending the patient's neck, to ensure an open airway.
   (b) reposition fingers and mask placement to prevent air escaping from under the mask, and to prevent airway occlusion from jaw compression.
   (c) evaluate for airway obstruction or obstruction of the BVM.
   (d) Answers (a) and (b).
   (e) Answers (a), (b), and (c).

58. When a spinal injury is suspected, and the patient's chest does not rise and fall with each BVM ventilation,

   (a) reposition the patient's head, gently hyperextending the patient's neck, to ensure an open airway. (An open airway can only be ensured by neck hyperextension, and ensuring an open airway is more important than responding to concerns for a potential spinal injury.)

   (b) reposition fingers and mask placement to prevent air escaping from under the mask, and to prevent airway occlusion from jaw compression.

   (c) evaluate for airway obstruction or obstruction of the BVM.

   (d) Answers (b) and (c).

   (e) Answers (a), (b), and (c).

59. After taking action to correct potential problems, if the chest still does not rise with each BVM ventilation,

   (a) continue repositioning the head or jaw and continue BVM ventilation attempts.

   (b) continue repositioning fingers and mask to obtain a better seal and continue BVM ventilation attempts.

   (c) use an alternative method of ventilation, such as mouth-to-mask or a manually triggered ventilation device.

   (d) Answers (a) and (b).

   (e) None of the above.

60. Which of the following statements regarding BVM ventilation of a patient via a stoma or tracheostomy tube is false?

   (a) Performance of the jaw-thrust or head-tilt, chin-lift maneuver is still required in order to keep the trachea in-line for effective stoma or tracheostomy tube ventilation.

   (b) The BVM can connect directly to a tracheostomy tube.

   (c) Use an adult bag with a pediatric mask when performing BVM-to-stoma ventilation of an adult.

   (d) Sealing the patient's mouth and nose closed may be required for adequate BVM tracheostomy tube ventilation.

   (e) If ventilation is still ineffective after suctioning the stoma or tracheostomy tube, seal the neck opening and attempt standard methods of BVM ventilation via the nose and mouth.

61. All of the following describe required features of a flow-restricted, oxygen-powered ventilation device (FROPVD), except

   (a) a peak flow rate of 100% oxygen at less than 40 lpm.

   (b) an activation trigger that allows the rescuer to maintain an adequate mask seal with both hands.

   (c) a pressure relief valve that closes to prevent the patient from exhaling excessively.

   (d) an audible alarm that sounds whenever the pressure relief valve is triggered.

   (e) standardized 15/22-mm fittings to fit face masks and endotracheal or tracheostomy tubes.

62. When using a FROPVD, ventilate the _____ patient every _____ seconds.
    (a) adult / 10
    (b) pediatric / 3
    (c) adult / 5
    (d) Answers (a) and (b).
    (e) Answers (b) and (c).

63. Which of the following statements regarding FROPVD operation is false?
    (a) Use of a FROPVD may make a chest injury worse.
    (b) The standard FROPVD is designed only for ventilation of adult patients.
    (c) Gastric distention is a common side effect of FROPVD use, and may lead to regurgitation and aspiration of stomach contents.
    (d) Simultaneous spinal immobilization is still required when ventilating a trauma patient with a FROPVD.
    (e) One of the greatest benefits of using a FROPVD is that the force of its ventilation-delivery makes it unnecessary to maintain jaw-thrust or head-tilt, chin-lift maneuvers.

64. Which of the following statements regarding the use of both oropharyngeal airway adjuncts (oral airways) and nasopharyngeal airway adjuncts (nasal airways) is false?
    (a) An oral or nasal airway should always be used for unconscious patients.
    (b) An oral or nasal airway should always be used when any form of artificial ventilation is employed.
    (c) Infection control practices are vital to the appropriate use of any airway adjunct.
    (d) If the patient begins to gag, immediately discontinue ventilation and remove whatever airway adjunct is in place.
    (e) Once an oral or nasal airway adjunct is in place, it is unnecessary to manually continue jaw-thrust or head-tilt, chin-lift maneuvers.

65. Oral airways should be used to assist an open airway
    (a) for all deeply unresponsive patients without a gag reflex.
    (b) whenever a BVM or FROPVD is required for ventilation.
    (c) for unconscious patients who have a gag reflex, but still need assistance keeping their tongue from obstructing their airway.
    (d) Answers (a) and (b).
    (e) Answers (a), (b), and (c).

66. Nasal airways may be used to assist an open airway
    (a) for all deeply unresponsive patients without a gag reflex.
    (b) whenever a BVM or FROPVD is required for ventilation.
    (c) for unconscious patients who have a gag reflex, but still need assistance keeping their tongue from obstructing their airway.
    (d) Answers (b) and (c).
    (e) Answers (a), (b), and (c).

67.   To select the appropriate size of an oral airway, measure from the
   (a) corner of the patient's lips to the bottom of the earlobe.
   (b) tip of the patient's nose to the bottom of the earlobe.
   (c) corner of the patient's lips to the angle of the jaw.
   (d) Answers (a) or (c).
   (e) Answers (b) or (c).

68.   To select the appropriate size of a nasal airway, measure from the
   (a) corner of the patient's lips to the bottom of the earlobe.
   (b) tip of the patient's nose to the bottom of the earlobe.
   (c) corner of the patient's lips to the angle of the jaw.
   (d) Answers (a) or (c).
   (e) Answers (b) or (c).

69.   Which of the following statements correctly describes the insertion technique for an oral airway?
   (a) Insert the airway upside down, with the tip facing toward the roof of the patient's mouth.
   (b) Insert the airway in the position of its function, with the tip facing the inferior oropharynx, and gently slide it behind the tongue.
   (c) Advance the airway gently, rotating it 180 degrees, so that it comes to rest with the flange on the patient's teeth.
   (d) Answers (a) and (c).
   (e) Answers (a) or (b), and (c).

70.   The preferred method for oral airway insertion in an infant or child is
   (a) no different from that of the adult insertion method.
   (b) using a tongue depressor to lift the tongue up and forward, while inserting the airway in the position of its function, with the tip facing the inferior oropharynx, and gently slide it behind the tongue.
   (c) the same as that of adult insertion, but only rotating the airway 90 degrees.
   (d) Answers (b) or (c).
   (e) None of the above.

71.   Which of the following statements regarding the insertion of a nasal airway is false?
   (a) Lubricate the airway with a petroleum-based (oil-based) lubricant to minimize the amount of trauma to the nasal mucosa.
   (b) Insert the airway with the bevel aimed toward the nasal septum.
   (c) Advance the airway until the flange rests against the nostril.
   (d) Gentle rotation from side to side may be required to completely insert the airway.
   (e) If the airway cannot be gently inserted into one nostril, try the other nostril.

72. When a gurgling sound is heard with the first ventilation of a patient, it indicates that
   (a) the patient requires immediate hyperventilation.
   (b) the patient needs immediate suction.
   (c) the ventilation device is not adequately sealing to the patient's face and should be repositioned and resealed before continuing ventilations.
   (d) the airway adjunct is an incorrect size and should be immediately removed.
   (e) the patient is being successfully ventilated.

73. The hard or rigid "Yankauer" suction catheter is also commonly called a
   (a) "tonsil sucker" or "tonsil tip."
   (b) "rigid sucker" or "rigid tip."
   (c) "French" catheter.
   (d) Answers (a) or (c).
   (e) Answers (b) or (c).

74. A soft suction catheter is also commonly called a
   (a) "tonsil sucker" or "tonsil tip."
   (b) "rigid sucker" or "rigid tip."
   (c) "French" catheter.
   (d) Answers (a) or (c).
   (e) Answers (b) or (c).

75. Which of the following statements regarding a Yankauer suction catheter is false?
   (a) It is useful for suctioning large particulate matter from the nasopharynx.
   (b) It is used to suction the mouth and oropharynx of an unresponsive patient.
   (c) It should be inserted only as far as you can see.
   (d) It may be used for pediatric patients, but caution should be exercised to avoid touching the back of the airway.
   (e) It should not be inserted farther than the base of the tongue.

76. Which of the following statements regarding a soft suction catheter is true?
   (a) It is useful for suctioning the nasopharynx.
   (b) When suctioning the oropharynx, the soft suction catheter should be measured so that it is inserted only as far as the base of the tongue.
   (c) It may be used to suction through an endotracheal tube.
   (d) Answers (b) and (c) are true.
   (e) Answers (a), (b), and (c) are true.

77. Which of the following statements regarding suctioning techniques is false?
   (a) Suction should only be applied during insertion of the catheter.
   (b) Suction an adult for no more than 15 seconds at a time.

(c) Rinse the catheter with water as needed, to prevent tubing obstruction.

(d) If secretions or emesis cannot be removed quickly and easily by suctioning, logroll the patient to his side for manual clearance of the oropharynx.

(e) When applying suction, move the catheter tip from side to side.

78. Vigorous suctioning at the posterior of the oropharynx may result in all of the following, except

(a) vagus nerve stimulation, causing a decrease in adult heart rate.

(b) vagus nerve stimulation, causing a decrease in pediatric heart rate.

(c) stimulation of the gag reflex, causing vomiting.

(d) stimulation of hypoxia, causing tachycardia or irregular heart rate in an adult.

(e) stimulation of the "rooting" reflex in infants, which will increase the effectiveness of suctioning.

79. Which of the following statements regarding suctioning is false?

(a) If the patient is producing secretions or vomitus faster than a suction catheter can effectively remove them, logroll the patient to his side to employ gravity and finger sweeps of the oropharynx.

(b) If the patient's heart rate suddenly changes during suctioning, immediately discontinue the suction and provide positive-pressure hyperventilation.

(c) Hyperventilation will force fluid or mucous into the lungs, and should only occur after all fluid or mucous is removed from the patient's airways. Repeat suctioning sessions may be required prior to performing any hyperventilation.

(d) If the patient is still producing frothy secretions after one suction session, do not repeat the suction until hyperventilation has been provided for at least 2 minutes.

(e) When suctioning a patient, residual air (oxygen) is also being removed.

80. At sea level, the atmosphere provides an adequately breathing person with _____ percent oxygen.

(a) 100

(b) 75

(c) 33

(d) 21

(e) 10

81. The medical term for an inadequate supply of oxygen to the tissues of the body is

(a) anoxia.

(b) hyperpnea.

(c) apnea.

(d) hypoxemia.

(e) hypoxia.

82. Even appropriately performed CPR is only _____ percent as effective as a patient's normal circulation.

    (a) 75 to 85

    (b) 55 to 75

    (c) 25 to 33

    (d) 10 to 15

    (e) 5 to 10

83. Which of the following statements regarding operational hazards associated with oxygen administration is false?

    (a) An increased risk of fire accompanies oxygen use, because oxygen causes fire to burn more rapidly.

    (b) Oxygen can be absorbed into fabric, saturating items such as towels, pillows, or sheets, and increasing their combustibility.

    (c) Oxygenation equipment must be oiled regularly to prevent dried connections from encouraging explosion.

    (d) If punctured, an oxygen tank may become a lethally destructive missile.

    (e) Because oxygen may cause it to combust, adhesive tape must never be used to protect an oxygen tank outlet, or to label an oxygen tank.

84. Which of the following statements regarding medical hazards occasionally associated with oxygen administration is false?

    (a) Because eye damage due to retinal-scarring of a premature newborn's eyes is a serious side effect of oxygen administration, only "blow-by" oxygen (at no more than 6 lpm) should be administered to premature infants with inadequate breathing.

    (b) COPD patients may lose their stimulus to breathe if high-flow oxygen is delivered over a long period of time.

    (c) Supplemental oxygen should never be withheld from a COPD patient experiencing an emergency.

    (d) Oxygen toxicity may cause collapse of alveoli, seriously reducing lung function.

    (e) Oxygen toxicity is only a concern when a patient who has been on supplemental oxygen for a long period of time requires transportation between facilities.

85. A full cylinder ("tank") of oxygen contains approximately _____ pounds of oxygen per square inch (psi).

    (a) 3,000

    (b) 2,000

    (c) 1,000

    (d) 500

    (e) None of the above. A full tank's psi varies, depending upon its size.

86. Oxygen cylinders come in many different sizes. The "D" cylinder contains
    _____ liters of oxygen.
    (a) 350
    (b) 625
    (c) 3,000
    (d) 5,300
    (e) 6,900

87. The "E" cylinder contains _____ liters of oxygen.
    (a) 350
    (b) 625
    (c) 3,000
    (d) 5,300
    (e) 6,900

88. The "M" cylinder contains _____ liters of oxygen.
    (a) 350
    (b) 625
    (c) 3,000
    (d) 5,300
    (e) 6,900

89. The "G" cylinder contains _____ liters of oxygen.
    (a) 350
    (b) 625
    (c) 3,000
    (d) 5,300
    (e) 6,900

90. The "H" cylinder contains _____ liters of oxygen.
    (a) 350
    (b) 625
    (c) 3,000
    (d) 5,300
    (e) 6,900

91. Which of the following statements regarding the nonrebreather mask is false?
    (a) The nonrebreather mask is the best means of providing oxygen to an
        emergency patient demonstrating a reasonably adequate respiratory rate.
    (b) A nonrebreather mask should never be used on premature newborns.
    (c) During an acute respiratory emergency, a nonrebreather mask should be
        employed to oxygenate a COPD patient.
    (d) The nonrebreather bag must be full before the mask is placed on the patient.
    (e) The oxygen flow rate must be high enough to ensure that the nonrebreather
        bag does not completely collapse when the patient inhales.

92. The optimal oxygen flow rate for a nonrebreather mask is _____ lpm.
   (a) 25 to 50
   (b) 12 to 15
   (c) 6 to 10
   (d) 5 to 8
   (e) 1 to 6

93. At the optimal flow rate of oxygen, a nonrebreather mask will deliver approximately _____ percent of oxygen.
   (a) 100
   (b) 80 to 90
   (c) 50 to 75
   (d) 24 to 44
   (e) 10 to 15

94. In the prehospital emergency setting, the nasal cannula oxygen delivery device
   (a) causes less anxiety, and thus is the best method of delivering supplemental oxygen to patients complaining of chest pain.
   (b) should be used only when the patient will not tolerate a nonrebreather mask.
   (c) is the only oxygen delivery device that should be used for COPD patients.
   (d) Answers (a) and (c).
   (e) Answers (b) and (c).

95. The maximum flow rate of oxygen when using a nasal cannula is _____ lpm.
   (a) 15
   (b) 10
   (c) 8
   (d) 6
   (e) 2

96. Depending upon the oxygen flow rate, the oxygen concentration delivered by a nasal cannula varies from _____ percent of oxygen.
   (a) 80 to 90
   (b) 50 to 75
   (c) 24 to 44
   (d) 13 to 22
   (e) 5 to 10

97. Which of the following special considerations regarding airway management and patients with facial injuries is false?
   (a) Because blood supply to the face is so rich, blunt injuries frequently result in severe swelling.
   (b) If facial injuries are present, no attempt should be made to insert an airway adjunct.

(c) Bleeding into the airway from facial injuries can be a challenge to manage.

(d) Frequent suctioning may be required in the presence of facial injuries.

(e) Advanced airway management may be required if severe facial injuries are present.

98. Which of the following special considerations regarding management of airway obstructions is false?

(a) Many suction units or catheters are inadequate for removing large solid objects, such as teeth or food, from the airway.

(b) Manual techniques for clearing the obstructed airway are important and include abdominal thrusts, chest thrusts, or finger sweeps.

(c) Logrolling the patient to a laterally recumbent position may be necessary to clear the airway.

(d) Because they prevent an adequate seal and pose an obstruction risk, dentures (especially "full" sets) should always be removed from an unconscious patient prior to providing artificial ventilation.

(e) If a foreign body airway obstruction persists, the EMT should transport the patient, continuing to perform manual techniques for clearing the obstructed airway enroute.

99. Which of the following special considerations regarding airway management of pediatric patients is false?

(a) The smaller mouth and nose of pediatric patients are more easily obstructed.

(b) The pediatric tongue takes up more space in the oropharynx than the adult's.

(c) Excessive hyperextension of the neck in pediatric patients should be avoided.

(d) Because pediatric patients are "belly breathers" (depending more on the diaphragm for breathing), what may appear to be "gastric distention" is actually an indicator of adequate ventilation and should be ignored.

(e) Children should be ventilated with only enough force and volume to produce a gentle chest rise.

100. A pulse oximeter is a small, photoelectric device that monitors

(a) the percentage of oxygen saturating the patient's blood.

(b) the patient's pulse rate.

(c) the amount of blood circulating in the patient's body.

(d) Answers (a) and (b), depending upon the pulse oximeter model.

(e) Answers (a), (b), and (c), depending upon the pulse oximeter model.

101. At sea level, a pulse oximeter (pulse-ox) reading of between _____ indicates that your patient's blood has a normal oxygen saturation.

(a) 76 and 80%

(b) 81 and 85%

(c) 86 and 90%

(d) 91 and 95%

(e) 96 and 100%

102. Which of the following statements about pulse-ox assessment is false?

    (a) Modern pulse-ox devices are highly sensitive to the difference between oxygen molecules and carbon monoxide molecules, and are especially helpful in evaluating the severity of a carbon monoxide poisoning.

    (b) Modern pulse-ox devices provide inaccurate readings when a patient is in shock.

    (c) If the patient is a chronic cigarette smoker, his pulse-ox reading will be falsely higher than his true oxygen saturation.

    (d) If the patient is hypovolemic, the pulse-ox reading will probably be inaccurate.

    (e) If the patient is hypothermic, the pulse-ox reading will probably be inaccurate.

103. Which of the following statements about pulse-ox assessment is false?

    (a) The pulse-ox reading for an anemic patient will probably be inaccurate.

    (b) Even if the patient's pulse-ox reading shows a normal saturation, high-flow oxygen should be administered if the patient is exhibiting signs or symptoms of respiratory distress.

    (c) If a COPD patient is in respiratory distress, it is vital to their ongoing care to determine their "room air" pulse-ox reading prior to providing any supplemental oxygen.

    (d) Pulse oximetry is helpful in evaluating the effectiveness of the emergency treatment provided to the patient.

    (e) Pulse oximetry is helpful in alerting you to a deterioration of the patient's status.

Questions 104 through 107 are related to the following scenario, as it develops:

104. You are eating at a restaurant with your family when you hear a woman start to yell, "Frank! Frank!" You observe the yelling woman sitting across from a conscious, medium-sized, middle-aged man. He is sitting in his chair and exhibiting the universal sign of choking. He is cyanotic, making no noise, and has a very distressed expression on his face. Upon reaching him, your first act should be to

    (a) perform 6 to 10 back blows.

    (b) perform 6 to 10 abdominal thrusts.

    (c) ask, "Are you choking? Can you speak? Can you cough?"

    (d) solicit information from bystanders (the yelling woman is hysterical and will be of little help).

    (e) direct a specific person to call 911, and perform finger sweeps of his oral airway.

105. Your treatment of Frank progresses according to protocol. After your delivery of a tenth abdominal thrust, Frank's airway status remains unchanged. He suddenly loses consciousness and begins to slide from his chair. You gently lower him to the floor. Your next act should be to

    (a) open his airway and attempt your first mouth-to-mouth ventilation.

    (b) perform 6 to 10 chest thrusts while he is supine.

(c) perform 6 to 10 abdominal thrusts while he is supine.

(d) direct a specific person to call 911.

(e) perform "blind" finger sweeps of his oral airway in case the object was dislodged while he was placed on the floor.

106. After your last action, Frank's airway status remains unchanged. Your next step should be to
(a) open his airway and attempt your first mouth-to-mouth ventilation.
(b) perform 6 to 10 chest thrusts while he is supine.
(c) perform 6 to 10 abdominal thrusts while he is supine.
(d) direct a specific person to call 911.
(e) perform "blind" finger sweeps of his oral airway in case the object was dislodged while he was placed on the floor.

107. Your last action was unsuccessful. Your next step should be to
(a) check to see if Frank has a pulse.
(b) perform 6 to 10 chest thrusts while he is supine.
(c) perform 6 to 10 abdominal thrusts while he is supine.
(d) direct a specific person to call 911.
(e) reposition his airway and again attempt mouth-to-mouth ventilation.

Questions 108 through 110 are related to the following scenario, as it develops:

108. A week later, you are eating at the same restaurant, when a woman runs out of the ladies' room, screaming, "She choked to death! She choked to death!" Upon entering the bathroom, you see an obese woman lying on the floor. There is no apparent trauma, and she is very cyanotic. You should immediately
(a) check for a pulse and direct a specific person to call 911.
(b) check for breathing and direct a specific person to call 911.
(c) check for level of consciousness and direct a specific person to call 911.
(d) perform 6 to 10 abdominal thrusts and direct a specific person to call 911.
(e) perform 6 to 10 chest thrusts and direct a specific person to call 911.

109. Your first attempt to ventilate this patient is unsuccessful. You should immediately
(a) perform 6 to 10 abdominal thrusts, perform "blind" finger sweeps of her oral airway, position for an open airway, and attempt to ventilate again.
(b) perform 6 to 10 chest thrusts, perform "blind" finger sweeps of her oral airway, position for an open airway, and attempt to ventilate again.
(c) reposition her airway and attempt to ventilate again.
(d) begin chest compressions (chest compression also acts as a "chest thrust" and may dislodge the airway obstruction).
(e) perform "blind" finger sweeps of her oral airway, position for an open airway, and attempt to ventilate again.

110. Your second attempt to ventilate this patient is also unsuccessful. Your next act should be to

    (a) perform 6 to 10 abdominal thrusts, perform "blind" finger sweeps of her oral airway, position for an open airway, and attempt to ventilate again.

    (b) perform 6 to 10 chest thrusts, perform "blind" finger sweeps of her oral airway, position for an open airway, and attempt to ventilate again.

    (c) reposition her airway and attempt to ventilate again.

    (d) begin chest compressions (chest compression also acts as a "chest thrust" and may dislodge the airway obstruction).

    (e) perform "blind" finger sweeps of her oral airway, position for an open airway, and attempt to ventilate again.

111. During normal breathing, a person's body uses only about 5 percent of the oxygen contained in the atmosphere. Because exhalation contains the remaining amount of atmospheric oxygen, when performing rescue breathing (without oxygen supplementation) the patient receives about _____ percent oxygen.

    (a) 95

    (b) 45

    (c) 21

    (d) 16

    (e) 5

112. When initiating rescue breathing for an unresponsive patient, perform

    (a) one quick breath, and then check for a pulse.

    (b) one slow breath before checking for a pulse.

    (c) two quick breaths, and then check for a pulse.

    (d) two slow breaths, and then check for a pulse.

    (e) a pulse check before providing two slow breaths.

113. To provide ongoing rescue breathing for an adult, perform _____ ventilations a minute.

    (a) 5 to 10

    (b) 10 to 12

    (c) 12

    (d) 20

    (e) 20 to 30

114. To accomplish this ventilation rate, ventilate the adult patient once every _____ seconds.

    (a) 2 to 3

    (b) 3

    (c) 5

    (d) 4 to 5

115. To provide ongoing rescue breathing for an 8-year-old, perform _____ ventilations a minute.

     (a) 5 to 10

     (b) 10 to 12

     (c) 12

     (d) 20

     (e) 20 to 30

116. To accomplish this ventilation rate, ventilate the 8-year-old patient once every _____ seconds.

     (a) 2 to 3

     (b) 3

     (c) 5

     (d) 4 to 5

     (e) 6 to 12

117. To provide ongoing rescue breathing for an infant, perform _____ ventilations a minute.

     (a) 5 to 10

     (b) 10 to 12

     (c) 12

     (d) 20

     (e) 20 to 30

118. To accomplish this ventilation rate, ventilate the infant once every _____ seconds.

     (a) 2 to 3

     (b) 3

     (c) 5

     (d) 4 to 5

     (e) 6 to 12

119. To provide optimal ventilation during ongoing rescue breathing for an adult, the duration of each ventilation (exhalation) should be

     (a) 1 to $1\frac{1}{2}$ seconds long.

     (b) 3 seconds long.

     (c) less than 1 second long.

     (d) 1 second long.

     (e) 2 seconds long.

120. To provide optimal ventilation during ongoing rescue breathing for a child, the duration of each ventilation (exhalation) should be

    (a) 1 to $1\frac{1}{2}$ seconds long.

    (b) 3 seconds long.

    (c) less than 1 second long.

    (d) 1 second long.

    (e) 2 seconds long.

The answer key for Test Section Two is on page 331.

3

DOT Module Three: Patient Assessment

Subjects:

- Scene Size-up
- The Initial Assessment
- The Focused History and Physical Exam of Trauma Patients
- The Focused History and Physical Exam of Medical Patients
- The Detailed Physical Exam
- Ongoing Assessment
- Communications
- Documentation
- An ELECTIVE Group of Medical Abbreviations and Symbols Questions

Test Section Three consists of 120 required questions and 60 elective. If only the 120 required questions are answered, Test Section Three is allotted 2 hours for completion. If all 180 questions are answered, Test Section Three is allotted 3 hours for completion.

1. Which of the following considerations are part of the EMT's *scene size-up* (assessment of the scene and surroundings)?
   (a) Scene safety considerations.
   (b) Consideration of the mechanism of injury or nature of illness.
   (c) Precautions required for body substance isolation.
   (d) Answers (a) and (b).
   (e) Answers (a), (b), and (c).

2. Which of the following statements regarding scene safety is false?
   (a) Scene safety considerations are focused only on ensuring patient safety.
   (b) Personal protection of the care providers is the first scene safety consideration.
   (c) Protection of bystanders is an important aspect of scene safety considerations.
   (d) Scene safety considerations are not limited to the initial scene size-up, but continue throughout the call.
   (e) If a scene is unsafe, it should not be entered for any reason until it is made safe by appropriately trained and equipped personnel.

3. Diseases are caused by _____, such as viruses and bacteria.
   (a) halogens
   (b) carcinogens
   (c) pathogens
   (d) biogens
   (e) chromogens

4. Infectious diseases may be spread by
   (a) direct contact with infected blood or other body fluids.
   (b) droplet infection from airborne organisms (coughing, sneezing, or breathing).
   (c) indirect contact via handling objects or materials contaminated with infectious secretions.
   (d) Answers (a) and (c).
   (e) Answers (a), (b), and (c).

5. Which of the following statements regarding personal protective equipment is false?
   (a) Hand washing before and after every patient contact is required only if protective gloves are not worn throughout the entire patient contact.
   (b) Protective gloves must be worn for every patient contact, and a separate pair must be used for each individual patient.

(c) Eye protection should be worn whenever airborne droplet (or fluid splashing) contact is anticipated.

(d) Masks should be worn whenever airborne droplet (or fluid splashing) contact is anticipated.

(e) A gown should be worn whenever spilling or splashing of infectious fluid is anticipated.

6. Which of the following statements regarding the EMT's consideration of the mechanism of injury (MOI) is true?

(a) Some injuries can be considered "common" to specific MOIs.

(b) Even though the patient's complaint is isolated to a single body part, the MOI may require suspicion of (and treatment for) "hidden" injuries in other body parts or areas.

(c) If the MOI appears superficial and the patient seems to be complaining of pain only in order to file a lawsuit against another party, the EMT may call his Medical Director to officially "rule-out" injuries to the patient, thus avoiding the necessity of expensive treatment and transportation.

(d) Answers (a) and (b) are true.

(e) Answers (a), (b), and (c) are true.

7. Determining whether or not adequate resources are immediately available to effectively deal with the emergency is part of every scene size-up. Upon arrival, if it appears that there are more than two seriously injured patients, the EMT should

(a) immediately begin treatment of the nearest seriously injured patient, and call for additional resources only after stabilizing all patients who have life-threatening conditions.

(b) immediately begin triage and call for additional resources only after identifying the specific number of patients who have life-threatening conditions.

(c) immediately call for additional resources, even before initiating triage or treatment.

(d) begin triage, initiate treatment for one minute, and then call for additional resources.

(e) perform an initial walk-through and obtain an accurate count of the patients present, prior to calling for additional resources.

8. Which of the following statements regarding the initial assessment of a patient's circulation is false?

(a) For patients of all ages, assess the radial pulse first.

(b) If no radial pulse is felt (on either side), palpate for a carotid pulse.

(c) If no carotid pulse is felt, start CPR.

(d) Assess for major bleeding and, if present, control the bleeding immediately.

(e) Only an approximate pulse rate needs to be determined.

9. The *initial assessment* of a patient consists of six specific steps. Of the following
    possible steps, select the six initial assessment steps and place them in correct
    order (from first-performed to last-performed).
    (1) Using the mnemonic "SAMPLE," assess the patient's medical history.
    (2) Using the mnemonic "AVPU," assess the patient's level of consciousness.
    (3) Form a general impression of the patient.
    (4) Assess the patient's circulation.
    (5) Identify the patient's priority.
    (6) Assess the patient's breathing.
    (7) Assess the patient's airway.

    (a) 7, 6, 4, 2, 3, 5.
    (b) 3, 2, 7, 6, 4, 5.
    (c) 7, 6, 4, 2, 1, 3.
    (d) 3, 7, 6, 4, 1, 5.
    (e) 5, 2, 7, 6, 4, 3.

10. When assessing the patient's medical history, the "S" of the mnemonic (memory
    aid) *SAMPLE* represents questions about
    (a) Signs and Symptoms—What are the patient's complaints and vital signs?
    (b) Size—What is the weight and height of the patient?
    (c) Speech—How well does the patient speak?
    (d) Snoring—Does the patient have an airway?
    (e) Surroundings—What is the patient environment like?

11. The "A" of a SAMPLE history stands for
    (a) Aftereffects—complaints following the incident.
    (b) Allergies—to medications, food, environmental substances.
    (c) Altered level of consciousness.
    (d) Affect—What does the patient look like?
    (e) Anxiety–Is the patient upset?

12. The "M" of a SAMPLE history stands for
    (a) Major—What are the patient's major complaints?
    (b) Minor—What are the patient's minor complaints?
    (c) Multiple—What is the number of the patient's complaints?
    (d) Married—Is the patient married, single, or divorced?
    (e) Medications—current and/or recent prescription, nonprescription drugs.

13. The "P" of a SAMPLE history stands for
    (a) Plan—your planned course of treatment.
    (b) Potential Problem—the suspected diagnosis.
    (c) Previous—the treatment already rendered.
    (d) Pertinent Past medical history—medical, surgical, and trauma.
    (e) Pulse—Does the patient have a pulse?

14. The "L" of a SAMPLE history stands for questions about the patient's
    (a) Likes and dislikes.
    (b) Last menstrual period.
    (c) Last meal or oral intake—time, quantity, and substance(s).
    (d) Looks—Does the patient appear sick or injured?
    (e) Late—developing signs and symptoms, if any.

15. The "E" of a SAMPLE history stands for
    (a) Equal—equality of grips, pupils, and movement.
    (b) Energy—Is the patient fatigued?
    (c) Events leading to the injury or illness.
    (d) Extra—What extra things can you think of asking?
    (e) Evaluation—the suspected diagnosis.

16. When assessing the patient's level of consciousness, the "A" of the mnemonic AVPU
    stands for
    (a) Alert.
    (b) Altered level of consciousness—the patient is confused.
    (c) Anxiety—Is the patient upset?
    (d) Awake and confused.
    (e) Alcohol—Has the patient been drinking?

17. The "V" of the mnemonic AVPU stands for your assessment that the patient is
    (a) Very unconscious.
    (b) Very alert (not confused).
    (c) responsive to Verbal stimuli.
    (d) unresponsive to Verbal stimuli.
    (e) Very Verbal (talkative) without any stimuli.

18. The "P" of the mnemonic AVPU stands for your assessment that
    (a) the patient responds to Painful stimuli.
    (b) the patient is Partially unconscious.
    (c) the patient is Partially conscious.
    (d) the patient is complaining of Pain.
    (e) Painful stimuli provoke no response in the patient.

19. The "U" of the mnemonic AVPU stands for your assessment that
    (a) Unusual circumstances are involved in this patient's situation.
    (b) an Unreliable history of the event or illness is being presented.
    (c) the patient is Unresponsive with an intact gag or cough reflex.
    (d) the patient is Unresponsive to verbal and painful stimuli.
    (e) the patient is Unhappy (has feelings of "impending doom").

20. A *general impression* of the patient must be developed. The general impression is first formed
    (a) after learning the exact nature of the patient's illness and/or injury, and the completion of a SAMPLE history.
    (b) after the patient's first set of vital signs are obtained.
    (c) immediately upon first observing the scene and the patient, and is based on the EMT's "gut" sense (or "sixth sense") for whether the patient's condition is critical or not.
    (d) immediately prior to delivering the patient to the emergency department.
    (e) after the emergency department has assumed patient care, during the writing of the patient care report.

21. The patient's skin color is assessed by looking at the patient's
    (a) nail beds.
    (b) lips or mucosal membranes.
    (c) conjunctiva of the eyes.
    (d) Answers (a) and (b).
    (e) Answers (a), (b), or (c).

22. Which of the following statements regarding capillary refill assessment is false?
    (a) Capillary refill should be assessed in patients of all ages.
    (b) Normal capillary refill takes less than two seconds.
    (c) Abnormal capillary refill takes greater than two seconds.
    (d) Capillary refill assessment is only required for pediatric patient assessment.
    (e) A capillary refill assessment can be performed on any extremity.

23. Which of the following statements regarding assessment of the conscious and responsive patient's airway status is true?
    (a) It is important to note if the patient is talking or crying.
    (b) If the patient is able to talk or cry (even if only weakly), adequate breathing is present and no further "airway" assessment is necessary.
    (c) Even when the patient is talking or crying, breathing may still be inadequate and require airway assistance.
    (d) Answers (a) and (c) are true.
    (e) None of the above are true.

24. Which of the following statements regarding assessment of breathing (and subsequent treatment) is false?
    (a) If a conscious patient is complaining of difficulty in breathing, but has a respiratory rate within normal limits, oxygen administration is not indicated.
    (b) All adult patients breathing faster than 24 times per minute should receive high flow oxygen (15 lpm by a nonrebreather mask).

(c) If the patient is unresponsive but with adequate breathing, open and maintain the airway, also providing high concentration oxygen.

(d) If the patient is unresponsive with inadequate breathing, open and maintain the airway, use ventilatory adjuncts and assist the patient's breathing, providing high concentration oxygen.

(e) If the patient is complaining of shortness of breath, oxygen should be administered no matter what the respiratory rate is.

25. When a life-threatening problem is encountered during the initial assessment of a patient,

(a) make a special mental note of the problem and quickly proceed to the next initial assessment step. It is important that all assessment steps are accomplished so that correct treatment can be determined.

(b) pause to treat the problem for up to one minute only. It is important that the full initial assessment be performed prior to spending large amounts of time on any single problem.

(c) stop the assessment procedure and treat each life-threatening problem as it is discovered. Additional assessment steps are only performed after a life-threatening problem is corrected.

(d) begin transport immediately (this is a critical patient), continuing the assessment until all steps are performed. Treatment may be initiated en route to the hospital, but only after all assessment steps have been performed.

(e) call for ALS assistance, but continue the assessment steps without treatment until all assessment steps have been performed, so as to provide a complete report upon ALS arrival.

26. Identification of the patient's *priority* means to identify whether or not the patient requires

(a) rapid transportation to the emergency department.

(b) the EMT to request that an ALS unit be dispatched.

(c) both a focused and a detailed physical examination, or only a focused physical examination.

(d) Answers (a) or (b).

(e) Answers (a), (b), or (c).

27. Identification of high-priority patients usually occurs very early in the assessment process. Of the following actions, which represents the "latest" point at which to identify a high-priority patient?

(a) After the initial assessment of mental status.

(b) After the initial assessment of airway and breathing status.

(c) After the initial assessment of circulatory status.

(d) After the performance of the focused physical examination.

(e) After the EMT's formation of a "general impression" of the patient.

28. Which of the following patients has the lowest-priority condition?
    (a) A patient who makes the EMT feel anxious because "he just doesn't look right!"
    (b) A patient with bleeding controlled by direct pressure.
    (c) A patient who is awake and responsive, but doesn't follow commands.
    (d) A patient complaining of severe pain in his right arm.
    (e) A patient complaining of chest pain, with a systolic blood pressure less than 100 mmHg.

29. For the trauma patient, the first step of the Focused History and Physical Examination (Focused Hx & PE) is
    (a) to begin treatment of any airway problems found during the initial assessment.
    (b) the reconsideration of the mechanism of injury.
    (c) to begin treatment of any breathing problems found during the initial assessment.
    (d) the reconsideration of the patient's sex or race.
    (e) None of the above.

30. According to the DOT-established order of performance, baseline vital signs should be obtained
    (a) at the end of the initial assessment.
    (b) at the very beginning of the Focused Hx & PE.
    (c) before beginning the focused physical exam.
    (d) after obtaining a SAMPLE history.
    (e) after completing the focused physical exam.

31. According to the DOT-established order of performance, a SAMPLE history should be obtained
    (a) at the end of the initial assessment.
    (b) at the very beginning of the Focused Hx & PE.
    (c) before beginning the focused physical exam.
    (d) after obtaining baseline vital signs.
    (e) after completing the focused physical exam.

32. An EMT's MOI consideration, by itself, is sufficient cause to treat a patient for all of the following conditions, except
    (a) spinal injury.
    (b) internal bleeding.
    (c) chest injury.
    (d) drug or alcohol abuse.
    (e) joint injuries.

33. Which of the following patients has the least-serious mechanism of injury?
    (a) Someone ejected from a vehicle during an auto accident.
    (b) The seat-belted passenger of a vehicle that crashed, killing the non-seat-belted driver, but who denies all complaints of injury.
    (c) A child who has fallen a distance of twice his height.
    (d) The seat-belted driver of a vehicle that rolled-over at least once, who denies all complaints of injury.
    (e) The seat-belted driver of a vehicle that collided with a bridge abutment at high-speed, who denies all complaints of injury, and reports, "I must have fallen asleep!"

34. Which of the following patients has the least-serious mechanism of injury?
    (a) The pedestrian victim of an auto–pedestrian accident.
    (b) A helmeted motorcycle operator who is well-oriented, ambulatory prior to your arrival, without any complaints, and reports that he avoided impact with an auto and other stationary structures because "I laid my bike down."
    (c) The restrained driver of an auto that struck an embankment at 20 miles per hour, who is ambulatory prior to your arrival, denies any complaints, but is confused about what happened and what's going on.
    (d) A patient who fell from approximately 20 feet.
    (e) A patient with a gunshot wound to his right hand.

35. Which of the following pediatric patients has the least-serious mechanism of injury?
    (a) A child without complaints or apparent injuries, who fell off his bicycle when rapidly riding through an empty lot filled with loose dirt.
    (b) A child without complaints or apparent injuries, who was unrestrained during a low-speed vehicular collision.
    (c) A child without complaints or apparent injuries, who was restrained during a medium-speed vehicular collision.
    (d) A child without complaints or apparent injuries, who fell from a window approximately 12 feet above a grass lawn.
    (e) A child with a stab wound to his right hand, without any other complaints or apparent injuries.

36. Which of the following statements regarding the use of seat belts during a motor vehicle accident are true?
    (a) When worn appropriately, seat belts save lives.
    (b) Even when worn appropriately, seat belts may cause serious injuries to abdominal organs.
    (c) If wearing an appropriately positioned seat belt, the patient will not have serious injuries.
    (d) Answers (a) and (b) are true.
    (e) All of the above are true.

37. Which of the following statements regarding the use of airbags during a motor vehicle accident are true?

   (a) Airbags save more lives than seat belts do.

   (b) Airbags are equally effective, with or without the use of seat belts.

   (c) Unseat-belted patients may impact the steering wheel after the airbag has deflated.

   (d) Answers (a) and (b) are true.

   (e) All of the above are true.

38. When assessing a motor vehicle accident where the patient's airbag has been deployed, the EMT should

   (a) recognize that serious trauma to the patient's head, chest, or abdomen is highly unlikely because of the efficiency of airbags.

   (b) "lift and look" under the airbag to determine if potentially serious patient injury may have occurred, as indicated by a dented dash or deformed steering wheel.

   (c) "lift and look" under the airbag, but remember that dash or steering wheel deformity is often caused by the normal deployment of airbags and is not a sign of patient injury.

   (d) treat the patient only for the minor abrasions that often accompany patient impact with airbags.

   (e) Answers (a) and (d).

39. The second step in the Focused Hx & PE for trauma patients with a significant mechanism of injury is to perform a Rapid Trauma Assessment. For the responsive patient this assessment section includes

   (a) continuing the spinal immobilization initiated in the initial assessment or after mechanism-of-injury re-evaluation.

   (b) determining the patient's chief complaint (what the patient most complains of or what prompted the emergency call).

   (c) considering the request for ALS support.

   (d) reconsidering the transport priority decision.

   (e) All of the above.

40. When performing a head-to-toe Rapid Trauma Assessment, the "D" of the mnemonic *DCAP-BTLS* represents examination for

   (a) a Disturbed area of skin.

   (b) a patient with Developmental Disabilities.

   (c) Degeneration of an area.

   (d) Disabled parts.

   (e) Deformities.

41. The "C" of a DCAP-BTLS assessment represents

   (a) examination for Contusions.

   (b) examination for Contraindications to treatment.

    (c) examination for Chief Complaint factors.

    (d) examination for Cold skin temperature.

    (e) Complications related to examination findings.

42. The "A" of a DCAP-BTLS assessment represents examination for

    (a) an Altered level of consciousness.

    (b) any Alcohol involvement.

    (c) Abrasions.

    (d) Alignment Alterations of the injured area or limb.

    (e) any Aggravating circumstances.

43. The "P" of a DCAP-BTLS assessment represents examination for

    (a) Partial avulsions or amputations.

    (b) Punctures or Penetrations.

    (c) Parietal skull injuries.

    (d) signs and symptoms of Probable injury.

    (e) the Presence of any injury findings.

44. The "B" of a DCAP-BTLS assessment represents examination for

    (a) a mechanism of injury involving Blunt injury.

    (b) Borderline findings for injury.

    (c) the Ballistic information required by gunshot wounds.

    (d) Burns.

    (e) Bulging anatomical parts.

45. The "T" of a DCAP-BTLS assessment represents examination for

    (a) Tenderness.

    (b) Tremulousness (shaking or shivering).

    (c) Total amputation of a part or area.

    (d) Tearing of a body part.

    (e) Tremendous (or devastating) evidence of injury.

46. The "L" of a DCAP-BTLS assessment represents examination for

    (a) Level of consciousness.

    (b) Location of injury.

    (c) Long bone injury findings (a potentially dire emergency).

    (d) Lacerations.

    (e) Loss of sensation or motor function.

47. The "S" of a DCAP-BTLS assessment represents examination for

    (a) loss of body-part Stability.

    (b) Swelling.

    (c) Significant injury.

    (d) Stable injury.

    (e) Soreness.

48. The discovery of *crepitation* (or *crepitus*) may be found in all of the following areas, except

    (a) the head.

    (b) the neck.

    (c) the chest.

    (d) the abdomen.

    (e) the pelvis.

49. The presence or absence of jugular vein distention should be evaluated in which of the following areas?

    (a) The neck.

    (b) The groin.

    (c) The forearms.

    (d) Answers (a) and (b).

    (e) Answers (a), (b), and (c).

50. The presence or absence of paradoxical motion should be evaluated in which of the following areas?

    (a) The abdomen.

    (b) The neck.

    (c) The chest.

    (d) Answers (a) and (c).

    (e) Answers (a), (b), and (c).

51. The presence or absence of distention should be evaluated in which of the following areas?

    (a) The head.

    (b) The neck.

    (c) The chest.

    (d) The abdomen.

    (e) All of the areas mentioned above require assessment for distention.

52. Which of the following statements regarding examination of the patient's pelvis is false?

    (a) Do not palpate the pelvis of any patient unless you are of the same gender as the patient.

    (b) If the patient complains of pelvic pain, do not palpate the pelvis.

    (c) If the conscious patient's pelvis appears deformed or otherwise injured, do not palpate the pelvis.

    (d) If the unconscious patient's pelvis appears deformed or otherwise injured, do not palpate the pelvis.

    (e) If the unconscious patient's pelvis appears free of deformity or injury, you must palpate it.

53.   The term _____ is defined as a permanent or temporary opening of some portion of the intestine, connected to the abdominal wall, where an external bag is attached to collect feces.

    (a) colonoscopy
    (b) colitis
    (c) colostomy
    (d) episiostomy
    (e) abdominal stoma

54.   The term _____ is used to describe the crackling or grating sound, or the crunchy palpation sensation, caused by movement of broken bone ends against each other.

    (a) pleuritis
    (b) crepitation
    (c) pronation
    (d) sonoration
    (e) osteopation

55.   The term _____ is defined as a condition of being larger than normal, stretched, or inflated.

    (a) hypervention
    (b) hyperbole
    (c) supernation
    (d) distention
    (e) hyperdration

56.   The phrase _____ motion (or movement) is used to describe when one part of the chest moves opposite to the rest of the chest during respiration.

    (a) paradoxical
    (b) hypothetical
    (c) paranormal
    (d) covert
    (e) pleuritic

57.   A spinal cord injury may produce a persistent erection of the penis. This condition is called

    (a) hypererection.
    (b) priapism.
    (c) penile hyperextension.
    (d) Cushing's erection.
    (e) Kusmall's erection.

58. When the patient is stable, vital signs should be assessed
    (a) after every medical intervention.
    (b) every 30 minutes.
    (c) every 15 minutes.
    (d) Answers (a) and (b).
    (e) Answers (a) and (c).

59. When the patient is unstable, vital signs should be assessed
    (a) after every medical intervention.
    (b) every 10 minutes.
    (c) every 5 minutes.
    (d) Answers (a) and (b).
    (e) Answers (a) and (c).

60. The mnemonic *OPQRST* is helpful for performing the first step of a medical patient's Focused Hx & PE. The "O" of the OPQRST assessment mnemonic stands for the word
    (a) Oxygen—"Do you use oxygen at home?"
    (b) Onset—"Describe the onset of this problem." (Time, activity during onset.)
    (c) Only—"Is this the only problem you have right now?"
    (d) Other or Old problems—"Do you have problems other than this one?" "Is this an old problem or a new one?"
    (e) Orientation—Does the patient know who he is, where he is, the day and the date?

61. The "P" of the OPQRST assessment mnemonic stands for the word
    (a) Plan—What treatment do you plan to provide to the patient?
    (b) Previous—"When have you had this problem before? What was it?"
    (c) Part—Which part of the patient does the problem involve?
    (d) Provocation—"What brought the problem on? What makes it worse?"
    (e) Payment—Does the patient have medical insurance? (If so, be sure to get the billing information.)

62. The "Q" of the OPQRST assessment mnemonic stands for the word
    (a) Qualify—Does the patient qualify for Medicare or Medicaid insurance?
    (b) Quit—"When did the problem stop bothering you? What made it better?"
    (c) Questions—"Do you have any questions for us or the doctor?"
    (d) Quick—Does the patient have a rapid heart rate or respiratory rate?
    (e) Quality—"Describe the quality of your pain, discomfort, or difficulty. What does it feel like?"

63. The "R" of the OPQRST assessment mnemonic stands for the word

    (a) Radiation of complaint—Does the patient have complaints that may be radiating from or related to the chief complaint? "Where else do you have discomfort or abnormal sensations?" (It is the EMT's job, not the patient's job, to determine whether or not other complaints are related to, or radiating from, the area of chief complaint.)

    (b) Relatives—"Have any of your relatives had these problems?" Determine family medical history.

    (c) Respirations—Does the patient complain of, or exhibit, any respiratory problems?

    (d) Religion—What is the patient's religious preference?

    (e) Reason—Why did the patient call?

64. The "S" of the OPQRST assessment mnemonic stands for the word

    (a) Severity—How does the patient rate the severity of this problem in relation to the most severe problem he's ever had?

    (b) Solution—"What would you like us to do for you today?"

    (c) Single—Is this a single problem, or does the patient also have other complaints?

    (d) Separate—"Is this a separate incidence of this problem, or have you had other incidents like this?"

    (e) Selection—"Which hospital would you like to go to?"

65. The "T" of the OPQRST assessment mnemonic stands for the word

    (a) Temperature—What is the patient's oral or rectal temperature?

    (b) Treatment Tried—Did the patient do or take anything to alleviate the problem, and did it work?

    (c) Time—What time did the problem start at or how long has it lasted?

    (d) Telephone—Has the patient called his private physician?

    (e) Talk—"Tell me all about this problem. Describe it."

66. The OPQRST history is immediately followed by obtaining

    (a) billing information to complete your patient care report.

    (b) a SAMPLE history.

    (c) an AVPU history.

    (d) Answers (a) and (c).

    (e) Answers (a), (b), and (c).

67. Which of the following statements regarding the performance of a focused, Rapid Physical Exam of the responsive (conscious) medical patient is true?

    (a) It is necessary to perform an in-depth physical examination only of body areas that directly relate to the patient's medical complaints (if the patient's only complaint is abdominal pain, a pupil exam is not necessary).

    (b) Every area of the patient's body must be thoroughly examined.

    (c) Areas where the patient complains of pain should be repeatedly palpated to determine consistency or inconsistency of the patient's response.

    (d) All of the above are true.

    (e) None of the above is true.

68. Which of the following statements regarding the performance of a focused, Rapid Physical Exam of the unresponsive (unconscious) medical patient is true?

    (a) It is necessary to perform an in-depth physical examination only of body areas that directly relate to the history provided by the calling party (if the patient's only complaint prior to becoming unconscious was abdominal pain, a pupil exam is not necessary).

    (b) Every area of the patient's body must be thoroughly examined.

    (c) Areas where the patient complains of pain should be repeatedly palpated to determine consistency or inconsistency of the calling party's report.

    (d) All of the above are true.

    (e) None of the above is true.

69. The Focused Hx & PE for all patients includes searching for medical ID devices that identify the patient's medical history and allergies. These devices can be found

    (a) on the patient's wrist or ankle (a bracelet ID).

    (b) around the patient's neck (a necklace ID).

    (c) in the patient's purse or wallet (a medical ID card).

    (d) Answers (a) and (b).

    (e) Answers (a), (b), and (c).

70. Another form of medical information that may be present in the patient's home is called a "Vial of Life." This is usually a small canister or baggie containing pertinent patient medical history information. The presence of a "Vial of Life" is usually identified by a sticker mounted on the

    (a) patient's refrigerator door.

    (b) main door of the patient's residence.

    (c) window closest to the main door.

    (d) Answers (b) or (c).

    (e) Answers (a), (b), or (c).

71. In addition to pertinent patient medical history information, a "Vial of Life" may contain

    (a) a picture of the patient.

    (b) Do Not Resuscitate (DNR) documentation.

    (c) a Living Will or its equivalent.

    (d) Answers (b) or (c).

    (e) Answers (a), (b), or (c).

72.   Which of the following statements regarding the Detailed Physical Exam (Detailed PE) are true?

    (a) The Detailed PE is performed only if time permits, usually while en route to the emergency department.

    (b) For patients with simple, isolated injuries, a Detailed PE of uninjured body areas is not required.

    (c) Treatment for critical or serious problems always precedes a Detailed PE.

    (d) Answers (a) and (c) are true.

    (e) Answers (a), (b), and (c) are true.

73.   The Detailed PE of the ear should include observing for

    (a) hearing deficits.

    (b) bleeding.

    (c) fluid drainage.

    (d) Answers (b) and (c).

    (e) Answers (a), (b), and (c).

74.   The Detailed PE of the eye should include observing for all of the following, except

    (a) contact lenses.

    (b) unequal pupils.

    (c) foreign bodies.

    (d) blood in the anterior chamber.

    (e) pupil color.

75.   The Detailed PE of the nose should include observing for

    (a) fluid drainage or bleeding.

    (b) paradoxical movement on respiration.

    (c) presence of mucous.

    (d) Answers (b) and (c).

    (e) Answers (a), (b), and (c).

76.   The Detailed PE of the mouth should include observing for

    (a) loose or broken teeth or other objects that may obstruct the airway.

    (b) wounds, discoloration, or edema of the tongue.

    (c) breath odor.

    (d) Answers (a) and (b).

    (e) Answers (a), (b), and (c).

77. The Ongoing Assessment phase of prehospital care can be best defined as a procedure for

(a) filling time until arrival at the patient's destination.

(b) detecting changes in the patient's clinical presentation, vital signs, and response to treatment that may identify or relate to underlying disease or injury processes.

(c) documenting several sets of vital signs to fulfill the legal requirements of basic examination documentation.

(d) Answers (a) and (c).

(e) Answers (a), (b), and (c).

78. The term *trending* is best defined as the process of

(a) assessing and documenting changes in the patient's clinical presentation, vital signs, and response to treatment that occur over a period of time, and may provide information that is important to identifying underlying disease or injury processes.

(b) identifying the patient's involvement in a specific "subculture," by assessing and documenting the patient's clothing and language patterns. (Identification of subculture trends may identify a patient at risk for specific illnesses or injuries.)

(c) following current protocols and trends of patient care, even when they are radically different from previously established, accepted protocols.

(d) Answers (b) and (c).

(e) Answers (a), (b), and (c).

79. Which of the following steps is not part of the Ongoing Assessment?

(a) Recheck the potential for life-threatening injury or illness by repeating the initial assessment.

(b) Reassess and record the patient's vital signs.

(c) Repeat the Focused Assessment regarding the patient's complaint or injuries.

(d) Assess and document the effectiveness of EMS interventions (adequacy of oxygen delivery or artificial ventilation, bleeding management, other medical interventions), and the patient's response to these interventions.

(e) Ensure that the patient's medical insurance and billing information is obtained prior to arrival at the emergency department.

80. All of the following determinations are part of the initial and ongoing phases of patient assessment, except for

(a) mental status assessment and monitoring.

(b) assessment/monitoring of airway and breathing status.

(c) assessment/monitoring of pulse presence, rate, and quality.

(d) assessment/monitoring of skin color and temperature.

(e) documentation of verbal comments that a patient makes regarding criminal activities.

81.   The best definition for the term (or phrase) _____ is a radio that is located at a stationary site, such as a hospital or public safety agency.

    (a) portable radio

    (b) base station

    (c) repeater

    (d) mobile two-way radio

    (e) cellular telephone

82.   The best definition for the term (or phrase) _____ is a transmitter/receiver that usually is mounted in a vehicle and typically transmits at 20 to 50 watts, with a general transmission range of 10 to 15 miles.

    (a) portable radio

    (b) base station

    (c) repeater

    (d) mobile two-way radio

    (e) cellular telephone

83.   The best definition for the term (or phrase) _____ is a radio that is handheld and typically transmits at power of 1 to 5 watts, with a limited general range of transmission.

    (a) portable radio

    (b) base station

    (c) repeater

    (d) mobile two-way radio

    (e) cellular telephone

84.   The best definition for the term (or phrase) _____ is a device that receives a transmission on one frequency and retransmits at a higher power on another frequency.

    (a) portable radio

    (b) base station

    (c) repeater

    (d) mobile two-way radio

    (e) cellular telephone

85.   The best definition for the term (or phrase) _____ is a device that transmits through the air instead of over wires so that its range is expanded; it has the advantage of simultaneous, two-way conversation (allowing for interruptions, questions, and answers during communication).

    (a) portable radio

    (b) base station

    (c) repeater

    (d) mobile two-way radio

    (e) cellular telephones

86. Radio frequencies are assigned, licensed, and monitored by
   - (a) the Federal Communication Commission (FCC).
   - (b) the County Communication Commission (CCC).
   - (c) the Federal Aviation Association (FAA).
   - (d) the County Aviation Association (CAA).
   - (e) the provider's local Communication Association [(city's initials) CA].

87. Communication with medical direction occurs when the EMT contacts
   - (a) the receiving facility regarding the patient's situation and time of facility arrival.
   - (b) a Medical Director regarding the patient, who then relays that information to the facility that will receive the patient.
   - (c) a Medical Director for consultation and receipt of patient care instructions or orders.
   - (d) Answers (b) or (c).
   - (e) Answers (a), (b), or (c).

88. The content of radio transmissions should be
   - (a) sketchy and nonspecific in order to conserve "air time," and can be provided in any order, as long as the patient's chief complaint and medical history is relayed.
   - (b) organized and concise, but complete; relaying all information pertinent to the patient's immediate medical condition, and any questions or concerns the EMT may have about the patient's care.
   - (c) as brief as possible, relaying only the patient's medical history and chief complaint (a well-trained EMT does not require radio consultations regarding patient care issues).
   - (d) Answers (a) and (c).
   - (e) Answers (a), (b), and (c).

89. Which of the following statements regarding EMT-physician radio communication is false?
   - (a) The Medical Director's orders and recommendations will be based solely upon the EMT's transmitted patient information, thus such information must be accurate.
   - (b) After receiving a medication or procedure order, the EMT should repeat that order back to the Medical Director.
   - (c) After receiving a denial of orders for medication or procedure performance, the EMT should repeat the denial of orders back to the Medical Director.
   - (d) Even if the Medical Director's orders are unclear or appear to be inappropriate, the EMT should never question such orders. The sole responsibility for performance of patient care lies with the Medical Director.
   - (e) EMTs' radio reports provide information that allows hospitals to prepare for a patient's arrival by having the right room, equipment, and personnel ready.

90. Which of the following statements regarding radio communication principles is false?

    (a) Ensure that the radio is on and the volume is properly adjusted.

    (b) Listen to the frequency before transmitting to ensure it is clear of other radio traffic.

    (c) Begin speaking immediately upon pushing the "press to talk" (PTT) button to avoid excessive obstruction of air time (or creation of "dead air").

    (d) Speak with your lips approximately two to three inches away from the microphone (too close, and your transmission becomes garbled – too far away and your transmission is too faint).

    (e) Address the unit being called, then give the name (and/or number) of the calling unit.

91. Which of the following statements regarding radio communication principles is false?

    (a) Speak clearly and slowly, using clear text, avoiding meaningless phrases like "Be advised."

    (b) Transmit as long as necessary to relay the entirety of your information before pausing to allow for other radio traffic. (If you pause, other radio transmissions may be aired, and will confuse the person to whom you are making your report.)

    (c) Avoid codes, using plain English (codes may confuse the person to whom you are making your report).

    (d) Courtesy is assumed when speaking on a radio, so there is no need to say "please," "thank you" and/or "you're welcome."

    (e) Stop transmitting approximately every 30 seconds to ensure that the person to whom you are making your report is receiving it, and to allow any other emergency radio traffic to regain use of the channel.

92. Which of the following statements regarding radio communication principles is false?

    (a) When transmitting a number that might be confused (for example, a number in the "teens," such as 15 being confused for 50), say the number first; then say the individual digits ("one-five").

    (b) To ensure appropriate reception of the patient, always transmit the patient's full name and the name of the patient's physician.

    (c) An EMT may be sued for slander for airing biased, derogatory, or injurious patient information over radio waves.

    (d) An EMT may be fined for using profanity over the air.

    (e) Avoid words that may be difficult to hear, such as "yes" or "no." Instead, use "affirmative" or "negative."

93. Which of the following statements regarding radio communication principles is false?

    (a) Standard formats of order for radio transmission of patient information are unnecessary as long as all important patient information is transmitted.

    (b) Indicate the end of radio transmission by saying, "over," and then get confirmation that the message was received.

    (c) Avoid identifying a "diagnosis" of the patient's problem.

    (d) Use EMS frequencies only for EMS communication.

    (e) Reduce background noise as much as possible before transmitting; for instance, close vehicle windows during transmission if you are en route.

Author's Note: *Question number 94 is more in-depth than any "standard" written examination question. If you are timing your test-taking performance, STOP timing NOW, and resume timing after you've completed this question.*

94. From the following list, select all the essential elements of a patient medical radio report and place them in the order in which they should be reported (from first-provided to last-provided).

    (1) Mental status

    (2) Chief complaint

    (3) Emergency medical care given

    (4) Estimated time of arrival (ETA) at the emergency department

    (5) The patient's age and sex

    (6) Brief, pertinent history of the patient's present illness or injury

    (7) Major past illnesses or injuries

    (8) Baseline vital signs

    (9) Pertinent physical exam findings

    (10) The patient's response to emergency medical care given

    (11) Identify your emergency unit and your level of care provision.

    (12) Identify the person/facility you are calling.

    (13) The patient's name

        (a) 12, 11, 4, 5, 2, 6, 7, 1, 8, 9, 3, 10.

        (b) 11, 12, 4, 13, 5, 2, 6, 7, 1, 8, 9, 3, 10.

        (c) 12, 11, 5, 2, 6, 8, 4.

        (d) 11, 12, 5, 2, 6, 8, 4.

        (e) 11, 12, 13, 5, 1, 2, 6, 7, 9, 8, 3, 10, 4.

[Resume Timing Now]

95. Which of the following statements regarding EMT activity following provision of a complete patient radio report is true?

    (a) If the radio report was made while en route to the emergency department, it is unnecessary to obtain any additional "sets" of the patient's vital signs. Only overall patient "condition" must be reassessed (at appropriate time intervals) prior to emergency department arrival.

    (b) When transporting a critical patient, the receiving emergency department personnel will be busy preparing for the patient's arrival. Do not distract them with any additional radio contacts about the patient's condition, for any reason, no matter how much time remains prior to emergency department estimated time of arrival (the ED ETA).

    (c) If the ED ETA permits, and as long as it doesn't distract the EMT from provision of vital patient care, any serious deterioration in the patient's condition should be relayed to the receiving facility via one or more additional radio contacts.

    (d) If the ED ETA is less than 30 minutes, no further radio contact should be made with the emergency department for any reason (repeat contacts are distracting to emergency department personnel).

    (e) If the ED ETA is greater than 30 minutes, the EMT must complete the written documentation of the patient's emergency prior to arrival, regardless of the patient's condition while en route.

96. Which of the following statements regarding the EMT's verbal report to the emergency department staff upon arrival is true?

    (a) The patient should be introduced by his first name (if known).

    (b) A summary of the same information relayed by radio should be given.

    (c) Any information obtained since your last radio transmission should be reported, such as additional vital signs, newly obtained medical history, treatment provided en route, or the patient's response to treatment en route.

    (d) Answers (b) and (c) are true.

    (e) Answers (a), (b), and (c) are true.

97. Which of the following statements regarding interpersonal communication with the patient is true?

    (a) Avoid causing patients emotional discomfort by avoiding direct eye contact.

    (b) As often as possible, position yourself above the patient. This identifies you as a figure of authority and provides the emotional relief that someone else is now in charge.

    (c) When you anticipate the truth being negative, frightening, or uncomfortable for the patient to hear, assure the patient of a pleasant and positive outcome.

    (d) All of the above are true.

    (e) None of the above is true.

98. Which of the following statements regarding interpersonal communication with the patient is true?

    (a) Use medical terminology as often as possible to demonstrate that you are an expert at emergency care. This will reassure frightened patients.

    (b) Use the patient's first name only after obtaining the patient's permission to do so.

    (c) It is often quite helpful to use pleasant nicknames for pediatric patients, such as "Sonny" (for boys) "Missy" (for girls), or the like. This reassures children that you are older, wiser, and able to take good care of them.

    (d) Both answers (a) and (c) are true.

    (e) All of the above are true.

99. Which of the following statements regarding the written prehospital patient care report (PCR) is false?

(a) The PCR provides for continuity of care. Although it may not be read immediately, it may be referred to later for important patient information.

(b) A good PCR documents what emergency medical care was provided and any changes in the patient's status.

(c) Because the PCR is a legal document, if it is thoroughly completed it can be submitted to lawyers, saving the PCR author from having to provide deposition or courtroom testimony.

(d) PCRs aid in EMT evaluation and quality improvement efforts.

(e) PCRs aid in billing the patient, are a source for service statistics, and are helpful for prehospital research.

100. Written documentation of every patient contact should include all of the following information, except the patient's

(a) chief complaint.

(b) level of consciousness (AVPU) and mental status.

(c) marital status and religious preference.

(d) skin color, condition, and temperature.

(e) respiratory rate and effort, and pulse rate and quality.

101. Documentation of things the EMT observes about an emergency scene (such as living conditions or motor vehicle damage) is called _____ information.

(a) approximated

(b) objective

(c) subjective

(d) pertinent negative

(e) unreliable

102. Documentation of things the EMT observes about a patient during the physical examination is called _____ information.

(a) approximated

(b) objective

(c) subjective

(d) pertinent negative

(e) unreliable

103. Documentation of symptoms or sensations the patient complains of is called _____ information.

(a) approximated

(b) objective

(c) subjective

(d) pertinent negative

(e) unreliable

104. Documentation of patient information reported by bystanders or family members is called _____ information.

(a) approximated

(b) objective

(c) subjective

(d) pertinent negative

(e) unreliable

105. Documentation of symptoms or sensations the patient denies having is called _____ information.

(a) approximated

(b) objective

(c) subjective

(d) pertinent negative

(e) unreliable

106. Documentation of the patient's vital signs or physical assessment findings is called _____ information.

(a) approximated

(b) objective

(c) subjective

(d) pertinent negative

(e) unreliable

107. The narrative section of a PCR

(a) supplements check box or "fill-in-the-blank" information sections by providing space to write any information the EMT considers important to patient care.

(b) consists of check boxes or "fill-in-the-blank" boxes regarding patient condition.

(c) consists of check boxes or "fill-in-the-blank" boxes for patient vital signs.

(d) consists of check boxes or "fill-in-the-blank" boxes for patient vital signs and patient condition information.

(e) is available only to EMTs who verbally dictate their reports over a telephone documentation system.

108. Which of the following statements regarding written documentation of patient condition, assessment, or treatment information is false?

    (a) To save space and allow room for complete documentation of important patient information, medical abbreviations and radio codes should be used on the PCR as often as possible.

    (b) Describe your findings in detail, but avoid drawing conclusions or documenting personal opinions.

    (c) Include all pertinent negatives regarding the patient's complaints and condition.

    (d) Record important scene observations, such as mechanism-of-injury descriptions, suicide notes, weapons, the presence of empty medication or alcohol containers, and the like.

    (e) Record pertinent statements made by the patient or another reporting party using their own words, placed between quotation marks.

109. Which of the following statements regarding the use of medical abbreviations is true?

    (a) Because the documenter must always appear in court along with the PCR, EMTs are free to compose their own, personal system of medical abbreviations.

    (b) Because even standard medical abbreviations may be confused for another meaning, use of medical abbreviations is discouraged. Always write it out!

    (c) Although medical abbreviations greatly improve the ability to document large amounts of patient information in small spaces, only standard medical abbreviations should be used (some services provide lists of acceptable abbreviations).

    (d) Radio codes are helpful in documenting patient information, but only standard radio codes may be used within a PCR (some services provide lists of acceptable PCR radio codes).

    (e) Both answers (a) and (d) are true.

110. Which of the following statements regarding written documentation of patient condition, assessment, or treatment information is true?

    (a) When information of a sensitive nature (such as communicable diseases) is documented, note the source of that information.

    (b) If you do not know how to spell a word, look up the correct spelling or use another word.

    (c) Spelling is not important to patient care; therefore, it is also not important to patient care documentation. As long as any reader can determine your intended message, spelling is not an issue.

    (d) Both answers (a) and (b) are true.

    (e) Both answers (a) and (c) are true.

111. Which of the following statements regarding written documentation of patient condition, assessment, or treatment information is true?

    (a) "If you didn't write it down, it wasn't done."

    (b) All of the information on the prehospital patient documentation form is considered to be confidential.

    (c) Only the patient's name, address, and billing information are considered to be confidential.

    (d) Both answers (a) and (b) are true.

    (e) Both answers (a) and (c) are true.

112. An error of omission is defined as

    (a) not doing something that should have been done.

    (b) not noticing something that should have been noticed.

    (c) performing a procedure that should not have been performed.

    (d) Answers (a) and/or (b).

    (e) Answers (a), (b), and/or (c).

113. An error of commission is defined as

    (a) not doing something that should have been done.

    (b) not noticing something that should have been noticed.

    (c) performing a procedure that should not have been performed.

    (d) Answers (a) and/or (b).

    (e) Answers (a), (b), and/or (c).

114. When an error of omission or commission occurs, the EMT should

    (a) document things as they should have been done, so that the PCR (the only legal record of the patient's prehospital care) cannot be used to punish or prosecute team members who committed the error.

    (b) carefully document only the correctly performed assessments or treatments, leaving information related to the error out of the written document.

    (c) document what did or did not happen, exactly as it occurred, and what steps were taken (if any) to correct the situation.

    (d) Answers (a) or (b).

    (e) Answers (a), (b), or (c).

115. Which of the following statements regarding falsification of information on the PCR is false?

    (a) Falsification of PCR information can lead to suspension or revocation of the EMT's certification or license.

    (b) Falsification of PCR information can lead to poor patient care because other health care providers will have a false impression of what was discovered or performed in the prehospital phase of the patient's illness or injury.

    (c) False prehospital vital sign documentation may detrimentally affect continuing patient care.

    (d) If a treatment was overlooked (such as application of oxygen) and then falsely documented as having occurred, such documentation may detrimentally affect continuing patient care.

    (e) PCRs are rarely actually read (simply filed in the patient's medical record); thus falsification of PCR information is rarely discovered.

116. If a patient refuses EMS treatment and transportation, the EMT should
   (a) try again to persuade the patient to allow treatment and transportation.
   (b) ensure that the patient is able to make a rational, informed decision. (Does the patient have an altered level of consciousness because of drugs or the effects of illness/injury?)
   (c) inform the patient specifically why he should allow treatment and transportation and what may happen to him if he does not.
   (d) consult medical direction as required by local protocol, perhaps allowing the Medical Director to speak directly with the refusing patient (via radio or phone contact).
   (e) perform all of the above actions.

117. Which of the following actions should be taken if the patient continues to refuse EMS treatment and transportation?
   (1) Document all assessment findings and any emergency medical care given.
   (2) Have the patient sign a refusal form, or the refusal section of the PCR.
   (3) Have a family member, bystander, or police officer sign beneath the patient's signature as a witness to the patient's refusal.
   (4) Document the care the EMT wished to provide.
   (5) Document the manner in which the EMT explained possible consequences of care refusal to the patient.
   (6) Encourage alternative methods of gaining care (such as a friend or family member transporting the patient to the emergency department).
   (7) Encourage the patient or family members to call the EMT back to the scene if the patient changes his mind.

     (a) 1 and 2 or 3.
     (b) 1, 2, and 3.
     (c) 1, 2 or 3, 5 and 7.
     (d) 1, 2, 3, 4, 5, and 7.
     (e) 1, 2, 3, 4, 5, 6, and 7.

118. When an error is made while writing the PCR, the EMT should
   (a) draw a single horizontal line through the error (so that the error can still be read), initial above the lined-through error, and write the correct information beside it.
   (b) carefully obliterate (darkly scribble over) all of the error, so that it cannot be read and will not confuse future readers of the report, then initial above the error.
   (c) carefully obliterate all of the error, write the word "error" above the obliteration, and then continue with the correct information.
   (d) leave the error as is, making a note at the end of the document regarding the error, and then supply the correct information.
   (e) perform any of the above actions; all that is important is that the error be corrected.

119. If a written error is discovered after a PCR has been submitted to the emergency department, the EMT should

    (a) take no action. Once a legal document has been submitted it cannot be changed.

    (b) write an entirely new PCR and have a supervisor substitute the corrected report for the one with the error, destroying the PCR with the error.

    (c) write an entirely new PCR, find and destroy all copies of the PCR with the error, and replace them with copies of the corrected form.

    (d) amend the EMT's PCR copy by drawing a single line though the error, initialing and dating the line, and writing a note with the correct information at the end of the report (initialing and dating the note). Then, copies of the corrected PCR should be distributed to all the appropriate personnel to be added to the previously submitted form.

    (e) simply find and destroy all copies of the PCR submitted with an error on it. Once submitted, a legal document cannot be changed, but an erroneous PCR should not remain in the patient's medical record.

120. Which of the following statements regarding multiple casualty incidents (MCIs) and PCR writing is false?

    (a) All prehospital patient care documentation requirements are exactly the same for MCIs as for any other patient contact.

    (b) There will probably not be enough time for the EMT to complete a PCR for each patient during MCIs. Thus, PCRs often must be completed at a later time.

    (c) The local MCI plan should include a means of temporarily recording important medical information (such as a triage tag), which can be used later to complete each patient's PCR.

    (d) Many details normally documented on a PCR will not be available when the MCI patient's PCR is finally written.

    (e) Local MCI preparedness plans should have altered guidelines established for what information is required on the final PCR for MCI patients.

The following 60 questions are an **elective** *group of* Medical Abbreviations *and* Symbols Questions. *All DOT-required medical terminology is presented in appropriate test sections of this text. However, the DOT does not list specific "standard" medical abbreviations or symbols.*

121. The medical abbreviation/symbol $\overline{a}$ means

    (a) before.

    (b) after.

    (c) every.

    (d) with.

    (e) without.

122. The medical abbreviation/symbol $\overline{s}$ means
    (a) before.
    (b) after.
    (c) every.
    (d) with.
    (e) without.

123. The medical abbreviation/symbol $\overline{c}$ means
    (a) before.
    (b) after.
    (c) every.
    (d) with.
    (e) without.

124. The medical abbreviation/symbol $\overline{p}$ means
    (a) before.
    (b) after.
    (c) every.
    (d) with.
    (e) without.

125. The medical abbreviation/symbol $\overline{q}$ means
    (a) before.
    (b) after.
    (c) every.
    (d) with.
    (e) without.

126. The medical abbreviation *abd* means
    (a) airway, breathing, disability.
    (b) always buy disposable items.
    (c) abdomen or abdominal.
    (d) abnormal appearance, bleeding, deformity.
    (e) alcohol, barbiturates, or other drugs.

127. The medical abbreviation for a sudden heart attack is
    (a) AMA (acute myocardial attack).
    (b) AHA (acute heart attack).
    (c) SHA (sudden heart attack).
    (d) AMI (acute myocardial infraction).
    (e) AMI (acute myocardial infarction).

128. The medical abbreviation for "two times a day" is
- (a) qd or q.d. (initials for the Latin, *quaque die*).
- (b) bid or b.i.d. (initials for the Latin, *bis in die*).
- (c) hs or h.s. (initials for the Latin, *hora somni*).
- (d) qid or q.i.d. (initials for the Latin, *quarter in die*).
- (e) tid or t.i.d. (initials for the Latin, *ter in die*).

129. The medical abbreviation for "everyday" is
- (a) qd or q.d. (initials for the Latin, *quaque die*).
- (b) bid or b.i.d. (initials for the Latin, *bis in die*).
- (c) hs or h.s. (initials for the Latin, *hora somni*).
- (d) qid or q.i.d. (initials for the Latin, *quarter in die*).
- (e) tid or t.i.d. (initials for the Latin, *ter in die*).

130. The medical abbreviation for "four times a day" is
- (a) qd or q.d. (initials for the Latin, *quaque die*).
- (b) bid or b.i.d. (initials for the Latin, *bis in die*).
- (c) hs or h.s. (initials for the Latin, *hora somni*).
- (d) qid or q.i.d. (initials for the Latin, *quarter in die*).
- (e) tid or t.i.d. (initials for the Latin, *ter in die*).

131. The medical abbreviation for "at bed time" is
- (a) qd or q.d. (initials for the Latin, *quaque die*).
- (b) bid or b.i.d. (initials for the Latin, *bis in die*).
- (c) hs or h.s. (initials for the Latin, *hora somni*).
- (d) qid or q.i.d. (initials for the Latin, *quarter in die*).
- (e) tid or t.i.d. (initials for the Latin, *ter in die*).

132. The medical abbreviation for "three times a day" is
- (a) qd or q.d. (initials for the Latin, *quaque die*).
- (b) bid or b.i.d. (initials for the Latin, *bis in die*).
- (c) hs or h.s. (initials for the Latin, *hora somni*).
- (d) qid or q.i.d. (initials for the Latin, *quarter in die*).
- (e) tid or t.i.d. (initials for the Latin, *ter in die*).

133. The medical abbreviation *BS* means
- (a) bovine scat.
- (b) breath sounds.
- (c) blood sugar.
- (d) Answers (b) or (c).
- (e) None of the above.

134. The medical abbreviation *BM* means
  (a) bowel movement.
  (b) basic mobility (of extremities).
  (c) basic movement (of extremities).
  (d) borderline mechanism.
  (e) blood measurement.

135. The medical abbreviation *BVM* means
  (a) basic voluntary movement (of extremities).
  (b) bag-valve-mask.
  (c) borderline vector of mobility (of extremities).
  (d) believable version of mechanism.
  (e) None of the above.

136. The medical abbreviation *CA* means
  (a) coronary attack.
  (b) cumulative assessment.
  (c) coronary artery.
  (d) cancer.
  (e) caught in the act.

137. The medical abbreviation *CHF* means
  (a) chronic heart failure.
  (b) coronary heart failure.
  (c) chronic heart fatigue.
  (d) cardiac/hepatic (kidney) failure.
  (e) congestive heart failure.

138. The medical abbreviation *CHI* means
  (a) congestive heart injury.
  (b) coronary heart injury.
  (c) chronic heart injury.
  (d) chronic head injury.
  (e) closed head injury.

139. The medical abbreviation *CNS* means
  (a) chronic nervous syndrome.
  (b) congested nervous syndrome.
  (c) central nervous system.
  (d) coronary node, sinus.
  (e) coughing, nausea, sputum.

140.   The medical abbreviation *COPD* means
    (a) cold or pneumonia disease.
    (b) coronary obstruction with pulmonary disease.
    (c) chronic obstructive pulmonary disease.
    (d) crazy old persons disease.
    (e) careful observation, palpation, and detection.

141.   The medical abbreviation *CVA* means
    (a) chronic ventricular activity.
    (b) cerebrovascular accident.
    (c) cardiovascular accident.
    (d) cerebrovascular activity.
    (e) chronic vascular accidents.

142.   The medical abbreviation *GI* means
    (a) grossly intact.
    (b) gastrointestinal.
    (c) gradually increasing (pain).
    (d) growth injury.
    (e) great injury.

143.   The medical abbreviation *GSW* means
    (a) growth spurt wound.
    (b) gradual signs of wounds (developing).
    (c) good sensation within (extremities).
    (d) gun shot wound.
    (e) gross signs of wounds.

144.   The medical abbreviation *GU* means
    (a) genitourinary.
    (b) grossly unwell.
    (c) growing upward.
    (d) gastrourinary.
    (e) growing underneath.

145.   The medical abbreviation *HA* means
    (a) helpful activity.
    (b) hardly any.
    (c) help arrives.
    (d) headache.
    (e) head accident.

146. The medical abbreviation *Hx* means
    (a) Hare traction (splint).
    (b) head exam.
    (c) history.
    (d) heart exam.
    (e) hasty exam.

147. The medical abbreviation *JVD* means
    (a) junior vascular disease.
    (b) jugular vein distention.
    (c) journeying vascular disease.
    (d) James Victor disease.
    (e) John Vincent disease.

148. The medical abbreviation *LBB* means
    (a) long back board.
    (b) little bundle branch.
    (c) long bone broken.
    (d) load-bearing buggy.
    (e) left brain barrier.

149. The medical abbreviation *LLQ* means
    (a) light or little quality (of pain).
    (b) long or lasting quality (of pain).
    (c) less lethal quality (of pain).
    (d) left lung quadrant.
    (e) left lower quadrant (of the abdomen).

150. The medical abbreviation *LMP* means
    (a) last menstrual period.
    (b) less movement with pain.
    (c) little movement (in response to) pain.
    (d) lower margin of parietal skull.
    (e) lower margin of peritoneum.

151. The medical abbreviation *lpm* means
    (a) little pain with movement.
    (b) liters per minute.
    (c) lower part of mediastinum.
    (d) lightly palpated motion.
    (e) last perceived memory.

152. The medical abbreviation *LUQ* means
- (a) less than usual quality (of pain).
- (b) lung upper quadrant.
- (c) lasting unusual quality (of pain).
- (d) left upper quadrant (of the abdomen).
- (e) lessening unusual quality (of pain).

153. The medical abbreviation *LOC* means
- (a) level of consciousness.
- (b) little of consequence.
- (c) loss of consciousness.
- (d) last observed (heard) comment.
- (e) location of crepitus.

154. The medical abbreviation *nc* means
- (a) nonchronic.
- (b) not counted (pulse or respiratory rate).
- (c) nasal cannula.
- (d) north corner.
- (e) no crepitus.

155. The medical abbreviation *NRB* means
- (a) no rotation or bulges (of the hip or leg).
- (b) normal return of breathing.
- (c) normal return of beats (pulse).
- (d) never returned to breathing.
- (e) nonrebreather mask.

156. The medical abbreviation *NTG* means
- (a) numbness and tingling.
- (b) nitroglycerine.
- (c) nontoxic gas.
- (d) normal teenage growth.
- (e) nontenting (skin condition).

157. The medical abbreviation *n/v* means
- (a) no volition.
- (b) nonvomiting.
- (c) nausea and vomiting.
- (d) nonviolent.
- (e) normal ventilations.

158. The medical abbreviation *n/v/d* means
- (a) normal ventilation and delivery (of oxygen).
- (b) nocturnal vascular disease.
- (c) normal ventricular delivery (of pulse).
- (d) nausea, vomiting, and dehydration.
- (e) nausea, vomiting, and diarrhea.

159. The medical abbreviation *PE* means
- (a) pulmonary embolism.
- (b) pulmonary edema.
- (c) partially eaten.
- (d) potential emergency.
- (e) pediatric emergency.

160. The medical abbreviation *PID* means
- (a) pulmonary interruption disease.
- (b) pediatric intelligence deficit.
- (c) partial intelligence disruption.
- (d) pelvic inflammatory disease.
- (e) pulmonary injury or disease.

161. The medical abbreviation *PNS* means
- (a) pulmonary nocturnal symptoms.
- (b) partially normal signs.
- (c) peripheral nervous system.
- (d) pain and numbness signs.
- (e) pain symptoms.

162. The medical abbreviation *PTOA* means
- (a) peripheral tingling or obstruction assessment.
- (b) previous times of assessments.
- (c) partial obstruction accident.
- (d) painful tingling or aches.
- (e) prior to our arrival.

163. The medical abbreviation *R/O* means
- (a) rule out.
- (b) rollover (motor vehicle accident).
- (c) renal obstruction (kidney stone).
- (d) relatives or others.
- (e) rings (and other jewelry) off.

164. The medical abbreviation *RLQ* means
    (a) relatively less in quality (of pain).
    (b) right lower quadrant (of the abdomen).
    (c) radiating and lasting quality (of pain).
    (d) right lung quadrant.
    (e) ridiculously low quality (of pain).

165. The medical abbreviation *RUQ* means
    (a) relatively unusual quality (of pain).
    (b) relatively usual quality (of pain).
    (c) right upper quadrant (of lungs).
    (d) radiating, unusual quality (of pain).
    (e) ridiculously unusual quality (of pain).

166. The medical abbreviation *SOB* means
    (a) shortness of breath.
    (b) signs of breathing.
    (c) symptoms of breathing.
    (d) Answers (b) or (c).
    (e) None of the above.

167. The medical abbreviation *TIA* means
    (a) tingling in abdomen.
    (b) times in accidents (previous MVA history).
    (c) transient ischemic attack.
    (d) telephoned-in assessment.
    (e) trauma injury assessment.

168. The medical abbreviation *URI* means
    (a) unknown reasons for injury.
    (b) upper respiratory infection.
    (c) unknown respiratory infection.
    (d) unreasonable reasons for injury.
    (e) urinary injury.

169. The medical abbreviation *UTI* means
    (a) unknown time of injury.
    (b) upper thoracic injury.
    (c) urinary tract infection.
    (d) unusual treatment of injury.
    (e) uterus intact.

170. The medical abbreviation *WNL* means
   (a) weeping, necrotic lesions.
   (b) with no loss (of).
   (c) wandering neural loss.
   (d) with normal length.
   (e) within normal limits.

171. The medical abbreviation *y/o* means
   (a) yellow.
   (b) yards of (travel).
   (c) yours/ours.
   (d) years old.
   (e) young or old.

172. The medical symbol ≈ stands for
   (a) change.
   (b) less than equal to.
   (c) approximately.
   (d) more than equal to.
   (e) unequal to.

173. The medical symbol Δ stands for
   (a) change.
   (b) sorority or fraternity member.
   (c) approximately.
   (d) angulated.
   (e) triangulated.

174. The medical symbol > stands for
   (a) less than.
   (b) greater than.
   (c) smaller than.
   (d) taller than.
   (e) above.

175. The medical symbol < stands for
   (a) less than.
   (b) greater than.
   (c) smaller than.
   (d) taller than.
   (e) above.

176. The medical symbol ♀ stands for a _____ patient.
- (a) pediatric
- (b) male
- (c) female
- (d) adult
- (e) psychiatric

177. The medical symbol ♂ stands for a _____ patient.
- (a) pediatric
- (b) male
- (c) female
- (d) adult
- (e) psychiatric

178. The medical symbol Ψ stands for a _____ patient.
- (a) pediatric
- (b) male
- (c) female
- (d) adult
- (e) psychiatric

179. The medical symbol ↑ stands for
- (a) above or taller than.
- (b) below or shorter than.
- (c) above or increased.
- (d) below or decreased.
- (e) up and away from.

180. The medical symbol ↓ stands for
- (a) above or taller than.
- (b) below or shorter than.
- (c) above or increased.
- (d) below or decreased.
- (e) down and away from.

The answer key for Test Section Three is on page 335.

4

DOT Module Four: Medical Emergencies

Subjects:

- General Pharmacology
- Respiratory Emergencies
- Metered-dose Inhalers
- Cardiac Emergencies
- Nitroglycerin
- Aspirin
- Automated External Defibrillation

(Other Medical Emergency subjects from DOT Module Four are addressed in Test Sections Five, Seven, and Nine.)

Test Section Four consists of 135 questions and is allotted 2 hours and 15 minutes for completion.

1.   The study of sources, characteristics, effects, and administration of medications (drugs) is called
   (a) medicology.
   (b) anatomy.
   (c) pharmacology.
   (d) physiology.
   (e) pharmacy.

2.   An EMT-Basic ambulance should be equipped with all of the drugs that an EMT is allowed to administer. These drugs include
   (a) activated charcoal, oral glucose, and aspirin.
   (b) oxygen.
   (c) nitroglycerin tablets or spray, common respiratory metered-dose inhalers, and epinephrine auto-injectors (for administration only to patients who have run out of their own prescribed medication).
   (d) Answers (a) and (b).
   (e) Answers (a), (b), and (c).

3.   With medical direction approval, EMT-Basics may assist patients in using their own prescribed
   (a) nitroglycerin.
   (b) epinephrine auto-injectors.
   (c) insulin.
   (d) Answers (a) and (b).
   (e) Answers (a), (b), and (c).

4.   When a drug is developed, its name is listed in the *U.S. Pharmacopoeia* with the initials "USP" following it. This USP name is the drug's
   (a) generic name.
   (b) chemical name.
   (c) trade name, or brand name.
   (d) slang or abbreviated name.
   (e) official name.

5.   When a manufacturer markets the drug, another name is created. This name is called the drug's
   (a) generic name (such as "epinephrine hydrochloride").
   (b) chemical name (such as "beta-(3,4-dihydroxyphenl)-a-methylaminoethanol").
   (c) trade name, or brand name (such as "Adrenalin®" or "Epi-Pen®").
   (d) slang or abbreviated name (such as "epi").
   (e) official name (such as "epinephrine").

6. The reasons for administering a medication (its most common uses) are called the drug's
    (a) contraindications.
    (b) contradictions.
    (c) side effects.
    (d) indications.
    (e) toxic effects.

7. Situations in which a medication should not be given (because it may cause harm to the patient or offer no improving effect) are called the drug's
    (a) contraindications.
    (b) contradictions.
    (c) side effects.
    (d) indications.
    (e) toxic effects.

8. A drug may cause predictable actions or effects other than those desired. Undesired drug actions or effects are called
    (a) contraindications.
    (b) contradictions.
    (c) side effects.
    (d) erroneous effects.
    (e) toxic effects.

9. Medications come in different forms. Activated charcoal is an example of a medication that comes in _____ form.
    (a) sublingual spray
    (b) compressed powder or tablet
    (c) suspension
    (d) Answers (a) or (b).
    (e) Answers (a), (b), and (c).

10. Nitroglycerin is an example of a medication that comes in _____ form.
    (a) sublingual spray
    (b) compressed powder or tablet
    (c) suspension
    (d) Answers (a) or (b).
    (e) Answers (a), (b), and (c).

11. Epinephrine is an example of a medication that comes in _____ form.
    (a) gel
    (b) injectable liquid
    (c) gas
    (d) a metered dose of fine liquid for sublingual spray
    (e) a metered dose of fine powder for inhalation

12. Glucose is an example of a medication that comes in _____ form.

   (a) gel
   (b) injectable liquid
   (c) gas
   (d) a metered dose of fine liquid for sublingual spray
   (e) a metered dose of fine powder for inhalation

13. An EMT-B may assist with the administration of a particular form of respiratory medication. This medication comes in _____ form.

   (a) gel
   (b) injectable liquid
   (c) compressed powder or tablet
   (d) a metered dose of fine liquid for sublingual spray
   (e) a metered dose of fine powder for inhalation

14. A sublingual medication is a drug that is administered by

   (a) spreading it on the skin.
   (b) injecting it just under the skin.
   (c) placing it under the armpit.
   (d) placing it on the skin.
   (e) placing it under the tongue.

15. Which of the following signs—by itself, or when accompanied by other signs or symptoms—may indicate a patient having serious difficulty breathing?

   (1) Restlessness.
   (2) Increased pulse rate.
   (3) Increased respiratory rate.
   (4) Decreased respiratory rate.
   (5) Frantically complaining of difficulty breathing in long, wordy sentences between gasps of air.
   (6) Retractions—the use of accessory muscles.
   (7) Altered level of consciousness.
   (8) Extreme fatigue.
   (9) Cyanotic skin color.
      (a) 1, 2, 3, 4, 6, 7, 8, and 9.
      (b) 2, 3, 4, 6, 7, 8, and 9.
      (c) 1, 2, 3, 4, 5, 6, 7, 8, and 9.
      (d) 2, 4, 5, 6, 7, and 9.
      (e) 2, 3, 6, 7, 8, and 9.

16.   The *tripod position* may be observed in children or adults and often indicates that they are having serious difficulty breathing. This position is best described as when the patient
   (a) lays on his side, bent at the waist, with legs straight out (also called the lateral "V" position).
   (b) leans forward while sitting upright, with arms straight, hands resting on knees (or another surface), and neck extended.
   (c) is slumped over in a large easy chair with his feet elevated.
   (d) assumes a semi-Fowler's position with legs straight out and elevated (also called the "V" position).
   (e) stands upright with legs spread apart, but bent over at the waist and dangling his head, while leaning one hand on a supportive surface (creating a "tripod" appearance).

17.   Observing that the patient has a *barrel chest* often indicates that the patient has a history of chronic lung disease. A barrel chest is best described as the observation that a patient has
   (a) an obesity problem (where the chest and abdomen are large and rounded, creating the impression that the patient's torso looks like a barrel).
   (b) an enlarged chest diameter with a shallow or minimal (fixed) amount of expansion/relaxation (creating the impression that the patient's chest looks like a barrel).
   (c) excessive chest expansion with inspiration and excessive chest deflation with expiration (creating the impression that the patient "blows up like a barrel" when he inhales).
   (d) Answers (a) or (b).
   (e) Answers (b) or (c).

18.   The medical term for the harsh, high-pitched "windy" type of sound characteristic of an upper airway obstruction caused by swelling in the larynx is
   (a) rhonchi.
   (b) wheezing.
   (c) rales.
   (d) crowing.
   (e) stridor.

19.   The medical term for the high- or low-pitched, musical noise characteristic of air being forced past swollen or mucous-filled lower airway structures (especially on expiration) is
   (a) rhonchi.
   (b) wheezing.
   (c) rales.
   (d) crowing.
   (e) stridor.

20.   Your patient has signs and symptoms of extreme trouble breathing, but does not
       have a prescribed respiratory medication inhaler. Which of the following treatment
       measures should be performed, and in what order (from first to last)?
       (1) Obtain baseline vital signs.
       (2) Administer oxygen by nonrebreather mask at 15 lpm.
       (3) Send someone to get the pulse oximeter from the ambulance, and then
            obtain a baseline "room air" reading.
       (4) Consult your medical director regarding assisted administration of a
            prescribed medication inhaler (one that is stocked in your ambulance,
            or one prescribed to another family member or close friend).
       (5) Repeat the inhaler administration as indicated.
       (6) Obtain a SAMPLE history.
       (7) Prepare the equipment necessary to assist the patient with ventilatory
            support and consider calling for ALS backup.
            (a) 3, 2, 1, 6, 4, 5, and 7.
            (b) 3, 2, 1, 6, and 7.
            (c) 2, 7, 1, and 6.
            (d) 2, 1, 6, 4, 5, and 7.
            (e) 2, 1, 6, 4, and 5.

21.   Your patient has signs and symptoms of extreme trouble breathing, and has a
       prescribed medication inhaler. Which of the following treatment measures should
       be taken, and in what order (from first to last)?
       (1) Obtain baseline vital signs.
       (2) Administer oxygen by nonrebreather mask at 15 lpm.
       (3) Send someone to get the pulse oximeter from the ambulance, and then
            obtain a baseline "room air" reading.
       (4) Consult your medical director regarding assisted administration of
            the patient's prescribed medication inhaler.
       (5) Repeat the inhaler administration as indicated.
       (6) Obtain a SAMPLE history.
       (7) Prepare the equipment necessary to assist the patient with ventilatory
            support and consider calling for ALS backup.
            (a) 3, 2, 1, 6, 4, 5, and 7.
            (b) 2, 1, 6, 4, 5, and 7.
            (c) 2, 4, 5, 1, 6, and 7.
            (d) 3, 1, 2, 7, 4, 5, and 6.
            (e) 7, 3, 2, 1, 6, 4, and 5.

22.   All of the following are generic names of prescribed metered-dose inhalers, except
       (a) albuterol and metaproteranol.
       (b) Alupent.
       (c) isoetharine.
       (d) bitolterol mesylate.
       (e) ipratropium.

23. All of the following are trade (or brand) names of prescribed metered-dose inhalers, except

   (a) Proventil and Ventolin.
   (b) Atrovent.
   (c) Bronkosol.
   (d) Metaprel.
   (e) salmeterol xinafoate.

24. Widening or opening of the bronchi or bronchioles (the tubes that lead from the trachea to the farthest portions of each lung's respiratory "tree") is called

   (a) bronchodilation.
   (b) bronchoalleviation.
   (c) bronchoexcursion.
   (d) bronchoconstriction.
   (e) bronchoscopy.

25. Narrowing or closing of the bronchi or bronchioles is called

   (a) bronchodilation.
   (b) bronchoalleviation.
   (c) bronchoexcursion.
   (d) bronchoconstriction.
   (e) bronchoscopy.

26. Most metered-dose inhalers prescribed for respiratory problems contain a beta agonist _____ medication that will increase airway size, reduce airway resistance, and improve the patient's ability to exchange oxygen and carbon dioxide.

   (a) bronchodilator
   (b) bronchoalleviator
   (c) bronchoexcursion
   (d) bronchoconstrictor
   (e) bronchoscopy

27. Anticipated side effects of prescribed metered-dose inhaler medication administration include

   (a) increased pulse rate.
   (b) tremors, especially of the extremities.
   (c) nervousness or restlessness.
   (d) Answers (a) and (c).
   (e) Answers (a), (b), and (c).

28. In order for the EMT to assist with the administration of a patient's prescription inhaler, which of the following criteria must be met?

   (a) The patient must exhibit signs and symptoms of a respiratory emergency.
   (b) The patient must have his own prescription inhaler present.
   (c) The EMT-B must contact the Medical Director and receive specific authorization to assist with the inhaler's administration.
   (d) Answers (b) and (c).
   (e) Answers (a), (b), and (c).

29. Contraindications for EMT assistance with the administration of a patient's prescription inhaler include all of the following situations, except when

   (a) the Medical Director denies the inhaler administration assistance request.
   (b) the patient already has used the inhaler the maximum times allowed.
   (c) the patient is unable to use the device, even with assistance (can't follow directions).
   (d) the patient has superficial wheezes that can be heard only with a stethoscope.
   (e) the inhaler is prescribed for a person other than the patient.

30. Which of the following statements regarding inhaler dosage (the number of times the inhaler can be used) is true?

   (a) The number of times an EMT can assist with inhaler use is based upon the number of doses the patient has already inhaled.
   (b) The number of times an EMT can assist with inhaler use is based upon the Medical Director's orders.
   (c) Only one EMT-assisted inhalation may be administered to any prehospital patient.
   (d) Answers (a) and (b) are true.
   (e) Answers (b) and (c) are true.

31. When assisting a patient with inhaler use, the EMT should do all of the following, except

   (a) check to be sure that the inhaler is prescribed for the patient.
   (b) check the expiration date of the inhaler.
   (c) avoid shaking or disturbing the inhaler's contents prior to inhalation.
   (d) assure that the inhaler is at room temperature or warmer.
   (e) assure that the patient is alert enough to use the inhaler.

32. A _____ is an attachment placed between the inhaler and the patient that allows for more effective use of the medication. If the patient has one, it should be used.

   (a) spirometer
   (b) bronchometer
   (c) spacer device
   (d) buff-cap
   (e) medimeter

33.   Even though they've used an inhaler for years, patients with difficulty breathing are often anxious or confused. If they neglect to correctly perform one or more steps for the appropriate use of an inhaler, the inhaler's effectiveness will be significantly minimized. Thus, the EMT should know how to coach the patient to best use the inhaler. From the following selection, choose the appropriate steps for effective inhaler use, and place them in their correct order (from first to last).

   (1) Have the patient exhale deeply.
   (2) Instruct the patient to hold his breath for as long as he comfortably can (so the medication can be absorbed as much as possible).
   (3) Assist the patient by pinching his nose closed (this prevents escape of medication through the nasal pharynx).
   (4) Have the patient depress the handheld inhaler as he begins to inhale deeply.
   (5) Have the patient put his lips around the opening of the inhaler.
   (6) If a second dose is to be administered, have the patient breathe normally a few times, and then repeat the administration steps.
   (7) Immediately after depressing the handheld inhaler, instruct the patient to exhale deeply (the patient should not be allowed to hold his breath, as too much medication will be retained).
   (8) Ensure that the patient holds the inhaler with the opening *directed at* his open mouth (not *in* his mouth) before depressing the inhaler. The medication should "shoot" into the patient's open mouth. Do not allow the nervous patient to actually place his lips on the inhaler and "suck" in the medication, as this may result in an overdose.

   (a) 1, 5, 4, 2, 6.
   (b) 8, 1, 3, 4, 7.
   (c) 1, 8, 4, 2, 6.
   (d) 5, 3, 4, 7, 6.
   (e) 3, 8, 4, 7.

34.   After assisting the patient with self-administration of a prescribed metered-dose inhaler medication, the EMT should

   (a) gather additional sets of vital signs and perform (or repeat) a focused assessment of the chest and respiratory function.
   (b) anticipate the potential for deterioration of the patient's condition in spite of the medication administration, and be prepared to perform positive pressure artificial ventilation.
   (c) continue high-flow oxygenation of the patient.
   (d) Answers (a) and (c).
   (e) Answers (a), (b), and (c).

35.   Which of the following illnesses is classified as chronic obstructive pulmonary disease (COPD)?

   (a) Emphysema
   (b) Chronic bronchitis
   (c) Asthma
   (d) Answers (a) and (b).
   (e) Answers (a), (b), and (c).

36.   Which of the following illnesses is considered an episodic (rather than a chronic) disease?
   (a) Emphysema
   (b) Chronic bronchitis
   (c) Asthma
   (d) All of the above.
   (e) None of the above.

37.   _____ is a respiratory disease that primarily restricts bronchial airflow in one direction, usually on exhalation.
   (a) Emphysema
   (b) Chronic bronchitis
   (c) Asthma
   (d) Answers (a) and (b).
   (e) Answers (a), (b), and (c).

38.   _____ is a respiratory disease that primarily affects middle-aged and older patients, rarely affecting children and teenagers.
   (a) Emphysema
   (b) Chronic bronchitis
   (c) Asthma
   (d) Answers (a) and (b).
   (e) Answers (a), (b), and (c).

39.   Normally, when bronchioles become inflamed and excess mucus is produced, the fine hairs along the interior lining of the bronchioles are able to "sweep" away the excess mucus, so it can be coughed out. These hairs are called
   (a) bronchia.
   (b) cilia.
   (c) silica.
   (d) pulmonary fibers.
   (e) bronchial fur.

40.   Because chronic bronchiole inflammation and mucus production is a primary aspect of _____, the fine hairs lining the bronchioles become damaged or destroyed, and then become unable to perform their sweeping, airway-clearing function.
   (a) emphysema
   (b) chronic bronchitis
   (c) asthma
   (d) Answers (a) or (b).
   (e) Answers (b) or (c).

41. Breakdown of alveolar wall surface, diminishing the functional surface area of the alveoli, is a common aspect of
    (a) emphysema.
    (b) chronic bronchitis.
    (c) asthma.
    (d) Answers (a) or (b).
    (e) Answers (b) or (c).

42. Loss of lung elasticity causing air to become "trapped" within the lungs is a common aspect of
    (a) emphysema.
    (b) chronic bronchitis.
    (c) asthma.
    (d) Answers (a) or (b).
    (e) Answers (b) or (c).

43. The respiratory disease _____ is often triggered by inhalation, ingestion, or injection of a substance the patient is allergic to (such as air pollutants, foods, or insect stings).
    (a) emphysema
    (b) chronic bronchitis
    (c) asthma
    (d) Answers (a) or (b).
    (e) Answers (b) or (c).

44. Rapid transport and consideration of ALS backup is required when someone has a prolonged and severe attack of asthma that doesn't respond to oxygen or medication. This kind of asthma attack is called
    (a) anaphylactic shock.
    (b) status asthmaticus.
    (c) status anaphylaxis.
    (d) status epilepticus.
    (e) hyperasthmaticus.

45. The right atrium receives blood from the _____ and directs (pumps) blood flow to the _____.
    (a) body and heart / left ventricle
    (b) lower extremities / upper extremities
    (c) pulmonary veins (the lungs) / left ventricle
    (d) body and heart / right ventricle
    (e) upper extremities / lower extremities

46.   The left atrium receives blood from the _____ and directs blood flow to the
_____ .
  (a) body and heart / left ventricle
  (b) lower extremities / upper extremities
  (c) pulmonary veins (the lungs) / left ventricle
  (d) body and heart / right ventricle
  (e) upper extremities / lower extremities

47.   The left ventricle directs blood flow to the
  (a) body, via the aorta.
  (b) lungs, via the pulmonary arteries.
  (c) lungs, via the pulmonary veins.
  (d) right ventricle.
  (e) right atrium.

48.   The right ventricle directs blood flow to the
  (a) body, via the aorta.
  (b) lungs, via the pulmonary arteries.
  (c) lungs, via the pulmonary veins.
  (d) left ventricle.
  (e) left atrium.

49.   The valves within the circulatory system (including the cardiac valves) serve to
  (a) pump blood forward.
  (b) pump blood upward.
  (c) propel blood backward.
  (d) stop too much blood from flowing forward.
  (e) prevent backflow of blood.

50.   All arteries
  (a) carry blood away from the heart.
  (b) carry blood back to the heart.
  (c) carry only oxygenated blood.
  (d) Answers (a) and (c).
  (e) Answers (b) and (c).

51.   All veins
  (a) carry blood away from the heart.
  (b) carry blood back to the heart.
  (c) carry only deoxygenated blood.
  (d) Answers (a) and (c).
  (e) Answers (b) and (c).

52. Pulmonary arteries
  (a) carry blood away from the heart.
  (b) carry blood back to the heart.
  (c) carry only deoxygenated blood.
  (d) Answers (a) and (c).
  (e) Answers (b) and (c).

53. Pulmonary veins
  (a) carry blood away from the heart.
  (b) carry blood back to the heart.
  (c) carry only oxygenated blood.
  (d) Answers (a) and (c).
  (e) Answers (b) and (c).

54. The medical abbreviation *ACLS* stands for
  (a) Always C-spine and Lay (the patient) Supine.
  (b) Advanced Controlled Lung Support (tracheal intubation with positive pressure ventilation).
  (c) Advanced Cardiac Life Support.
  (d) Alpha, Charly, Lima, Sierra.
  (e) Anxiousness, Clammy skin, Low blood pressure, Sweating (the cardinal signs of shock).

55. The medical abbreviation *CHF* stands for
  (a) Cardiac Heart Function.
  (b) Compromised Heart Function.
  (c) Coronary Heart Failure.
  (d) Complex Heart Fluctuation (another term for irregular heart beat).
  (e) Congestive Heart Failure.

56. The medical abbreviation *CAD* stands for
  (a) Carotid Artery Dysfunction.
  (b) Coronary Artery Disease.
  (c) Chronic Atherosclerosis Disease.
  (d) Congestive Artery Disease.
  (e) Complex Arterial Dysfunction.

57. The condition that results from the buildup of fatty deposits on the inner walls of arteries, causing them to become narrowed (restricting blood flow), is called
  (a) arteriosclerosis.
  (b) ascites.
  (c) asystole.
  (d) atherosclerosis.
  (e) arterial petrification.

58.   The condition that results from the buildup of calcium deposits on the inner walls of arteries, causing them to become hard and unable to dilate or constrict well, is often called "hardening of the arteries." The medical term for this condition is

   (a) arteriosclerosis.
   (b) ascites.
   (c) asystole.
   (d) atherosclerosis.
   (e) arterial petrification.

59.   When a section of an artery's wall becomes weakened, the layers of the wall may split, allowing blood to enter between them and causing the section to "balloon" (expand) with blood and become weakened. This condition is called

   (a) an aortic bypass.
   (b) an embolism.
   (c) an aneurysm.
   (d) a cardiac bypass.
   (e) grafting.

60.   A blood clot attached to the wall of an artery that grows in size as it collects plaque and other debris is called

   (a) a thrombophlebitis.
   (b) an aneurysm.
   (c) an embolism.
   (d) a coronary.
   (e) a thrombus.

61.   An object composed of fat or plaque that breaks loose from the wall of an artery and travels through the circulatory system is called

   (a) a thrombophlebitis.
   (b) an aneurysm.
   (c) an embolism.
   (d) a coronary.
   (e) a thrombus.

62.   The term _____ is used when referring to clotted blood, fat, or plaque completely obstructing blood flow through a blood vessel.

   (a) occlusion
   (b) aneurysm
   (c) coronary
   (d) asystole
   (e) arrhythmia

63.   The phrase *cardiac compromise* may be used to describe the condition of patients who

   (a) complain of dyspnea.
   (b) have low blood pressure.

(c) have irregular heart beats.

(d) complain of chest pain.

(e) demonstrate signs or symptoms indicative of any form of heart problem.

64. Which of the following symptoms—*by itself*—may indicate that a patient is experiencing cardiac compromise?

(1) Complaint of dull and/or squeezing pressure in the chest.

(2) Complaint of jaw pain.

(3) Complaint of nausea, with vomiting.

(4) Complaint of nausea, without vomiting.

(5) Complaint of epigastric pain.

(6) Complaint of difficulty breathing (dyspnea).

(7) Description of a feeling of "impending doom."

(a) 1, 6, or 7.

(b) 1, 3, 5, or 6.

(c) 1, 3, 4, 5, or 6.

(d) 1, 2, 3, 4, 5, or 6.

(e) 1, 2, 3, 4, 5, 6, or 7.

65. Which of the following signs—*by itself*—may indicate that a patient is experiencing cardiac compromise?

(1) Extreme anxiety or irritability.

(2) An altered level of consciousness.

(3) A regular tachycardia.

(4) An irregular tachycardia.

(5) A regular bradycardia.

(6) An irregular bradycardia.

(7) An abnormally low blood pressure.

(8) An abnormally high blood pressure.

(9) A sudden onset of profuse sweating.

(a) 1, 2, 3, 4, 5, 6, 7, 8, or 9.

(b) 2, 3, 4, 5, 6, 7, or 8.

(c) 2, 4, 6, 7, or 8.

(d) 2, 3, 5, 7, or 8.

(e) 2, 3, 5, or 8.

66. The literal translation of the Latin medical phrase *angina pectoris* is

(a) heart palpitations.

(b) heart pain.

(c) pain in the chest.

(d) a heart attack.

(e) agony of the breast.

67. Angina is caused by the heart tissue being deprived of oxygen. Heart tissue oxygen deprivation can result from

   (a) narrowed or obstructed coronary arteries.

   (b) the increased cardiac workload that accompanies psychological (emotional) stress, if the patient has coronary artery disease.

   (c) the increased cardiac workload that accompanies physical exertion, if the patient has coronary artery disease.

   (d) Answers (a) or (c).

   (e) Answers (a), (b), or (c).

68. Which of the following statements regarding "stable angina" is true?

   (a) Stable angina is often relieved by rest.

   (b) Normal attacks of stable angina usually last for two to four hours.

   (c) If a patient has a prescription for nitroglycerin, it probably means that the patient has a history of stable angina attacks.

   (d) Answers (a) and (c) are true.

   (e) Answers (a), (b), and (c) are true.

69. Which of the following statements regarding "unstable angina" is false?

   (a) Unstable angina is not something that a basic EMT can recognize in the field.

   (b) If a patient reports being awakened from sleep by angina, the patient definitely has unstable angina.

   (c) If the angina is not relieved by nitroglycerin, it is probably unstable angina.

   (d) Unstable angina is angina that occurs during rest.

   (e) If an angina attack continues for longer than the patient is used to experiencing it, it is probably unstable angina.

70. Acute myocardial infarction (AMI) may occur when

   (a) a portion of the heart dies from lack of oxygen.

   (b) the narrowing or obstruction of a coronary artery prevents enough oxygenated blood from reaching an area of heart tissue.

   (c) a coronary artery ruptures.

   (d) Answers (a) or (b).

   (e) Answers (a), (b), or (c).

71. Cardiac arrest may result from CAD or an acute respiratory problem. Additional causes of cardiac arrest include

   (a) high levels of emotional stress.

   (b) COPD.

   (c) unusual exertion.

   (d) Answers (b) or (c).

   (e) Answers (a), (b), or (c).

72. Since obstruction of a coronary artery by a clot is a frequent cause of AMI, _____ medications have been developed to correct this problem. The nickname for these medications is "clot busters," because they dissolve clots.

   (a) hemodialysis
   (b) hemorrhagic
   (c) thrombolytic
   (d) blood-clotting
   (e) antibleeding

73. Aspirin (acetylsalicylic acid—abbreviated as ASA) is a drug that accomplishes which of the following actions?

   (a) Decreases the ability of platelets to clump together.
   (b) Reduces the size of blood clots that are blocking coronary arteries.
   (c) Relieves the muscular pain of myocardial infarction.
   (d) Answers (a) and (b).
   (e) Answers (a), (b), and (c).

74. Before an EMT may administer ASA to a patient, which of the following conditions must be met?

   (1) The medical director must authorize ASA administration, via an on-line order or an off-line standing protocol.
   (2) The patient must be able to swallow without choking or coughing.
   (3) The patient must be complaining of chest discomfort.
   (4) The patient must be complaining of a headache.
   (5) The patient must have high blood pressure.
   (6) The patient must have no history of asthma.
   (7) The patient must not be allergic to ASA.
   (8) The patient must not be regularly taking other medications that prevent clotting.
       (a) 1, 2, 3, 4, 5, 6, 7, and 8.
       (b) 1, 2, 3, 5, 6, 7, and 8.
       (c) 1, 2, 3, 6, 7, and 8.
       (d) 1, 2, 5, 6, 7, and 8.
       (e) 1, 2, 4, 7, and 8.

75. All of the following may contraindicate ASA administration, except

   (a) a history of gastrointestinal ulcer or recent GI bleeding.
   (b) recent ingestion of Viagra®, or any other drug prescribed for erectile dysfunction.
   (c) pregnancy.
   (d) a history of recent major surgery.
   (e) a history of a bleeding disorder.

76.   The dosage of a single ASA administration for cardiovascular emergencies is
   (a) 243 mg (no more than three tablets).
   (b) 162 to 324 mg (two to four tablets).
   (c) 162 to 405 mg (two to five tablets).
   (d) 162 mg (no more than two tablets).
   (e) 81 mg (no more than one tablet).

77.   Which of the following statements regarding ASA administration is false?
   (a) Obtain a baseline set of vital signs prior to administering ASA.
   (b) Be sure to tell the patient to swallow (not chew) the ASA, to ensure proper drug delivery.
   (c) Perform a focused history and cardiac patient exam prior to calling for ASA administration orders.
   (d) Perform a focused history and cardiac patient exam prior to administering ASA according to standing orders (off-line protocols).
   (e) Only one ASA administration should be performed by the EMT.

78.   The medical term *edema* is best defined as
   (a) an accumulation of stagnant blood in the legs, making them swollen.
   (b) the "goose-egg" swelling caused by blunt injury.
   (c) a localized or general accumulation of excessive fluid within body tissues.
   (d) a localized or general accumulation of excessive blood within body tissues.
   (e) an accumulation of stagnant blood in the lungs, causing dyspnea.

79.   Edema that accumulates in the feet, ankles, and/or lower legs is called
   (a) orthopedic edema.
   (b) pedal edema.
   (c) pediatric edema.
   (d) gout.
   (e) pregnancy edema.

80.   Edema that accumulates in the abdomen is called
   (a) obesity.
   (b) abdominal rigidity (or a "hot abdomen").
   (c) ascites.
   (d) peritonitis.
   (e) None of the above; edema does not accumulate in the abdomen.

81.   Edema that accumulates in the lungs is called
   (a) pulmonary edema.
   (b) pleurisy.
   (c) COPD.
   (d) peripheral edema.
   (e) pneumonia.

82. CHF is a condition that can result in edema of
    (a) the feet and/or ankles.
    (b) the lungs.
    (c) a variety of body organs or parts.
    (d) Answers (a) or (b).
    (e) Answers (a), (b), or (c).

83. Which of the following statements regarding CHF is false?
    (a) One of the earliest signs and symptoms of CHF is chronic nasal congestion (hence, the term "congestive").
    (b) CHF may be caused by lung function failure.
    (c) Lung function failure may be caused by CHF.
    (d) CHF may be caused by heart function failure.
    (e) Heart function failure may be caused by CHF.

84. A *diuretic* medication is best defined as one that
    (a) decreases urine output so as to retain the body's fluid volume.
    (b) normalizes the body's fluid volume. (If the patient is hypovolemic, the agent acts to retain fluid, decreasing urine output. If the patient has too much body fluid, the agent increases urine output.)
    (c) increases urine output, decreasing the body's fluid volume.
    (d) Answers (a) or (b), depending upon the type of diuretic.
    (e) Answers (b) or (c), depending upon the type of diuretic.

85. Which of the following statements regarding placing the cardiac compromise patient in a position of comfort is false?
    (a) Especially for cardiac compromise patients with shortness of breath, the position of comfort most often will be sitting up.
    (b) The vast majority of cardiac compromise patients prefer to lie flat (supine) with their feet elevated eight to ten inches. This "shock" positioning reduces the workload of the heart, diminishing chest pain and relieving shortness of breath.
    (c) Hypotensive cardiac compromise patients (those with a systolic blood pressure less than 90 mmHg) may feel dizzy or become confused when sitting up. These patients may feel better lying down (supine).
    (d) If the cardiac compromise patient is both hypotensive and complaining of dyspnea, a position of comfort may be difficult to find.
    (e) Ask the patient what position feels most comfortable.

86.   Nitroglycerin (NTG) reduces or relieves angina by
   (a)   anesthetizing (numbing) injured areas of the heart.
   (b)   dilating coronary arteries, thus increasing oxygenated blood flow to injured areas of the heart.
   (c)   dilating coronary arteries, thus increasing oxygenated blood flow past areas of obstruction.
   (d)   Answers (a) and (c).
   (e)   Answers (b) and (c).

87.   Nitroglycerin also reduces or relieves angina by
   (a)   dilating the body's blood vessels and decreasing the amount of blood the heart must pump.
   (b)   constricting the body's blood vessels and decreasing the amount of blood the heart must pump.
   (c)   decreasing the amount of oxygen demanded by the heart muscle.
   (d)   Answers (a) and (c).
   (e)   Answers (b) and (c).

88.   Nitroglycerin is available in several forms, including
   (a)   tablet or spray form, which is placed or sprayed under the patient's tongue, where it is absorbed into the circulatory system.
   (b)   patches that stick to the patient's skin, slowly releasing nitroglycerin into the patient's system throughout the day.
   (c)   gelatin capsule form, which the patient breaks open with his teeth before pushing it under his tongue, where it is allowed to dissolve and is absorbed into the circulatory system.
   (d)   Answers (a) and (b).
   (e)   Answers (a), (b), and (c).

89.   Which of the following conditions must be met before an EMT-B may assist the patient with taking NTG?
   (1)   The patient must be complaining of chest pain.
   (2)   The patient must be complaining of nausea.
   (3)   The patient must be complaining of shortness of breath.
   (4)   The EMT must have on-line or off-line authorization from the Medical Director to assist the patient with nitroglycerin administration.
   (5)   The patient must have his own prescribed nitroglycerin with him.
   (6)   The ambulance nitroglycerin stock must be fresh (patients' NTG often isn't).
   (7)   The patient must be alert.
   (8)   The patient's diastolic blood pressure must be greater than 100 mmHg.
   (9)   The patient's systolic blood pressure must be greater than 100 mmHg.
      (a)   1, 3, 4, 5, 6, 7, and 9.
      (b)   1, 4, 5, 7, and 9.
      (c)   1, 2, 4, 5, 6, 7 and 8.
      (d)   1, 4, 5, 7, and 8.
      (e)   1, 2, 3, 4, 5, 7, and 9.

90.   Which of the following situations does not contraindicate NTG administration?
     (a) The patient has recently taken Viagra® or any other erectile dysfunction drug.
     (b) The patient has a head injury.
     (c) The patient has already taken the maximum number of prescribed doses.
     (d) The patient's systolic blood pressure is 90 mm Hg.
     (e) The patient's diastolic blood pressure is 90 mm Hg.

91.   The EMT may assist the patient with taking up to a maximum of ___ dose(s) of NTG,
     as long as _____.
     (a) one / the patient has only taken one dose prior to the EMT's arrival
     (b) two / the patient has taken no doses prior to the EMT's arrival
     (c) three / the patient has only taken two doses prior to the EMT's arrival
     (d) three / the patient has taken no doses prior to the EMT's arrival
     (e) five / the patient has taken no doses prior to the EMT's arrival

92.   The administration of one NTG is considered successful when
     (a) the patient reports approximately a 25% decrease in chest pain.
     (b) the patient reports complete relief from the chest pain.
     (c) the patient reports approximately a 50% decrease in chest pain.
     (d) Answers (a) or (b).
     (e) Answers (b) or (c).

93.   If no contraindications have developed, with the Medical Director's permission, the
     EMT may assist the patient to take another NTG dose ___ minutes after the first
     dose.
     (a) 2
     (b) 3
     (c) 4
     (d) 5
     (e) 10

94.   Which of the following statements regarding reassessment of the patient's blood
     pressure after nitroglycerin administration is true?
     (a) Recheck the patient's blood pressure within 2 minutes of NTG administration.
     (b) Because NTG is a strong and fast-acting medication, the patient's blood
          pressure should be rechecked every 30 seconds for the first 5 minutes
          following administration (leave the blood pressure cuff on the patient's arm).
     (c) The patient's system must become adjusted to the effects of NTG. Wait for
          at least 5 minutes following administration before rechecking the patient's
          blood pressure (readings taken earlier will be falsely low).
     (d) The patient's system must become adjusted to the effects of NTG. Wait for
          at least 10 minutes following administration before rechecking the patient's
          blood pressure (readings taken earlier will be falsely low).
     (e) Every system rechecks blood pressures at different times. There is no set
          standard for the timing of blood pressure rechecks when administering NTG.

95.   Side effects of nitroglycerin administration may include all of the following, except
(a) hypotension (nitroglycerin lowers blood pressure).
(b) headache.
(c) increased pulse rate.
(d) hypertension (increased circulation often increases cardiac output).
(e) decreased pulse rate.

96.   The American Heart Association (AHA) has identified a sequence of specific events vital to prehospital survival of cardiac arrest; the "Chain of Survival." Which of the following represents all of the Chain of Survival "links"?
(a) Early access, Early defibrillation, Early nitroglycerin administration, Early aspirin administration, Early oxygen, Early CPR, and Early advanced care.
(b) Early access, Early defibrillation, Early oxygen, Early CPR, and Early advanced care.
(c) Early access, Early oxygen, Early nitroglycerin administration, Early aspirin administration, and Early defibrillation.
(d) Early access, Early CPR, Early defibrillation, and Early advanced care.
(e) Early access, Early CPR, and Early advanced care.

97.   Biological death begins when
(a) the patient stops breathing.
(b) the patient's heart stops beating.
(c) brain cells begin to die.
(d) Answers (a) and (b).
(e) Answers (a), (b), and (c).

98.   Clinical death begins when
(a) the patient stops breathing.
(b) the patient's heart stops beating.
(c) brain cells begin to die.
(d) Answers (a) and (b).
(e) Answers (a), (b), and (c).

99.   If deprived of oxygen, brain cells begin to die in about
(a) 1 minute.
(b) 1 to 2 minutes.
(c) 3 minutes.
(d) 4 to 6 minutes.
(e) 10 minutes.

100.   The two most critical factors to successful resuscitation are
(a) delivery of high-quality chest compressions.
(b) early defibrillation.

(c) early endotracheal intubation.

(d) Answers (a) and (b).

(e) Answers (b) and (c).

101. Completely disorganized and chaotic electrical activity best describes the cardiac rhythm called

(a) ventricular tachycardia.

(b) ventricular fibrillation.

(c) asystole.

(d) Answers (a) or (b).

(e) Answers (a) or (c).

102. The absence of electrical activity (sometimes called "flatline") best describes the cardiac rhythm called

(a) ventricular tachycardia.

(b) ventricular fibrillation.

(c) asystole.

(d) Answers (a) or (b).

(e) Answers (a) or (c).

103. The cardiac rhythm _____ can be described as the presence of organized electrical activity that shows unusually wide and very rapid complexes.

(a) ventricular tachycardia

(b) ventricular fibrillation

(c) asystole

(d) Answers (a) or (b).

(e) Answers (a) or (c).

104. The cardiac rhythm _____ is always an indication for delivery of an electrical shock.

(a) ventricular tachycardia

(b) ventricular fibrillation

(c) asystole

(d) Answers (a) or (b).

(e) Answers (a) or (c).

105. The cardiac rhythm _____ is a rhythm that should never be shocked.

(a) ventricular tachycardia

(b) ventricular fibrillation

(c) asystole

(d) Answers (a) or (b).

(e) Answers (a) or (c).

106. The cardiac rhythm _____ may occur while the patient is still breathing and responsive, and should not be shocked.
   (a) ventricular tachycardia
   (b) ventricular fibrillation
   (c) asystole
   (d) Answers (a) or (b).
   (e) Answers (a), (b), or (c).

107. The cardiac rhythm called pulseless electrical activity (PEA) is best described as
   (a) any cardiac rhythm with or without a pulse.
   (b) ventricular tachycardia, with a pulse.
   (c) any organized, coordinated (usually slow) cardiac rhythm that generates no pulse.
   (d) any cardiac electrical activity without a pulse.
   (e) ventricular fibrillation, with a pulse.

108. If EMS responders arrive within 8 minutes of the patient's cardiac arrest, 50 to 60 percent of the time the patient will be in
   (a) ventricular tachycardia.
   (b) ventricular fibrillation.
   (c) asystole.
   (d) Answers (a) or (b).
   (e) Answers (a) or (c).

109. A patient in the cardiac rhythm _____ may have a pulse.
   (a) ventricular tachycardia
   (b) ventricular fibrillation
   (c) asystole
   (d) Any of the above.
   (e) None of the above (patients in these rhythms never have a pulse).

110. There are two types of automated external defibrillators (AEDs). The _____ operates without the EMT's participation (apart from turning on the power and placing the monitor-defibrillation pads on the patient).
   (a) fully automated defibrillator
   (b) incompletely automated defibrillator
   (c) semiautomated defibrillator
   (d) EMT-Basic defibrillator
   (e) cardiac autodefibrillator

111. The _____ has a computer voice synthesizer that advises the EMT whether or not to press the button for a shock delivery. A shock is not delivered unless the EMT pushes the button.
   (a) fully automated defibrillator
   (b) incompletely automated defibrillator

    (c) semiautomated defibrillator

    (d) EMT-Basic defibrillator

    (e) cardiac autodefibrillator

112. AEDs use _____ monitor-defibrillation pads to sense the electrical activity of the patient's heart and to deliver an electrical shock.

    (a) 12

    (b) 5

    (c) 3

    (d) 2

    (e) 1

113. The reasons for an AED inappropriately recommending or delivering a shock include all of the following, except

    (a) application of the AED to a patient with a pulse.

    (b) inaccurate placement of the third monitor-defibrillation pad.

    (c) application of the AED to a patient who is breathing.

    (d) poorly charged AED batteries.

    (e) improper AED maintenance.

114. An AED is a very sensitive device. All of the following forms of stimulus may be sensed by the AED during cardiac rhythm analysis and may produce a false interpretation or inappropriate shock recommendation, except

    (a) excessively loud crowd noise or vehicle horns.

    (b) engine vibrations during patient transportation.

    (c) movement of any part of the patient's body by others.

    (d) spontaneous patient body movement.

    (e) some radio transmissions.

115. The most important rule to remember when considering the application of any AED model or type is that

    (a) every medical patient should have an AED applied for cardiac rhythm diagnosis.

    (b) every unconscious patient should have an AED applied for cardiac rhythm diagnosis.

    (c) any apneic patient should have an AED applied for cardiac rhythm diagnosis.

    (d) any conscious patient with no palpable radial pulse should have an AED applied for cardiac rhythm diagnosis.

    (e) only unconscious, apneic, pulseless patients should have an AED applied for cardiac rhythm diagnosis.

116. Which of the following statements regarding the use of an AED is true?

  (a) Modern AEDs are capable of accurately analyzing cardiac rhythms and appropriately indicating "shock" or "no shock" when being used during transportation of a patient in an ambulance.

  (b) When the AED defibrillates a patient, it delivers an electrical shock that travels along a straight line between the monitor-defibrillation pads. As long as no responders are actually touching these pads (or the space between them), no harm will come to a person in contact with the patient's body during defibrillation.

  (c) When the AED defibrillates a patient, it delivers an electrical shock only to the patient's body. If the patient receiving a shock is lying in a pool of water or on a metal surface, as long as no responders are actually touching the patient's body, no harm will come to them during defibrillation.

  (d) Both answers (a) and (c) are true.

  (e) None of the above is true.

117. Artificial cardiac pacemakers are implanted in patients whose natural pacemaker no longer functions appropriately. Which of the following statements regarding implanted artificial pacemakers and AED use is true?

  (a) If a patient in cardiac arrest has an implanted artificial pacemaker, the AED should not be used. The patient's implanted device will interfere with the AED's ability to correctly analyze the patient's cardiac rhythm and safely deliver appropriate shocks.

  (b) The battery that powers the patient's artificial pacemaker is most commonly imbedded beneath the patient's skin, below the right or left clavicle.

  (c) If a lump that feels like an artificial pacemaker's battery is found in the area where you normally would put an AED pad, place the pad several inches away from the battery lump. Then continue operation of the AED as usual.

  (d) Both answers (a) and (b) are true.

  (e) Both answers (b) and (c) are true.

118. Although not as commonly seen as patients with pacemakers, patients with surgically implanted automatic cardiac defibrillators (AICDs or ICDs) may be encountered by EMTs. These patients have had a tiny defibrillator implanted in their bodies because they have a high risk for developing ventricular tachycardia or ventricular fibrillation. Which of the following statements regarding emergency care, CPR, and AED use for these patients is true?

  (a) Since they already have a defibrillator implanted, an AED should never be used on these patients, even when they are in cardiac arrest.

  (b) It is extremely dangerous for anyone to be in contact with these patients when their defibrillator shocks them. Avoid all physical contact with these patients at all times.

(c) Because of the physical contact danger, a voice synthesizer is also implanted in the patient (usually in the abdomen, where there is more room). Just prior to administering a shock, the implanted defibrillator will activate the voice synthesizer, and the message, "Stand back!" will be broadcast three times before the shock is given.

(d) All of the above are true.

(e) None of the above is true.

119. Which of the following statements regarding AED use and cardiac arrest patients with transdermal medication patches is false?

(a) The warning that nitroglycerine patches may ignite or "explode" if left on the patient's chest during defibrillation is a myth! NTG patches should remain in place so that the patient continues to receive the benefits of this medication during treatment for cardiac arrest.

(b) Any transdermal medication patch may melt or ignite if the AED's monitor-defibrillator pads are placed on top of it, and a shock is delivered into the patch.

(c) AED monitor-defibrillator pads should not be placed over any form of transdermal medication patch because the patch may block the pads' sensing or defibrillating effects.

(d) All forms of transdermal medication patches must be removed prior to AED use. Wear gloves to do so, thoroughly wipe the area the patch was removed from with a towel or gauze pad, and avoid placing an AED monitor-defibrillator pad on any site where any medication patch was previously affixed.

(e) If you touch the medication-side of any transdermal medication patch with your ungloved fingers, the medication may enter your system through your skin and adversely affect you.

120. Which of the following statements regarding AED use and interruption of CPR is false?

(a) CPR should be stopped before a shock is delivered.

(b) Chest compressions should be stopped when the patient's rhythm is being analyzed by the AED.

(c) No person should be touching the patient when a shock is delivered.

(d) Artificial ventilations must be stopped when the patient's rhythm is being analyzed by the AED.

(e) Because it is entirely plastic, it is safe to hold a BVM attached to an endotracheal tube (or similar airway device) during a shock delivery, as long as no other portion of the patient is contacted.

121. Which of the following statements regarding initial AED use and interruption of CPR is false?

   (a) For EMS-witnessed cardiac arrests with an AED immediately available, the AED should be used as soon as possible.

   (b) When EMS personnel did not witness an out-of-hospital cardiac arrest, up to 5 cycles of CPR should be performed prior to AED analysis and defibrillation.

   (c) When a shock is indicated, CPR should be stopped only long enough to deliver one shock.

   (d) After being cued by the AED to deliver a shock, the rescuer should deliver 1 shock and then immediately resume CPR, beginning with chest compressions.

   (e) If the AED has signaled a shock delivery, up to 3 shocks should be delivered before CPR is resumed.

122. Which of the following statements regarding biphasic and monophasic AEDs is false?

   (a) To operate a biphasic AED, the power should be turned on before the monitor-defibrillation pads are placed on the patient.

   (b) Biphasic AEDs can deliver lower energy shocks than monophasic AEDs.

   (c) Monophasic AEDs deliver a shock in one direction, only: from the negative pad to the positive pad.

   (d) A monophasic AED's monitor-defibrillation pads are interchangeable (it doesn't matter which one is placed where—neither has a specifically "positive" or "negative" polarization).

   (e) A biphasic AED's monitor-defibrillation pads are interchangeable (it doesn't matter which one is placed where—neither has a specifically "positive" or "negative" polarization).

123. Which of the following statements regarding correct monitor-defibrillation pad placement is false?

   (a) If bilateral anterior-chest placement is being used, the negative monitor-defibrillation pad should be placed just below the right clavicle, midway between the sternum and the right anterior axillary line.

   (b) If bilateral anterior-chest placement is being used, the negative monitor-defibrillation pad should be placed just below the patient's left nipple, and slightly toward the patient's left anterior axillary line.

   (c) If posterior/anterior pad placement is being used, the negative monitor-defibrillation pad is also known as the posterior pad.

   (d) If posterior/anterior pad placement is being used, the positive monitor-defibrillation pad is also known as the anterior pad, and is placed over the apex of the heart, just medial to the patient's left nipple.

   (e) If bilateral anterior-chest placement is being used, the positive monitor-defibrillation pad should be placed just below the patient's left nipple, and slightly toward the patient's left anterior axillary line.

124. Rescuer fatigue has been shown to result in inadequate performance of chest compression rates and/or depth. In 2010, the AHA mandated that when 2 or more rescuers are available to perform adult CPR, the chest-compressor should switch roles with the ventilator, or be replaced by another chest-compressor, after performing

    (a) 5 cycles of CPR.
    (b) 5 minutes of chest compression.
    (c) 10 cycles of CPR.
    (d) 10 minutes of chest compression.
    (e) 15 minutes of chest compression.

125. In 2010, the AHA mandated that when 2 or more trained rescuers are available to perform CPR for a child aged 8 to 13 years old, the chest-compressor should switch roles with the ventilator, or be repalced by another chest-compressor, after performing

    (a) 1 minute of chest compression (approximately 5 cycles of CPR).
    (b) 2 minutes of chest compression (approximately 5 cycles of CPR).
    (c) 5 minutes of chest compression.
    (d) 10 minutes of chest compression.
    (e) 15 minutes of chest compression.

126. Up to _____ AED shocks may be delivered without pulse checks or CPR between them.

    (a) 2
    (b) 3
    (c) 5
    (d) 6
    (e) None of the above. Two minutes of CPR should be performed after each shock.

127. Some AEDs have built-in tape recorders. These tape recorders are designed to

    (a) catch EMTs making mistakes so that they can be reprimanded.
    (b) assist in documentation of the event's activities as well as shock delivery and CPR performance.
    (c) represent the EMT's actions in a court of law, so that the EMT will not have to appear (the AED record is considered a "real-time deposition").
    (d) Answers (a) and (c).
    (e) Answers (a), (b), and (c).

128. If your AED is equipped with a tape recorder, which of the following statements regarding when you should begin providing a "narrative report" by speaking directly to the tape recorder is true?

   (a) Begin your narrative report en route to the call; providing the call number, responding unit number, names of responding crew, and so on.

   (b) Record your narrative report after the call is over (before you have forgotten the circumstances and activities).

   (c) Begin your narrative report after turning on the AED's power button (if your AED has one, the tape recorder comes on automatically after its use is initiated).

   (d) Begin your narrative report after turning off the AED's power button (if your AED has one, the tape recorder comes on automatically after its use is terminated).

   (e) The EMT should never speak directly to the AED tape recorder. Doing so would distract the EMT from performing important assessments and treatments, and would sound suspicious.

129. When the AED provides a "no shock" message after an analysis, the EMT should immediately

   (a) call his Medical Director to pronounce the patient "DOA" (dead on arrival).

   (b) resume CPR.

   (c) check the patient's pulse and breathing.

   (d) have CPR resumed by others while calling his Medical Director to pronounce the patient "DOA" (dead on arrival).

   (e) switch the monitor-defibrillation pad placement, to ensure that the positive and negative pads are in the right place.

130. Which of the following statements regarding coordination of ALS personnel (EMT-Intermediates or Paramedics) with BLS care-provision is false?

   (a) Upon discovery of an unconscious patient in cardiac arrest, ALS personnel should not be summoned by BLS personnel until after they have applied and initiated their AED, unless both tasks can be done simultaneously.

   (b) The use of an AED does not require the presence of ALS personnel on scene.

   (c) Upon discovery of an unconscious patient in cardiac arrest, BLS personnel should not apply the AED until after they have summoned ALS personnel.

   (d) If ALS personnel are responding from a significant distance, a cardiac arrest patient may be transported by BLS personnel to a rendezvous point.

   (e) If ALS personnel are not available, a cardiac arrest patient may be transported to the emergency department by BLS personnel.

131. If no on-scene ALS assistance is available, the patient should be transported to the emergency department by BLS personnel when which of the following occurs?

   (a) The patient regains a pulse.
   (b) After two sets of three shocks have been administered without success.
   (c) After the AED has given three consecutive "no shock" messages (with two minutes of CPR performed after each).
   (d) Answers (a) or (b).
   (e) Answers (a) or (c).

132. The universal single-rescuer CPR compression-to-ventilation ratio for cardio-pulmonary arrest victims of all ages (except newborns) is

   (a) 5:1 (1 ventilation for every 5 chest compressions).
   (b) 15:2 (2 ventilations for every 15 chest compressions).
   (c) 30:2 (2 ventilations for every 30 chest compressions).
   (d) 15:1 (1 ventilation for every 15 chest compressoins).
   (e) 30:1 (1 ventilation for every 30 chest compressions).

133. The compression-to-ventilation ratio 2 trained rescuers should perform for adult CPR is

   (a) 5:1 (1 ventilation for every 5 chest compressions).
   (b) 15:2 (2 ventilations for every 15 chest compressions).
   (c) 30:2 (2 ventilations for every 30 chest compressions).
   (d) 15:1 (1 vetilation for every 15 chest compressions).
   (e) 30:1 (1 ventilation for every 30 chest compressions).

134. The compression-to-ventilation ratio 2 trained rescuers should perform for cardio-pulmonary arrest victims aged 1 year old to puberty is

   (a) 5:1 (1 ventilation for every 5 chest compressions).
   (b) 15:2 (2 ventilations for every 15 chest compressions).
   (c) 30:2 (2 ventilations for every 30 chest compressions).
   (d) 15:1 (1 ventilation for every 15 chest compressions).
   (e) 30:1 (1 ventilation for every 30 chest compressions).

135.   The compression-to-ventilation ratio a single lay or trained rescuer should perform
for the newborn infant in cardiopulmonary arrest is

    (a)   3:1 (1 ventilation for every 3 chest compressions).
    (b)   5:2 (2 ventilations for every 5 chest compressions).
    (c)   30:2 (2 ventilations for every 30 chest compressions).
    (d)   15:1 (1 ventilation for every 15 chest compressions).
    (e)   5:1 (1 ventilation for every 5 chest compressions).

The answer key for Test Section Four is on page 341.

5

DOT Module Four: Medical Emergencies

Subjects:

- Altered Mental Status
- Diabetes
- Stroke
- Allergies
- Ingested Poisoning and Overdose
- Environmental Emergencies
- Behavioral Emergencies
- Patient Restraint

(Other Medical Emergency subjects from DOT Module Four are addressed in Test Sections Four, Seven, and Nine.)

Test Section Five consists of 150 questions and is allotted 2 hours and 30 minutes for completion.

1.   The rapid onset of an altered mental status or altered level of consciousness (LOC) may be caused by all of the following, except
   (a) hypoglycemia.
   (b) hyperglycemia.
   (c) poisoning.
   (d) head trauma.
   (e) hypoxia.

2.   The condition of *hypoglycemia* can be determined by a routine blood test, and is defined as a
   (a) high level of sugar in the blood.
   (b) low level of sugar in the blood.
   (c) low level of insulin in the blood.
   (d) high level of insulin in the blood.
   (e) low level of hormones in the blood.

3.   The condition of *hyperglycemia* can be determined by a routine blood test, and is defined as a
   (a) high level of sugar in the blood.
   (b) low level of sugar in the blood.
   (c) low level of insulin in the blood.
   (d) high level of insulin in the blood.
   (e) low level of hormones in the blood.

4.   The specific condition of *diabetes mellitus* is often referred to, simply, as diabetes. Thus, *diabetes* is most often defined as a disorder caused by the
   (a) inadequate production or utilization of the hormone insulin.
   (b) inadequate production of the polysaccharide glycogen.
   (c) inadequate production of the hormone glucose.
   (d) overproduction of the hormone insulin.
   (e) overproduction of the polysaccharide glycogen.

5.   Because _____ cannot move from the blood into the cells of the body without assistance (a "key" to "unlock" the cell door), _____ must be present to allow its entrance.
   (a) insulin / oxygen
   (b) glucose / insulin
   (c) oxygen / insulin
   (d) glucose / oxygen
   (e) insulin / glucose

6.   The most common diabetes-related medical emergency is often also known as "insulin shock." The medical term for this emergency is
      (a) hypoinsulinemia.
      (b) hyperinsulinemia.
      (c) hyperglycemia.
      (d) hypoglycemia.
      (e) gluconeogenesis.

7.   Which of the following statements regarding hyperglycemia is false?
      (a) A fruity or nail-polish-remover-like breath odor ("acetone breath" or "ketone breath") may accompany hyperglycemia.
      (b) Deep inhalations with a rapid respiratory rate often accompany hyperglycemia.
      (c) Extreme thirst with excessive fluid intake and frequent urination often accompanies hyperglycemia.
      (d) Hyperglycemia has a very rapid onset of signs and symptoms.
      (e) Hyperglycemia may progress to unconsciousness and/or death.

8.   A diabetes-related altered LOC may occur without any identifiable factors preceding the event. However, which of the following situations would not normally cause a sudden onset of diabetes-related altered LOC?
      (a) The patient took his daily prescribed insulin and then missed a single meal.
      (b) The patient took his daily prescribed insulin, ate a normal meal, but then vomited and did not eat again before engaging in normal activities.
      (c) After normal insulin administration and eating a normal meal, the patient engaged in an unusual amount of physical exercise or work.
      (d) The patient ate normally and engaged in normal activities, but forgot to take his daily prescribed insulin.
      (e) The patient forgot to take his prescribed insulin the previous evening, so he doubled his morning dose, ate a normal breakfast, and engaged in normal daytime activities.

9.   Most often, the first sign of insulin shock is
      (a) tachycardia.
      (b) hypotension.
      (c) nausea, with or without vomiting.
      (d) unusual behavior (altered level of consciousness).
      (e) extreme pallor.

10.   All of the following signs and symptoms are associated with insulin shock, except
      (a) slurred speech and staggering (as though intoxicated by alcohol or drugs).
      (b) tachycardia with cool, pale, and/or clammy skin.
      (c) abnormal thirst, with increased fluid intake and frequent urination.
      (d) seizures.
      (e) anxiousness, combativeness, or other uncharacteristic behaviors.

11. All of the following medications may be prescribed to a patient with diabetes mellitus, except

    (a) the oral medication insulin (Humulin®, Novolin®, Lente®).

    (b) the oral medication Orinase®.

    (c) the oral medications Micronase® or Diabeta®.

    (d) the subcutaneously injected medication insulin (Humulin®, Novolin®, Lente®).

    (e) the oral medications Diabinese® or Glucamide®.

12. The prescription drug insulin (Humulin®, Novolin®, Lente®) is most often found in the diabetic patient's

    (a) refrigerator.

    (b) pant pocket.

    (c) bathroom medicine cabinet.

    (d) purse or wallet.

    (e) dresser drawer or on a bedside table.

13. Oral glucose administration acts to

    (a) increase the patient's blood sugar levels.

    (b) decrease the patient's blood sugar levels.

    (c) increase the patient's insulin levels.

    (d) Answers (b) and (c).

    (e) Answers (a) and (c).

14. Even with off-line ("standing orders") permission from the Medical Director for administration of oral glucose to a patient with a history of diabetes, oral glucose may only be administered if the patient also

    (a) is conscious.

    (b) is unconscious.

    (c) can swallow.

    (d) Answers (a) or (b).

    (e) Answers (a) and (c).

15. Which of the following methods of oral glucose administration is contraindicated?

    (a) Have the patient squeeze the tube between his own cheek and gum.

    (b) Place the gel on a tongue depressor and hold it between the conscious patient's cheek and gum.

    (c) After properly inserting an oral airway into the unconscious patient's mouth, squeeze the gel into the pocket between the patient's cheek and gum.

    (d) Place the gel on a tongue depressor and have the conscious patient hold it between his own cheek and gum.

    (e) None of the above is contraindicated (all are acceptable methods of oral glucose administration).

16.   Which of the following statements regarding the use of glucometers (blood glucose meters) to measure a patient's blood glucose level, when the patient's condition permits the time to use one, is false?

    (a)   If the EMT has a glucometer, the EMT should measure the blood glucose level of any patient with an altered LOC, even if the patient is not known to have a diabetic medical history.

    (b)   If a patient with an altered LOC has a history of diabetes and the EMT has a glucometer, the EMT should measure the patient's blood glucose level.

    (c)   If the EMT does not have a glucometer, but the patient or the patient's family member has just obtained a glucometer reading using the patient's glucometer, the patient's glucometer reading should be reported to the Medical Director when requesting advice or orders for the patient's treatment.

    (d)   If the EMT does not have a glucometer, but the patient or the patient's family member has just obtained a glucometer reading using the patient's glucometer, no glucometer reading should be reported to the Medical Director when requesting advice or orders for the patient's treatment. Glucometers owned and used by patients (or their family members) are notoriously inaccurate.

    (e)   If a diabetic patient is acting "drunk" and clearly smells like he's been drinking alcohol, and the EMT has a glucometer, the EMT should measure the patient's blood glucose level.

17.   Glucometer operational procedures should be performed according to the device manufacturer's instructions. However, some operational rules are common to all glucometers. Which of the following statements regarding common operational rules for glucometer operation is false?

    (a)   In order to obtain the most accurate reading, all glucometers must be calibrated and stored according to the manufacturer's recommendations.

    (b)   Always cleanse the patient's finger before using a lancet to perform a finger stick and obtain a blood sample for testing.

    (c)   If cleansing the patient's finger with alcohol, always allow the patient's finger to dry before using a lancet to perform a finger stick to obtain a blood sample.

    (d)   Answers (a), (b), and (c) are true.

    (e)   None of the above is true.

18.   When a diabetic patient is merely confused, a glucometer reading of _____ indicates the need to rapidly obtain orders (or act on standing orders) for the administration of glucose.

    (a)   100 or less

    (b)   80 or less

    (c)   60 or less

    (d)   Answers (b) or (c).

    (e)   Answers (a), (b), or (c).

19.   When a diabetic patient is exhibiting any signs or symptoms possibly indicating insulin shock, a glucometer reading of _____ indicates the need to rapidly obtain orders (or act on standing orders) for the administration of glucose.
  (a) 100 or less
  (b) 80 or less
  (c) 60 or less
  (d) Answers (b) or (c).
  (e) Answers (a), (b), or (c).

20.   When a patient without a known history of diabetes is exhibiting any signs or symptoms possibly indicating insulin shock, a glucometer reading of _____ indicates the need to rapidly obtain orders (or act on standing orders) for the administration of glucose.
  (a) 100 or less
  (b) 80 or less
  (c) 60 or less
  (d) Answers (b) or (c).
  (e) Answers (a), (b), or (c).

21.   The medical term *idiopathic* means
  (a) a condition or disease that causes the patient to pathologically deteriorate in level of intelligence (becoming an "idiot").
  (b) a person with a very low level of intelligence (idiocy), but who abnormally excels in one or two areas of function (such as math or the arts).
  (c) a condition or disease that occurs because of an unknown cause.
  (d) a condition or disease that causes severe mental deficiency (idiocy).
  (e) a mentally impaired person with a pathological fixation on perversion.

22.   Seizures may be caused by all of the following, except
  (a) infections (especially when accompanied by fever).
  (b) insulin shock.
  (c) poisoning (chemical or plant toxic exposures).
  (d) excessive oxygen administration (most often caused by using a nonrebreather mask to treat patients who are merely hyperventilating).
  (e) any form of head trauma.

23.   Seizures may be caused by all of the following, except
  (a) excessive water ingestion (causing a body chemistry imbalance).
  (b) missing a single dose of seizure medication.
  (c) missing a single dose of hyperglycemia medication.
  (d) a brain tumor or congenital brain defect.
  (e) hypoxia caused by a medical or traumatic event.

24. Seizures may be caused by all of the following, except
    (a) pregnancy.
    (b) extremely low blood pressure.
    (c) extremely high blood pressure.
    (d) excessive candy ingestion (children who overdose on sugar products).
    (e) measles, mumps, or other childhood diseases.

25. Seizures may be caused by all of the following, except
    (a) a nondiabetic who goes without eating an entire day.
    (b) cerebrovascular accidents (strokes).
    (c) transient ischemic accidents ("little strokes").
    (d) excessive heat exposure.
    (e) drug or alcohol withdrawal.

26. Seizures may be caused by all of the following, except
    (a) cardiac rhythm abnormalities.
    (b) ingestion of more than 5 Crayola® crayons (in children).
    (c) an entirely unknown or undetermined cause.
    (d) a condition known as eclampsia.
    (e) hyperglycemia.

27. *Idiopathic seizures* are defined as seizures produced by
    (a) an entirely unknown or undetermined cause.
    (b) severe mental retardation (idiocy).
    (c) missing a dose of diabetic medication.
    (d) excessive oxygen administration (most often caused by using a nonrebreather mask to treat patients who are merely hyperventilating).
    (e) a prolonged lack of oxygen (causing the patient to pathologically deteriorate in the level of intelligence, and become an "idiot").

28. The most common cause of seizures in an adult is
    (a) an idiopathic cause.
    (b) hypoglycemia.
    (c) cardiac dysrhythmias.
    (d) failure to take prescribed anticonvulsant (antiseizure) medication.
    (e) excessive oxygen administration (most often caused by using a nonrebreather mask to treat patients who are merely hyperventilating).

29. The most common cause of seizure in an infant or child (especially between the ages of 6 months and 3 years) is
    (a) hypoxia.
    (b) high fever.
    (c) poisoning.
    (d) failure to take prescribed anticonvulsant (antiseizure) medication.
    (e) excessive oxygen administration (most often caused by using a nonrebreather mask to treat children who don't need the extra oxygen).

30. The medical term *epilepsy* is used to describe

(a) any patient who has any kind of seizure, for any reason.

(b) a patient who has had seizures since birth, or since suffering a traumatic head injury.

(c) a patient who has seizures whenever excessive oxygen is administered.

(d) any patient who experiences a "first-time" seizure (the term is only used as a temporary diagnosis).

(e) people who have seizures due to blood sugar problems.

31. Which of the following statements regarding a patient who is still seizing when you arrive on scene is false?

(a) Unless your response time was less than 2 or 3 minutes, the patient is probably in status epilepticus.

(b) You should immediately restrain the patient (three or more people may be required to hold all extremities still) and apply high-flow oxygen via a nonrebreather mask.

(c) Move any hard or sharp objects away from the patient.

(d) If nearby hard or sharp objects are immovable, gently move the patient away from the objects, or place cushions of some sort between the patient and the objects.

(e) Remove anything that a bystander may have put in the patient's mouth to "keep him from biting his tongue."

32. Which of the following statements regarding activities that occur while a patient is seizing is false?

(a) If the patient's urinary sphincter seized, the patient will be incontinent of urine.

(b) If the patient's anal sphincter seized, the patient will be incontinent of feces.

(c) The patient may bite his tongue or the inside of his cheeks, resulting in one or more superficial lacerations that generally will not interfere with breathing or care provision after the seizure.

(d) If a "bite block" is not inserted between the patient's teeth, the patient may "swallow his tongue" and occlude his own airway.

(e) Never put your fingers inside the mouth of a seizing patient.

33. If a patient is cyanotic when his seizure stops,

(a) do not be concerned; this is a normal phase of seizures.

(b) immediately perform an airway maneuver and artificially ventilate the patient.

(c) roll the patient to his side and wait at least 3 minutes for his color to improve (allowing normal recovery) before performing any other form of emergency treatment.

(d) roll the patient to his side and provide suction for at least 1 minute, then apply oxygen via a nonrebreather mask.

(e) Answers (a) and (c).

34. Which of the following statements regarding positioning of a patient immediately after a full-body seizure is true?

(a) Roll the patient to his side to allow for fluid drainage and airway protection only if there is no mechanism of injury that suggests spinal trauma.

(b) If there is a mechanism of injury that suggests spinal trauma, keep the patient supine and manually suction the airway.

(c) The patient must not remain supine (even if the mechanism of injury suggests spinal trauma) because the patient may swallow his tongue and choke. Roll him to his side as a unit and place a bite block between his teeth before suctioning.

(d) Answers (a) and (b) are true.

(e) Answers (a) and (c) are true.

35. Your trauma patient has been immobilized to a long backboard and is receiving oxygen via a nonrebreather mask. Suddenly he loses consciousness and begins to have a full-body seizure. You should

(a) rapidly remove all straps or other devices used to secure the patient to the long backboard.

(b) leave the nonrebreather mask in place.

(c) tighten each strap or other device used to secure the patient to the long backboard if any becomes loose as the patient seizes.

(d) Answers (a) and (b).

(e) Answers (b) and (c).

36. There are several different kinds of seizures that usually are grouped into two different types: partial seizures and generalized seizures. Which of the following would be classified as partial seizures?

(a) "Jacksonian" or "focal motor" seizures, which involve only one body part or one side of the body. They consist of tingling sensation, stiffening, or uncontrollable jerking of that body portion. There is no loss of consciousness unless the seizure progresses to involve the entire body.

(b) "Psychomotor" or "temporal lobe" seizures, which involve various forms of uncontrollable abnormal behavior. The patient may act as though intoxicated or on drugs, may struggle or fight with responders, may scream and cry out while running around, disrobing or engaging in other bizarre behavior. There is no loss of consciousness unless the seizure progresses to involve the entire body.

(c) "Petit mal" seizures, which are also called "absence seizures." They usually are very brief in duration (1 to 10 seconds) and involve only temporary loss of concentration or awareness. Because no dramatic physical movement, slumping, or falling accompanies them, they often go unnoticed by the patient, or those around the patient.

(d) Answers (a) and (b).

(e) Answers (b) and (c).

37.   Which of the following would be classified as generalized seizures?

(a) "Jacksonian" or "focal motor" seizures (see description in question 36).

(b) "Psychomotor" or "temporal lobe" seizures (see description in question 36).

(c) "Tonic-clonic" or "grand mal" seizures, which produce unconsciousness and involve uncontrollable motor activity of the entire body. Tongue or cheek biting and/or incontinence of bladder or the bowels may occur. The clonic phase consists of violent flexion/contraction and extension of the body, and may last for 1 to 3 minutes.

(d) Answers (a) and (b).

(e) Answers (b) and (c).

38.   Some patients describe experiencing an *aura* before having a seizure. Which of the following describes a sensation that could be considered an aura?

(a) The sensation of a strange taste experienced just prior to the seizure.

(b) A hallucination of bright bursts of colors or lights just prior to the seizure.

(c) An odd or out-of-place odor smelled just prior to the seizure.

(d) Answers (a) or (b).

(e) Answers (a), (b), or (c).

39.   Which of the following treatment and transportation considerations related to specific seizure incidents is true?

(a) When a child with a history of chronic seizure disorder has a seizure, it is rarely a life-threatening situation, and only requires emergency treatment and ambulance transportation when the parent (or guardian) specifically requests it, or if some kind of trauma occurred during the seizure.

(b) No matter what the patient's seizure history, all pediatric seizures (including "febrile seizures") should be considered a life-threatening event, and the EMT should do everything possible to ensure that emergency treatment and ambulance transportation are accomplished.

(c) Persons with chronic seizure disorders may have very brief seizures (10 seconds to 3 minutes), or somewhat prolonged seizures (5 to 10 minutes), depending upon each individual's personal history. If the patient's seizure was not of an unusual length, and no injury occurred during the seizure, emergency treatment and ambulance transportation are not needed.

(d) Answers (a) and (c) are true.

(e) None of the above answers is true.

40.   All of the following are generic names of medications commonly prescribed to patients with seizure disorders, except

(a) Dilantin.

(b) carbamazepine.

(c) phenytoin.

(d) valproic acid.

(e) clonazepam.

41. All of the following are trade (or brand) names of medications commonly prescribed to patients with seizure disorders, except
    (a) Tegretol or Epitol.
    (b) primidone.
    (c) Depakene or Depakote.
    (d) Mysoline and Clonopin.
    (e) Zarontin and Neurontin.

42. Which of the following statements regarding the condition *status epilepticus* is false?
    (a) Status epilepticus is a life-threatening condition. Immediately begin transportation, providing care en route, and call for an ACLS intercept en route to the emergency department (if available).
    (b) Any patient who has two or three seizures within a 24-hour period is in status epilepticus.
    (c) Any patient in status epilepticus requires immediate and ongoing airway control and artificial ventilation, and occasional suctioning.
    (d) Any patient who has two or more seizures in a row without regaining consciousness between them is in status epilepticus.
    (e) Any single seizure that continues beyond 10 minutes indicates a patient in status epilepticus.

43. The _____ phase or state begins after all of a generalized seizure's physical activity has stopped.
    (a) tonic
    (b) clonic
    (c) preictal
    (d) postictal
    (e) peri-ictal

44. Once the seizure stops, the patient may complain of, or demonstrate, which of the following signs and symptoms?
    (1) Physical exhaustion and weakness.
    (2) An altered level of consciousness.
    (3) A rapid return to consciousness, with only minor confusion.
    (4) An unresponsive state of sleep, with or without snoring.
    (5) A significantly confused, excited or agitated state of excessive physical activity.
    (6) Complaint of a headache.
    (7) Complaint of drowsiness, or an abnormal lack of interest in his environment.

    (a) 1, 2, 3, 4, 5, 6, or 7.
    (b) 1, 2, 3, 4, 6, or 7.
    (c) 1, 2, 4, 6, or 7.
    (d) 1, 4, 6, or 7.
    (e) 1, 5, or 7.

45. The phase or state that begins after all of a generalized seizure's physical activity has stopped (when the patient exhibits the signs and symptoms described in the previous question)

  (a) lasts no longer than 1 minute.

  (b) lasts no longer than 10 minutes.

  (c) continues for at least 30 minutes.

  (d) lasts no longer than 1 hour.

  (e) may resolve after 30 seconds, or last over an hour.

46. Your patient complains, "The room is spinning!" This complaint indicates a disturbance of the patient's sense of balance and may be a symptom of inner ear trauma or infection. The medical term used to indicate the patient's "The room is spinning!" complaint is

  (a) WADAO ("Weak And Dizzy All Over").

  (b) psychiatric dizziness.

  (c) the vapors.

  (d) syncope.

  (e) vertigo.

47. Syncope is the medical term for

  (a) fainting (a transient loss of consciousness).

  (b) an episode of dizziness, without loss of consciousness.

  (c) the sudden sensation of weakness, without loss of consciousness.

  (d) a patient experiencing psychiatric difficulties.

  (e) Answers (b) or (c).

48. Which of the following statements regarding syncope is true?

  (a) Syncope can occur in patients of any age.

  (b) Unless the patient is a head trauma victim, syncope occurs only in adult patients.

  (c) Unless the patient is a head trauma victim, syncope usually occurs only in the elderly (patients over 50 years old).

  (d) If the "syncope" patient is a child, it indicates that the child has psychiatric problems or is a victim of child abuse. (In case it was the result of abuse, every pediatric syncopal event requires a social services report.)

  (e) Answers (c) and (d) are true.

49. Syncope can be caused by all of the following, except

  (a) excessive oxygen administration (such as high-flow oxygen being administered via a nonrebreather mask to a hyperventilating patient).

  (b) a hypovolemic patient suddenly standing up from a sitting position.

  (c) a hypotensive patient suddenly standing up from a sitting position.

  (d) a hypoglycemic patient suddenly standing up from a sitting position.

  (e) anything that causes a sudden episode of diminished blood flow or oxygen to the brain.

50. Syncope can also be caused by (or be a sign of) which of the following?

(1) Dehydration.
(2) Tachycardia.
(3) Alcohol intoxication.
(4) A sudden fright.
(5) Gastrointestinal bleeding.
(6) Head trauma.
(7) Bradycardia.
(8) Drug intoxication.
(9) A brain tumor.
(10) An irregular heartbeat.
(11) Inner or middle ear infection or trauma.
(12) A cerebrovascular accident.
(13) Someone bearing down too hard to have a bowel movement.

    (a) 1, 2, 3, 4, 5, 6, 7, 8, 9, 10, 11, 12, or 13.
    (b) 1, 2, 4, 5, 6, 7, 9, 10, 11, 12, or 13.
    (c) 1, 2, 5, 6, 7, 9, 10, 11, or 12.
    (d) 1, 2, 5, 6, 7, 9, 10, or 12.
    (e) 1, 2, 5, 6, 7, 9, 10, or 11.

51. Which of the following statements regarding EMT assessment and treatment of syncope is false?

(a) If the syncopal patient is still unconscious or disoriented upon your arrival (after having been supine for 1 minute or longer), provide high flow oxygen via a nonrebreather mask and consider calling for ALS backup or providing immediate rapid transport before performing any further assessment or evaluation.

(b) If the victim of syncope is not supine on your arrival, and is still confused, immediately place him supine and administer high flow oxygen via a nonrebreather mask while you perform further assessment.

(c) Be careful to assess for possible trauma having occurred during a syncopal episode, even if the supine patient is alert, well oriented, and denies all complaints.

(d) If trauma does not appear to be associated with the event, do not strip the syncope victim of all clothing – but, you still must look at all parts of the patient's body (in case multiple nitroglycerin patches are on the patient's back, or the like).

(e) If the syncope victim is alert and well oriented upon your arrival, denies all complaints, and refuses treatment and transportation, no assessment or emergency medical treatment need be performed. Simply document the call as a "not needed," and return to service.

52. Which of the following statements regarding syncope is false?

(a) Because a few seconds of jerky muscle movement may accompany an episode of syncope, bystanders may report that a syncope victim had a seizure or "convulsion."

(b) A victim of syncope returns to full consciousness and is reasonably well oriented, almost immediately after becoming supine.

(c) Victims of syncope may have cool, pale, and moist skin.

(d) Most often, syncope victims remain unconscious for 20 to 30 minutes after falling to the floor.

(e) Bladder or bowel incontinence may accompany a syncopal episode.

53. An *allergen* is best defined as

(a) an exaggerated but non-life-threatening immune response.

(b) a severe and life-threatening, exaggerated immune response, causing dilation of the body's blood vessels (low blood pressure), edema of the respiratory tissues, and bronchoconstriction (both of which threaten the patient's airway).

(c) something that causes an exaggerated immune response.

(d) a hormone produced by the body that constricts blood vessels and dilates respiratory passages.

(e) an electrolyte produced by the body that dilates blood vessels and constricts respiratory passages.

54. An *allergic reaction* is best defined as

(a) an exaggerated but non-life-threatening immune response.

(b) a severe and life-threatening, exaggerated immune response, causing dilation of the body's blood vessels (low blood pressure), edema of the respiratory tissues, and bronchoconstriction (both of which threaten the patient's airway).

(c) something that causes an exaggerated immune response.

(d) a hormone produced by the body that constricts blood vessels and dilates respiratory passages.

(e) an electrolyte produced by the body that dilates blood vessels and constricts respiratory passages.

55. *Anaphylaxis* (or *anaphylactic shock*) is best defined as

(a) an exaggerated but non-life-threatening immune response.

(b) a severe and life-threatening, exaggerated immune response, causing dilation of the body's blood vessels (low blood pressure), edema of the respiratory tissues, and bronchoconstriction (both of which threaten the patient's airway).

(c) something that causes an exaggerated immune response.

(d) a hormone produced by the body that constricts blood vessels and dilates respiratory passages.

(e) an electrolyte produced by the body that dilates blood vessels and constricts respiratory passages.

56. Epinephrine (adrenalin) is best defined as
    (a) an exaggerated but non-life-threatening immune response.
    (b) a severe and life-threatening, exaggerated immune response, causing dilation of the body's blood vessels (low blood pressure), edema of the respiratory tissues, and bronchoconstriction (both of which threaten the patient's airway).
    (c) a substance that causes an exaggerated immune response.
    (d) a hormone produced by the body that constricts blood vessels and dilates respiratory passages.
    (e) an electrolyte produced by the body that dilates blood vessels and constricts respiratory passages.

57. Which of the following can trigger an allergic reaction or anaphylactic shock?
    (1) Food ingestion, such as nuts (especially peanuts), shellfish, milk, or the like.
    (2) Insect bites or stings (bees, wasps, and the like).
    (3) Prescription medications.
    (4) Over-the-counter medications.
    (5) Latex products (such as gloves).
    (6) Vitamins.
    (7) Plant pollen.
    (8) Animal fur or dander.

    (a) 1, 2, 3, 4, 5, 6, 7, 8.
    (b) 1, 2, 3, 5, 6, 7, 8.
    (c) 1, 2, 3, 5, 7, 8.
    (d) 1, 2, 5, 7, 8.
    (e) 1, 2, 7, 8.

58. The medical term *erythema* is best described as
    (a) a localized or generalized redness of the skin.
    (b) a sensation of heat and/or tingling in the face, mouth, chest, feet, and hands.
    (c) a generalized itching sensation.
    (d) itchy, reddened bumps or bulges.
    (e) generalized tissue swelling of the face, neck, hands, feet, or tongue.

59. The medical term *urticaria* (also called *hives*) is best described as
    (a) a localized or generalized redness of the skin.
    (b) a sensation of heat and/or tingling in the face, mouth, chest, feet, and hands.
    (c) a generalized itching sensation.
    (d) itchy, reddened bumps or bulges.
    (e) generalized tissue swelling of the face, neck, hands, feet, or tongue.

60. Which of the following statements regarding allergic reactions or anaphylactic shock is true?

   (a) When an individual is allergic to a foreign substance, it means that their body created antibodies specifically to attack that substance, the first time they were exposed to it.

   (b) First exposure to an allergen results in an immediate allergic reaction.

   (c) An allergic reaction rarely ever occurs until the second exposure to an allergen.

   (d) Answers (a) and (b) are true.

   (e) Answers (a) and (c) are true.

61. Which of the following statements regarding allergic reactions and anaphylactic shock is false?

   (a) Localized allergic reactions do not present a life-threat to the patient and are not commonly treated by EMT-assisted epinephrine auto-injector use in the field.

   (b) Anaphylaxis may include any or all of the signs of a localized allergic reaction.

   (c) Localized allergic reactions often cause seriously low blood pressure. That is why low blood pressure is not an indication for EMT-assisted epinephrine auto-injector use in the field.

   (d) Wheezing (or any other signs of respiratory compromise) indicates an anaphylactic reaction, and justifies seeking an order for EMT-assisted epinephrine auto-injector use in the field.

   (e) With an allergic reaction, if the patient also begins to develop an altered mental status or (simply) a profound sense of impending doom, this indicates the possibility of an anaphylactic reaction. These symptoms justify seeking an order for EMT-assisted epinephrine auto-injector use in the field.

62. Skin signs and symptoms of anaphylaxis may include

   (a) a warm, tingling sensation in the face, mouth, chest, feet, and hands.

   (b) itching, hives, or erythema.

   (c) edema of the face, neck, hands, feet, or tongue.

   (d) Answers (b) or (c).

   (e) Answers (a), (b), or (c).

63. Respiratory signs and symptoms of anaphylaxis may include all of the following, except

   (a) the patient's complaint of hoarseness or a "tightness" in his throat or chest.

   (b) coughing or labored breathing.

   (c) slow, relaxed, and even respiratory patterns.

   (d) stridor.

   (e) wheezing (audible with or without a stethoscope).

64. Cardiac signs and symptoms of anaphylaxis include

   (a) tachycardia.

   (b) bradycardia.

    (c) hypotension.

    (d) Answers (a) and (c).

    (e) Answers (b) and (c).

65. Generalized signs and symptoms of anaphylaxis include all of the following, except

    (a) euphoria and increased energy.

    (b) complaint of itchy, watery eyes and/or a runny nose.

    (c) complaint of headache.

    (d) report of a sense of impending doom.

    (e) deteriorating mental status.

66. Which of the following questions is not required for the focused history interview of an allergic reaction or anaphylaxis patient?

    (a) Does the patient have a history of allergies? To what?

    (b) When was the patient's last tetanus shot?

    (c) What was the patient exposed to, and how did exposure occur?

    (d) What are the patient's complaints and how have they changed since exposure?

    (e) What has the patient already done to seek relief, and how successful was it?

67. Prior to contacting the Medical Director to request an order to assist a patient with the use of an epinephrine auto-injector, the EMT must determine that the patient is eligible for assisted epinephrine administration. Which of the following criteria must be met prior to EMT-assisted epinephrine administration?

    (a) The patient must have a history of previous allergic reactions to the same substance causing this exposure incident.

    (b) The patient must be complaining of respiratory distress or exhibiting signs and symptoms of shock (hypoperfusion).

    (c) The patient must have a prescribed epinephrine auto-injector with him.

    (d) Answers (a) or (b).

    (e) Answers (a), (b), and (c).

68. Your patient has a history of previous allergic reactions to the same substance causing this exposure incident, has his prescribed epinephrine auto-injector present, but does not have signs and symptoms of respiratory distress or shock. The EMT should

    (a) contact the Medical Director for a consultation. If the Medical Director orders it, assist the patient with administration of his epinephrine auto-injector.

    (b) contact the Medical Director only to report the situation and provide your ETA. If the Medical Director orders it, remind him of protocol and refuse to assist with administration of the patient's epinephrine auto-injector until the patient develops respiratory distress or shock signs and symptoms.

    (c) continue with oxygen treatment and the focused assessment.

    (d) Answers (a) and (c).

    (e) Answers (b) and (c).

69. Your patient has a history of previous allergic reactions to the same substance causing this exposure incident and has signs and symptoms of shock, but he has left his prescribed epinephrine auto-injector at another location. A bystander offers the use of her prescribed epinephrine auto-injector, and the patient identifies the bystander's auto-injector brand and dose as being the same as his own prescription. The EMT should

   (a) contact the Medical Director and request an order to assist the patient with administration of the bystander's prescribed epinephrine auto-injector.

   (b) request an ALS intercept and transport the patient immediately, treating the patient for shock en route to the intercept (or the emergency department), without administering the bystander's auto-injector to the patient.

   (c) transport the patient to the location of his prescribed epinephrine auto-injector, if it is less than 10 minutes away, and then proceed with the normal assisted-administration of a patient's prescribed epinephrine auto-injector protocol.

   (d) consider the fact that the patient is in a life-threatening situation. Since the patient reports having the same prescription as the bystander, do not tell the Medical Director that the auto-injector present on scene is not actually the patient's auto-injector when calling to request administration orders.

   (e) immediately assist the patient with administration of the bystander's auto-injector, and contact the Medical Director only after the fact.

70. If the adult patient continues to deteriorate after the first EMT-assisted epinephrine auto-injector use, and the patient has another prescribed auto-injector with him, the EMT should

   (a) remember that only one EMT-assisted auto-injector use (0.3 mg of medication) is allowed, and refuse to assist in the administration of a second dose.

   (b) remember that two simultaneous auto-injector uses (0.6 mg of medication) must be given for a second injection administration, and refuse to assist in the administration of only one auto-injector as a second dose.

   (c) contact the Medical Director and obtain an order for another assisted auto-injector use (a second administration of 0.3 mg of medication).

   (d) automatically assist with the administration of another single-dose auto-injector, without contacting medical direction to obtain another assisted-administration order.

   (e) remember that only one EMT-assisted auto-injector use (0.3 mg of medication) is allowed and should prevent the patient from self-administering another epinephrine auto-injector.

71. Which of the following statements indicates the correct protocol and dosage for EMT-assisted infant or child epinephrine auto-injector use?

   (a) Assist with only one infant/child auto-injector use (0.15 mg of medication).

   (b) If the patient has both respiratory distress and signs and symptoms of shock, assist with two simultaneous infant/child auto-injector uses (0.3 mg of medication, total).

(c) Assist with one infant/child auto-injector use (0.15 mg of medication), followed by another assisted injection (if ordered) every 5 minutes until the patient's injectors are all used or you arrive at the emergency department.

(d) If the patient has both respiratory distress and signs and symptoms of shock, assist with two simultaneous infant/child auto-injector uses (0.6 mg of medication) every 5 minutes, until the patient's injectors are all used or you arrive at the emergency department.

(e) None of the above. Infants and children are not prescribed epinephrine auto-injectors.

72. What is the location for epinephrine auto-injector administration?
(a) On the patient's right or left hip, alternating sites with subsequent administrations (every 5 minutes).
(b) On the patient's right or left shoulder, alternating sites with subsequent administrations (every 5 minutes).
(c) On the lateral portion of the patient's right or left thigh, midway between the waist and the knee.
(d) On the medial portion of the patient's right or left thigh, midway between the waist and the knee.
(e) Any of the above locations, depending on local protocol.

73. Common side effects of epinephrine auto-injector administration include any of the following, except
(a) dizziness, excitement, or anxiousness.
(b) hypotension (systolic blood pressure of less than 90 mmHg).
(c) tachycardia and/or pale skin color.
(d) chest pain and/or nausea and vomiting.
(e) headache.

74. Which of the following questions is not required for the focused history interview of a poisoning or overdose patient?
(a) What was the patient exposed to, and how did exposure occur?
(b) How much of the substance was taken, and over what time period?
(c) When was the patient's last tetanus shot?
(d) How much does the patient weigh?
(e) What has the patient already done to seek relief, and how successful was it?

75. Indications for the administration of activated charcoal include
(a) overdose of medications in tablet or capsule form.
(b) ingestion of liquid poison.
(c) ingestion of poisonous plant material.
(d) Answers (a) or (b).
(e) Answers (a), (b), or (c).

76.   Which of the following are common trade names for activated charcoal?

      (1) SuperChar®
      (2) InstaChar®
      (3) Actidose®
      (4) Actidose-Aqua®
      (5) LiquiChar®
      (6) Charcoaid®

         (a) 1, 2, 3, 4, 5, 6.
         (b) 1, 2, 4, 6.
         (c) 1, 2, 4, 5.
         (d) 1, 2, 5, 6.
         (e) 1, 2, 3.

77.   Which of the following are contraindications to the administration of activated charcoal?

      (1) The patient has an altered LOC.
      (2) The patient is having difficulty swallowing, or is unable to swallow.
      (3) Acid or alkali ingestion.
      (4) Bleach or ammonia ingestion.
      (5) Cyanide ingestion.
      (6) Gasoline ingestion.

         (a) 1 or 2.
         (b) 2 or 3.
         (c) 2, 3, or 4.
         (d) 1, 2, 3, 4, or 6.
         (e) 1, 2, 3, 4, 5, or 6.

78.   Activated charcoal is available

    (a) premixed in an alcohol solution (a better dilution solution than water) containing 12.5 or 25 grams of the medication.
    (b) premixed in a water solution containing 12.5 or 25 grams of the medication.
    (c) in a powder form that should not be stocked on an ambulance.
    (d) Answers (a) and (b).
    (e) Answers (b) and (c).

79.   The universal administration dose of activated charcoal is 1 gram of the medication per kilogram of body weight. However, the commonly accepted dose range for a single adult administration is

    (a) 50 to 100 grams of medication.
    (b) 25 to 50 grams of medication.
    (c) 12.5 to 25 grams of medication.
    (d) Answers (a) or (b), depending upon the poison ingested.
    (e) Answers (a) or (c), depending upon the poison ingested.

80. The commonly accepted dose range for a single pediatric activated charcoal administration is

    (a) 50 to 100 grams of medication.

    (b) 25 to 50 grams of medication.

    (c) 12.5 to 25 grams of medication.

    (d) Answers (a) or (b), depending upon the poison ingested.

    (e) Answers (b) or (c), depending upon the poison ingested.

81. Which of the following statements regarding administration of activated charcoal is false?

    (a) An on-line or off-line order for administration must be obtained from medical direction.

    (b) The medication container must be shaken thoroughly before administration.

    (c) If the patient takes too long to drink the medication it may lose its potency. Open a new container and have the patient resume drinking until the appropriate dose is ingested.

    (d) If the patient takes too long to drink the medication, the charcoal may settle to the bottom of the container. Shake or stir it again, and have the patient resume drinking.

    (e) A covered container with a straw may improve the patient's speed at drinking the medication, since he will not be able to see it.

82. Which of the following statements regarding the actions of activated charcoal is true?

    (a) Activated charcoal binds to certain poisons and prevents them from being absorbed into the body.

    (b) Activated charcoal deactivates most poisons, turning them into nontoxic substances.

    (c) Activated charcoal coats the stomach, blocking all ingested poison absorption.

    (d) Answers (a) and (b) are true.

    (e) Answers (a), (b), and (c) are true.

83. Which of the following statements regarding the side effects of activated charcoal is true?

    (a) The medication may cause black stools.

    (b) Some patients may vomit, especially if they have ingested poisons that cause nausea.

    (c) If the patient vomits, the dose should be repeated one time.

    (d) Answers (a) and (b) are true.

    (e) Answers (a), (b), and (c) are true.

84. Administration of activated charcoal to a patient with an altered level of consciousness

(a) may be accomplished by having the patient open his mouth so you can squirt very small amounts at a time under his tongue. This form of administration will take much longer than preferred, so it should be accomplished en route to the emergency department.

(b) may be accomplished by using a tongue depressor to open the patient's mouth and squirting very small amounts at a time under his tongue. This form of administration will take much longer than preferred, so it should be accomplished en route to the emergency department.

(c) is always contraindicated.

(d) is contraindicated only if small amounts squirted under the patient's tongue make him cough or spit.

(e) is contraindicated only if the patient is unconscious.

85. The medical term *hypothermia* is best defined as having

(a) a body temperature below normal.

(b) the sensation of chills or shivering.

(c) a body temperature above normal.

(d) a headache.

(e) the sensation of a fever.

86. The medical term *hyperthermia* is best defined as having

(a) a body temperature below normal.

(b) the sensation of chills or shivering.

(c) a body temperature above normal.

(d) a headache.

(e) the sensation of a fever.

87. Heat loss that occurs by simply losing heat to the atmosphere (space) around you is called

(a) radiation.

(b) convection.

(c) conduction.

(d) evaporation.

(e) breathing (respiration).

88. Heat loss that occurs because perspiration or a moist body surface acts to cool the body as it dries is called

(a) radiation.

(b) convection.

(c) conduction.

(d) evaporation.

(e) breathing (respiration).

89.   Warm air being expelled by the body (and not being returned) describes the process
        of heat loss from
        (a) radiation.
        (b) convection.
        (c) conduction.
        (d) evaporation.
        (e) breathing (respiration).

90.   Heat loss that occurs because of direct contact with a cold object, drawing heat out
        of the body is called
        (a) radiation.
        (b) convection.
        (c) conduction.
        (d) evaporation.
        (e) breathing (respiration).

91.   Heat loss that occurs because of moving air or flowing liquids passing over the
        body, carrying away the body's heat, is called
        (a) radiation.
        (b) convection.
        (c) conduction.
        (d) evaporation.
        (e) breathing (respiration).

92.   Body temperature is measured by degrees (°), and based upon one of two scales:
        the Fahrenheit (F) scale or the Celsius (C) scale. The normal body temperature for
        an adult is considered to be
        (a) 99.2° F (37.3° C).
        (b) 98.8° F (37.1° C).
        (c) 98.6° F (37° C).
        (d) 96.8° F (36° C).
        (e) 90.6° F (32.5° C).

93.   The normal body temperature for a child is considered to be
        (a) 99.2° F (37.3° C).
        (b) 98.8° F (37.1° C).
        (c) 98.6° F (37° C).
        (d) 96.8° F (36° C).
        (e) 90.6° F (32.5° C).

94. The medical phrase *generalized hypothermia* is best defined as

  (a) the presence of a freezing injury on any single body part (if one part is frozen, the entire body must be hypothermic).

  (b) the cooling of the entire body (with or without localized freezing injuries).

  (c) any body temperature different from the normal body temperature.

  (d) Answers (a) or (b).

  (e) Answers (a) or (c).

95. Which of the following statements regarding factors that increase a patient's susceptibility to generalized hypothermia is false?

  (a) Atmospheric temperatures at or below freezing temperature are required before generalized hypothermia can occur in a dry adult.

  (b) Elderly patients often exist on low incomes and cannot afford to adequately heat their environment. Thus, they are more susceptible to generalized hypothermia.

  (c) Chronic illness will increase a patient's susceptibility to generalized hypothermia.

  (d) A poor diet may increase a patient's susceptibility to generalized hypothermia.

  (e) Certain medications may increase a patient's susceptibility to generalized hypothermia.

96. Which of the following statements regarding factors of an infant's or pediatric patient's susceptibility to generalized hypothermia is false?

  (a) Infants and children are small in size, but their body surface area is larger when compared to their entire body mass. Thus, they are more susceptible to generalized hypothermia than adults.

  (b) Children actually have a larger muscle mass (compared to total body mass) than adults. Thus they are better able to effectively generate heat by shivering. This is the one factor that makes them less susceptible to generalized hypothermia than adults.

  (c) Children have a smaller muscle mass than adults. Thus, they are less able to effectively generate heat by shivering and more susceptible to generalized hypothermia than adults.

  (d) Infants may be unable to shiver at all. Thus, they are even more susceptible to generalized hypothermia than children.

  (e) Infants and children have less body fat to insulate them from heat loss. Thus, they are more susceptible to generalized hypothermia than adults.

97. Which of the following conditions may increase any patient's susceptibility to generalized hypothermia?

  (a) Outdoor resuscitation.

  (b) Water immersion.

  (c) Presence of high winds.

  (d) Answers (b) and (c).

  (e) Answers (a), (b), and (c).

98. Which of the following conditions may increase any patient's susceptibility to generalized hypothermia?

    (1) Shock (hypoperfusion).
    (2) Head injury.
    (3) Burns.
    (4) Generalized infections.
    (5) Diabetes and hypoglycemia.
    (6) Spinal cord injury.
    (7) Alcohol ingestion.
    (8) Overdose or poisoning.
    (9) Chest or abdominal trauma.

        (a) 1, 3, 7, or 8.
        (b) 1, 3, 5, 7, or 8.
        (c) 1, 2, 3, 4, 5, 7, or 8.
        (d) 1, 2, 3, 4, 5, 6, 7, or 8.
        (e) 1, 2, 3, 4, 5, 6, 7, 8, or 9.

99. Which of the following statements regarding the signs and symptoms of increasing degrees of hypothermia is false?

    (a) Mental status progressively deteriorates as a patient develops a lower body temperature. Poor judgment may cause the hypothermic patient to remove his clothing.

    (b) Motor function progressively deteriorates as a patient develops a lower body temperature.

    (c) In the early stages of hypothermia, a patient's pulse may range from normal to slow. As the patient develops a lower body temperature, his pulse gradually increases (in an effort to generate heat) until it becomes so fast that ventricular fibrillation develops and causes his heart to stop.

    (d) Muscular rigidity becomes progressively worse as a patient develops a lower body temperature. Stiff or rigid postures may develop.

    (e) The lower the patient's body temperature, the less able he is to attempt generation of heat by shivering. Thus, the absence of shivering is a dire sign in cases of hypothermia.

100. Which of the following statements regarding the signs and symptoms of increasing degrees of hypothermia is true?

    (a) In the early stages of hypothermia, a patient's respiratory rate will usually be slow and shallow (in an effort to retain body heat). As the patient develops a lower body temperature, his rate and depth of breathing gradually increase, hyperventilating until just before respiratory arrest occurs.

    (b) In the early stages of hypothermia, the patient's skin may appear red. It is only in later stages of hypothermia that the patient's skin may become pale or cyanotic.

    (c) In the most extreme cases of hypothermia, some of a patient's body parts may feel stiff or hard, as though the patient is almost completely frozen.

    (d) Both answers (a) and (c) are true.

    (e) Both answers (b) and (c) are true.

101. Which of the following statements regarding emergency medical care for a victim of generalized hypothermia is false?
    (a) Immediately remove the patient from the environment and protect the patient from further heat loss.
    (b) Remove all of the patient's wet clothing and wrap him with blankets.
    (c) Handle the patient gently. Rough handling may cause the patient's heart to go into ventricular fibrillation.
    (d) If the patient is conscious, assist him to his feet and begin forced exercise (walk the patient for at least 5 minutes prior to transportation). This activity will increase circulation of warm body-core blood to the patient's near-frozen extremities, and will also help the patient begin to generate heat again.
    (e) Administer oxygen, preferably warmed and humidified.

102. Which of the following statements regarding the pulse assessment for a victim of extreme generalized hypothermia is true?
    (a) Carotid pulse assessment should be performed for as long as 30 to 45 seconds. If any pulse is felt during that time (even a heart rate as low as 10 per minute), chest compressions should not be performed.
    (b) Carotid pulse assessment should be performed for no longer than 30 seconds. If the patient's detectable pulse rate is slower than 60 beats per minute, begin chest compressions.
    (c) If a radial pulse is not present, begin CPR.
    (d) Carotid pulse assessment should be performed for no longer than 15 seconds. If the patient's detectable pulse rate is slower than 60 beats per minute, begin chest compressions.
    (e) If a radial pulse is present, but less than 60 beats per minute, begin chest compressions.

103. Which of the following statements describe *passive rewarming* techniques?
    (a) Apply heated blankets.
    (b) Turn the ambulance patient compartment heater to a high setting.
    (c) Apply heat packs or hot water bottles to the patient's groin, axillary, and cervical regions.
    (d) Answers (a) and (b).
    (e) Answers (a) and (c).

104. Which of the following statements describe *active rewarming* techniques?
    (a) Apply heated blankets.
    (b) Turn the ambulance patient compartment heater to a high setting.
    (c) Apply heat packs or hot water bottles to the patient's chest, axillary, groin, and cervical regions.
    (d) Answers (a) and (b).
    (e) Answers (b) and (c).

105. If allowed by local protocols, active rewarming techniques are indicated for hypothermic patients who are

    (a) alert and responding appropriately.

    (b) alert, but do not respond in an appropriate manner.

    (c) unconscious.

    (d) Answers (a) or (b).

    (e) Answers (b) or (c).

106. Even when active rewarming techniques are allowed by local protocols, only passive rewarming techniques are indicated for hypothermic patients who are

    (a) alert and responding appropriately.

    (b) alert, but do not respond in an appropriate manner.

    (c) unconscious.

    (d) Answers (a) or (b).

    (e) Answers (b) or (c).

107. Local cold injuries are now classified as early (or superficial) and late (or deep) local cold injuries. Early or superficial local cold injuries were once called

    (a) frostbite.

    (b) frostnip.

    (c) first-degree frostnip.

    (d) second-degree frostnip.

    (e) third-degree frostbite.

108. Late or deep local cold injuries were once called

    (a) frostbite.

    (b) frostnip.

    (c) first-degree frostnip.

    (d) second-degree frostnip.

    (e) third-degree frostbite.

109. All of the following are signs and symptoms of early or superficial local cold injuries, except

    (a) the skin in the area remains soft to palpation.

    (b) the patient reports loss of feeling and sensation in the injured area.

    (c) there is a swelling of the injured area.

    (d) the skin in the area "blanches" when touched and the color does not return.

    (e) the patient may complain of a tingling or burning sensation, if the part has been rewarmed.

110. All of the following are signs and symptoms of late or deep local cold injuries, except
    (a) the area's skin is red and icy-looking.
    (b) the area feels firm or frozen when palpated.
    (c) there is a swelling of the injured area.
    (d) there are blisters on the injured area.
    (e) the patient complains of moderate to severe pain in a part that has been partially or completely thawed.

111. Which of the following statements regarding general emergency care measures for all local cold injuries is false?
    (a) Remove the patient from the cold environment.
    (b) Remove all wet or restrictive clothing.
    (c) Protect the cold injured extremity from further injury.
    (d) Administer oxygen.
    (e) If transportation will require re-exposure of the patient to the cold, minimize the risk of increasing the amount of injury by performing active rewarming (thawing) measures before re-exposure.

112. Which of the following statements regarding emergency care measures for early or superficial local cold injuries is true?
    (a) Encourage the patient to vigorously exercise his superficially cold injured hands and fingers to stimulate circulation of warm blood to those parts.
    (b) Encourage the patient to gently massage his superficially cold injured nose and/or ears (or massage them for the patient) to stimulate circulation of warm blood to those parts.
    (c) Encourage the patient to gently massage his superficially cold injured toes and/or feet (or massage them for the patient) to stimulate circulation of warm blood to those parts.
    (d) If in a warm environment and if dry socks or slippers are available, put them on the patient and encourage gentle pacing to stimulate circulation of warm blood to his superficially cold injured toes and/or feet.
    (e) If an extremity is involved, splint and cover it after passive warming.

113. Which of the following statements regarding emergency care.measures for late or deep local cold injuries is true?
    (a) Remove any jewelry that is present and cover the injured area with dry clothing or dressings.
    (b) Since the patient is unlikely to be able to exercise or massage the part himself, gently massage the part for him to stimulate circulation of warm blood to the injured areas.
    (c) Apply hot packs to all deeply cold-injured parts as soon as possible (especially if re-exposure to cold will occur before or during transport).
    (d) Both answers (a) and (b) are true.
    (e) Both answers (a) and (c) are true.

114. Active, rapid rewarming of late or deep local cold injuries is

    (a) never recommended during prehospital care, for any reason.

    (b) recommended only when an extremely delayed transport is inevitable.

    (c) important to accomplish if re-exposure to cold is inevitable.

    (d) a primary recommended treatment for any local cold injury.

    (e) a procedure that should only be initiated during prehospital care if transport time is less than 15 minutes.

AUTHOR'S NOTE: *Several of the next few questions (115–125) may require an unusual amount of time to answer. If you are timing your test performance, make a note of the time already elapsed, and stop timing now. (Your time at this point should not be over 1 hour and 54 minutes.)*

If you could use a break, take a break NOW. When you return to the test, do not resume timing until cued to do so.

AUTHOR'S TIP: *When faced with a long list of numbered activities and statements requiring a true or false determination, just read through them first, noting the number of each activity or statement you KNOW to be TRUE on your scrap paper. (It is also helpful to simultaneously make a list of the numbered options you KNOW to be FALSE!) Then, compare your known-TRUE-number set with the number sets offered in the answer options. Select the answer option containing the number set that matches yours. If none of them matches, you should probably study that question's subject. However, you can also "rule out" answer options that contain one or more numbered activities or statements you KNOW to be FALSE.*

115. Which of the following statements regarding heat injuries are true?

    (1) High ambient temperature reduces the body's ability to lose heat by radiation.

    (2) High ambient temperature increases the body's ability to lose heat by conduction.

    (3) High relative humidity (especially in a still environment) reduces the body's ability to lose heat through evaporation.

    (4) In a still environment, high relative humidity increases the body's ability to lose heat through convection.

    (5) Exercise and activity can cause the loss of more than 1 L of sweat per hour and will increase heat production, which can cause hypovolemia and/or heat injury.

    (6) Exercise and activity can cause a loss of fluid, but will protect the body from heat injury because the airflow created by rapid movement facilitates heat loss via convection.

        (a) 1, 2, 3, 4, 6.

        (b) 1, 4, 6.

        (c) 2, 3, 6.

        (d) 1, 3, 5.

        (e) 1, 4, 5.

116. Which of the following activities and statements related to providing active, rapid rewarming for a late or deep local cold injury are true?

    (1) Immerse the affected part in a warm water bath (100° to 105° F). The water should not be so hot that the heat feels uncomfortable when placing *your* finger in it.

    (2) Immerse the affected part in a hot water bath (105° to 110° F). The water should be too hot for you to put *your* finger in it. (By the time the patient's part has thawed enough to feel the hot water, the water will have significantly cooled. You can't "burn" a frozen body part.)

    (3) Immerse the affected part in cool water first, then gradually add warmer and warmer water until the temperature reaches 105° to 110° F. It is important to slowly and gradually thaw a frozen part.

    (4) The water bath container must be large enough to allow the injured area to be fully immersed without touching the bottom or sides of the container.

    (5) Continuously stir the water, replacing it when it cools below the desired water bath temperature.

    (6) Expect the patient to complain of moderate to severe pain throughout the thawing process.

    (7) Continue the water bath until the part is soft, with return of color and sensation.

    (8) After thawing, gently dry the area and dress with dry, sterile dressings.

    (9) After thawing, keep the part moist by covering with sterile saline-soaked dressings.

  (10) If the hands or feet are involved, place dressings between fingers or toes.

  (11) Protect against refreezing of the injured part.

    (a) 2, 4, 5, 6, 7, 9, 10, 11.
    (b) 3, 4, 6, 7, 9, 10, 11.
    (c) 1, 4, 5, 6, 7, 8, 10, 11.
    (d) 1, 4, 5, 6, 7, 9, 10, 11.
    (e) This is a "trick question." Active, rapid rewarming of late or deep local cold injuries is never recommended during prehospital care, for any reason.

Use the following list of statements to answer both questions 117 and 118.

    (1) These patients often cause their own heat injuries, because they are always turning up the thermostat of the furnace.

    (2) These patients cannot remove their own clothing to compensate for (alleviate the effects of) increased heat.

    (3) Because they have a poor ability to sense temperature, these patients are always complaining of feeling "too hot." If they are in a cool environment, they do not have a heat-related problem or injury.

    (4) The bodies of these patients have poor thermoregulation abilities.

    (5) These patients may be on medications that inhibit their body's ability to respond to temperature regulation needs.

    (6) Lack of mobility may prevent these patients from escaping a hot environment.

    (7) These patients always should be considered to be seriously susceptible to heat injury.

117. Which of the previous 7 statements are true about elderly patients' susceptibility to heat injuries?

    (a) 1, 4, 5, 6, and 7.

    (b) 1, 2, 3, 5, and 6.

    (c) 4, 5, 6, and 7.

    (d) 1, 5, 6, and 7.

    (e) 1, 3, and 5.

118. Which of the 7 statements preceding question 117 are true about newborns and infants' susceptibility to heat injuries?

    (a) 2, 6, and 7.

    (b) 2, 4, 6, and 7.

    (c) 2, 5, 6, and 7.

    (d) 1, 3, and 5.

    (e) 2, 3, 6, and 7.

119. The signs and symptoms that accompany the condition commonly called "Heat Cramps" have caused it to now be officially classified as a medical heat emergency called

    (a) "Patient with Warm, Dry, Pink skin."

    (b) "Patient with Moist, Pale, Normal-to-Cool Skin."

    (c) "Patient with Hot Skin, Moist or Dry."

    (d) "Patient with a Muscle Cramp."

    (e) Answers (b) or (c).

120. The signs and symptoms that accompany the condition commonly called "Heat Exhaustion" have caused it to now be officially classified as a medical heat emergency called

    (a) "Patient with Warm, Dry, Pink skin."

    (b) "Patient with Moist, Pale, Normal-to-Cool Skin."

    (c) "Patient with Hot Skin, Moist or Dry."

    (d) "Patient who is Tired."

    (e) Answers (b) or (c).

121. The signs and symptoms that accompany the condition commonly called "Heat Stroke" have caused it to now be officially classified as a medical heat emergency called

    (a) "Patient with Warm, Dry, Pink skin."

    (b) "Patient with Moist, Pale, Normal-to-Cool Skin."

    (c) "Patient with Hot Skin, Moist or Dry."

    (d) "Patient with Cold Skin, Moist or Dry."

    (e) Answers (b) or (c).

122. Which of the following signs and symptoms may be exhibited by a patient suffering from the condition commonly called "Heat Exhaustion?"

    (1) Altered mental status.
    (2) Dizziness or faintness.
    (3) Excitement and euphoria.
    (4) Heavy perspiration (pronounced diaphoresis).
    (5) Hot skin.
    (6) Dry or moist skin (little to no perspiration).
    (7) Moist, pale skin of normal-to-cool temperature.
    (8) Muscular cramping (most often in the legs or abdomen).
    (9) Rapid pulse.
    (10) Rapid, shallow respirations.
    (11) Seizure activity.
    (12) Shivering.
    (13) Unconsciousness.
    (14) Warm, dry, and pink skin.
    (15) Weakness or exhaustion.

        (a) 1, 2, 3, 4, 5, 6, 7, 8, 9, 10, 11, 12, 13, 14, or 15.
        (b) 1, 2, 5, 6, 9, 10, 11, 13, or 15.
        (c) 2, 3, 4, 5, 7, 8, 9, 10, 11, 12, 13, or 15.
        (d) 1, 2, 4, 7, 8, 9, 10, 13, or 15.
        (e) 1, 2, 3, 5, 6, 9, 10, 11, 12, 13, 14, or 15.

123. Which of the numbered signs and symptoms listed for question 122 may be exhibited by a patient suffering from the condition commonly called "Heat Stroke?"

    (a) 1, 2, 3, 4, 5, 6, 7, 8, 9, 10, 11, 12, 13, 14, or 15.
    (b) 1, 2, 5, 6, 9, 10, 11, 13, or 15.
    (c) 2, 3, 4, 5, 7, 8, 9, 10, 11, 12, 13, or 15.
    (d) 1, 2, 4, 7, 8, 9, 10, 13, or 15.
    (e) 1, 2, 3, 5, 6, 9, 10, 11, 12, 13, 14, or 15.

124. Which of the following emergency care actions should be employed for a patient suffering from the condition commonly called "Heat Exhaustion?"

    (1) Remove the patient from the hot environment and place him in a cool environment (such as an air-conditioned ambulance).
    (2) Withhold oxygen administration; none is needed.
    (3) Apply cold packs to the patient's forehead while keeping the patient lightly covered with warm blankets to prevent a rebound hypothermic reaction.
    (4) Apply cold packs to both armpits of the patient, both sides of his neck, and his groin area.
    (5) Employ only light fanning to cool the patient.
    (6) Employ aggressive fanning to cool the patient.
    (7) Delay transport to immerse the patient in ice water, keeping his head and neck above the water line. (Rapid cooling is more important than rapid transport.)

   (8) If rapid transport cannot be immediately accomplished, find a tub or similar container and immerse the patient in cool water, keeping his head and neck above the water line.

   (9) Even when the patient's mechanism of injury does not suggest spinal trauma, immobilize the patient to a long backboard. Total body immobilization improves the effectiveness of cooling techniques.

  (10) If the patient is not nauseated, have him drink sips of tepid or cool water. But, stop ALL oral water administration if the patient becomes nauseated.

  (11) If the patient is unresponsive or has an altered LOC, carefully trickle small amounts of tepid or cool water under his tongue.

  (12) If the patient is nauseated, has an altered LOC, or is unresponsive, withhold ALL oral fluids and transport with the patient on his left side.

  (13) Cool the patient's skin by sponging it with cool water or applying wet towels to his entire body.

  (14) Loosen or remove any constrictive or warm clothing.

  (15) Place the patient in a supine position with his feet elevated and keep him at rest.

  (16) Administer oxygen by nonrebreather mask at 15 lpm.

  (17) Remove all of the patient's clothing.

  (18) Transport the patient without any delay.

    (a) 1, 4, 6, 8, 12, 13, 15, 16, 17, and 18.
    (b) 2, 3, 6, 9, 13, 16, and 18.
    (c) 2, 3, 10, 12, 14, 15, 16, and 18.
    (d) 1, 4, 6, 7, 9, 12, 16, and 18.
    (e) 1, 5, 10, 12, 14, 15, 16, and 18.

125. Which of the emergency care actions listed for question 124 should be employed for a patient suffering from the condition commonly called "Heat Stroke?"

    (a) 1, 4, 6, 8, 12, 13, 14, 15, 16, 17, and 18.
    (b) 2, 3, 6, 9, 13, 16, and 18.
    (c) 2, 3, 10, 12, 15, 16, and 18.
    (d) 1, 4, 6, 7, 9, 12, 16, and 18.
    (e) 1, 5, 10, 12, 14, 15, 16, and 18.

AUTHOR'S NOTE: *ADD 10 minutes to your previous time-elapsed record, and* resume timing your performance NOW. *(Had the previous 10 questions not been so time-consuming, your test-taking-time should not be over 2 hours and 4 minutes at this point.)*

126. The phrase "near drowning"

    (a) is no longer considered a valid diagnosis or victim description. Anyone who survives or dies following a submersion / immersion emergency should be considered a "drowning" incident victim.

    (b) indicates that death did not occur following a submersion / immersion event.

    (c) describes a death that occurred more than 24 hours after the submersion / immersion event.

    (d) describes a death that occurred more than 48 hours after the submersion / immersion event.

    (e) Answers (b) and (c) or (d), depending upon the local medical examiner's opinion.

127. Drowning can be caused by any kind of liquid submersion / immersion event, and is

    (a) usually an entirely preventable cause of accidental (unintentional) injury or death.

    (b) legally defined as a death that occurs within 24 hours of a submersion / immersion event.

    (c) usually survived with a good outcome if the victim spontaneously regains circulation and breathing before reaching the ED.

    (d) Answers (a) and (c).

    (e) Answers (a), (b), and (c).

128. Which of the following statements regarding drowning emergencies is false?

    (a) If you have not been trained in (and/or are not equipped for) deep water rescue, do not, under any circumstances, attempt a deep water rescue.

    (b) To rescue a victim, untrained personnel may enter shallow ponds or pools (for example, rescuer-waist-deep only) that have a known depth and a uniform bottom.

    (c) Full-body submersion is not required for drowning to occur.

    (d) Children and infants can drown in only a few inches of water.

    (e) At least 1 foot depth of water is required for an adult to drown. If you find a drowned adult in less than 12 inches of water, the death is probably a homicide and you should report it to the police.

129. Which of the following statements regarding emergency medical care of drowning and near-drowning victims is false?

    (a) Every unconscious drowning or near-drowning patient should be considered to have a spinal injury, especially one retrieved from a shallow pond or pool.

    (b) If associated with a diving or boating accident, every conscious or unconscious drowning or near-drowning patient should be considered to have a spinal injury.

    (c) All unconscious patients who require water rescue also require in-line immobilization and use of a long backboard (or the like) during removal.

    (d) During a water rescue, an apneic victim should receive rescue breathing while still in the water.

    (e) During a water rescue, a pulseless victim should receive chest compressions while still in the water (as soon as he is placed on a long backboard).

130. An unconscious near-drowning victim

    (a) may only have a small amount of water in his lungs.

    (b) will always have a large amount of water in his lungs.

    (c) may or may not have a large amount of water in his stomach.

    (d) Answers (a) and (c).

    (e) Answers (b) and (c).

131. Which of the following statements regarding emergency medical care of drowning and near-drowning victims is false?

    (a) If there is no suspected spinal injury, place the conscious patient on his left side to allow water, vomitus, and secretions to drain away from the upper airway.

(c) Abdominal pressure to manually relieve gastric distention is always contraindicated (forcing the evacuation of stomach contents will result in aspiration of the contents and cause death).

(d) If gastric distention interferes with artificial ventilation, the patient should be logrolled to his left side. With suction immediately available, the EMT should place his hand over the epigastric area of the patient's abdomen and apply firm pressure to relieve the distention.

(e) Every apneic, pulseless patient who has been submerged in cold water should receive all possible resuscitation efforts.

132. A patient who became apneic and pulseless during submersion in

(a) cold water also will have severe hypothermia. Thus, it is highly unlikely that the patient will be successfully resuscitated.

(b) cold water for up to 30 minutes has a better chance of successful resuscitation than a victim submerged in warm water for an equal duration of time.

(c) warm water for up to 30 minutes has a better chance of successful resuscitation than a victim submerged in cold water for an equal duration of time.

(d) cold water for greater than 15 minutes is unlikely to be successfully resuscitated unless he is less than 5 years old.

(e) cold or warm water for longer than 15 minutes will have brain damage.

133. Which of the following statements are true about the SCUBA diving emergency called *decompression sickness* ("the bends")?

(1) This occurs when ascent to the surface too rapidly from a dive causes nitrogen bubbles to form in the victim's blood and body tissues.

(2) This occurs when air leaving damaged lung tissue enters the bloodstream.

(3) This may occur during an ascent from only 3 to 6 feet below the water surface.

(4) This is not only a "SCUBA diving emergency." An auto accident victim with chest trauma could develop it when freed from a partially submerged vehicle.

(5) Onset of S/Sx are abrupt and severe, usually beginning within 10 to 15 minutes of occurrence.

(6) Onset of S/Sx may be delayed and the patient may wait for up to 12 to 24 hours after occurrence before seeking treatment.

(7) For the best possible outcome, victims of this should be transported to a facility with a hyperbaric oxygen chamber ("decompression" chamber).

(8) Hyperbaric oxygen is not helpful to victims of this.

    (a) 1, 3, 4, 5, and 7.
    (b) 2, 3, 6, and 7.
    (c) 2, 3, 6, and 8.
    (d) 1, 6, and 7.
    (e) 1, 6, and 8.

134. Which of the statements listed in the previous question (133) are true about the SCUBA diving emergency called *arterial gas embolism* (AGE)?

    (a) 1, 3, 6, and 7.
    (b) 1, 3, 5, and 8.
    (c) 1, 3, 4, 6, and 7.
    (d) 2, 3, 4, 5, and 7.
    (e) 2, 3, 4, 5, and 8.

135. From the following list of signs and symptoms, select all those that are common to decompression sickness victims.

    (1) "Sharp" or "tearing" pain in one or more central parts of the body, especially the chest.
    (2) Extreme pain and stiffness in the joints.
    (3) Tingling or numbness in the extremities.
    (4) Weakness or paralysis of the extremities.
    (5) Itchy, red skin blotches.
    (6) Bloody froth from mouth or nose.
    (7) Dyspnea.
    (8) Altered level of consciousness.

        (a) 1, 2, 5, 6, 7, and 8.
        (b) 1, 3, 4, 6, 7, and 8.
        (c) 2, 5, 6, 7, and 8.
        (d) 1, 4, 5, 6, and 7.
        (e) 2, 3, 4, 5, 7, and 8.

136. From the list of signs and symptoms in the previous question (135), select all those that are common to victims of arterial gas embolism emergencies.

    (a) 1, 2, 5, 6, 7, and 8.
    (b) 1, 3, 4, 6, 7, and 8.
    (c) 2, 5, 6, 7, and 8.
    (d) 1, 4, 5, 6, and 7.
    (e) 2, 3, 4, 5, 7, and 8.

137. Which of the following statements represent a definition of a *behavioral emergency*?

    (a) When a person is acting in a manner that may be dangerous to himself or others.
    (b) When a person is acting in a manner that his family reports is abnormal for him.
    (c) When a person has an altered level of consciousness and is acting in a manner that the general community considers to be abnormal.
    (d) Answers (a) and (c).
    (e) Answers (a), (b), and (c).

138. Medical or traumatic causes of an altered LOC that may be confused for a "psychiatric" behavioral emergency include all of the following, except

    (a) low blood sugar.
    (b) mania or severe depression.

(c) head trauma or stroke.

(d) drug or alcohol abuse.

(e) hypothermia or hyperthermia.

139. If a patient has no medical (physical) illness, but is experiencing a psychological crisis, which of the following signs and symptoms is he least likely to exhibit?

(a) A slow heart rate or low blood pressure.

(b) Panic or agitation.

(c) Bizarre behavior or comments suggesting bizarre thinking (delusions).

(d) Comments or activities suggesting suicidal or self-destructive ideas.

(e) Comments or activities suggesting homicidal ideas.

140. Which of the following factors or life situations are considered to be things that may contribute to someone developing self-destructive behavior or suicidal ideas?

(1) An individual over the age of 40.

(2) An unmarried individual.

(3) Persons who have lost their spouse through divorce or death.

(4) A person with an alcohol-abuse problem.

(5) A person who can verbalize a specific, lethal plan of action.

(6) A person who purchases a gun or hoards large volumes of pills.

(7) A patient with a previous history of self-destructive behavior.

(8) A patient who has been recently diagnosed with a serious illness.

(9) A person who has recently lost a loved one.

(10) Someone who has recently lost his job.

(11) A person recently placed under arrest or imprisoned.

    (a) 3, 4, 5, 6, 7, 8, 9, and 10 only.

    (b) 3, 5, 6, 7, 8, 9, and 11 only.

    (c) 1, 2, 3, 4, 5, 6, 7, 8, 9, 10, and 11.

    (d) 1, 3, 5, 6, 7, 8, 9, and 11 only.

    (e) 2, 3, 5, 6, 7, 8, 9, and 11 only.

141. Which of the following approaches to behavioral emergency patients are rarely ever calming or helpful?

(a) Specifically verbalize your observations to the patient and repeatedly assure him you are there to help him. For example, if the patient appears upset you should say something to the effect of, "I can hear (or see) that you are upset. How can I help you?"

(b) Avoid saying anything that you believe might upset or further agitate the patient. If this means having to lie to a patient, then a small amount of lying is acceptable (but only to avoid conflict).

(c) Always inform a patient of what you intend to do before you do it.

(d) Maintain a comfortable distance from the patient.

(e) Do not make any rapid or quick moves.

142. Which of the following statements about effectively dealing with behavioral emergency patients is false?

  (a) Do not threaten, challenge, or argue with emotionally disturbed patients.

  (b) Tell the truth at all times. Never lie to a patient.

  (c) If the patient seems to be experiencing visual or auditory hallucinations, "play along" with his abnormal perceptions. This provides a sense of "agreement" on your part and quickly wins the patient's confidence and cooperation.

  (d) When family members or friends are present (if they are calm and in control of their own emotions), encourage their participation in convincing the patient to consent to treatment and transport.

  (e) Be prepared to remain on scene for an extended length of time. Unless your safety is threatened, you should always remain with the patient.

143. Which of the following statements regarding behavioral emergency medical and legal considerations is false?

  (a) Any person acting in any type of unusual manner should be arrested by the police so that you can provide them with medical treatment and transport (generating a 911 call constitutes "disturbance of the peace").

  (b) If you can convince an emotionally disturbed patient to consent to treatment, the risk of legal difficulties will be greatly reduced.

  (c) To provide care against a patient's will, you must be able to explain why you believed that the patient would harm himself or others if he wasn't treated.

  (d) A patient who is acting in a manner that suggests a threat to himself or others may be transported and treated against his will after contacting medical direction or after obtaining law enforcement's assistance.

  (e) Emotionally disturbed adult patients often resist treatment but may only be treated or transported against their will if they have an altered LOC or are demonstrating behavior that may pose a threat to themselves or others.

144. Which of the following statements regarding the use of force when restraining a patient for the purpose of treatment and transportation without consent is false?

  (a) EMTs may use any reasonable force to defend against a patient who is attacking them.

  (b) EMTs should make every effort to avoid the use of physical force that may result in patient injury.

  (c) Once a patient becomes calm and begins acting rationally, all restraints must be removed (it is unlawful to continue the use of restraints once someone becomes cooperative).

  (d) EMTs should always seek medical direction when considering the use of restraints on a patient.

  (e) Handcuffs or plastic criminal restraints (Flex Cuffs®, or Tuff-Cuffs®, or the like) are contraindicated for the restraint of any emergency patient being transported in an ambulance to the emergency department prior to initial incarceration.

145. Which of the following statements regarding patient restraint application is false?

    (a) You may only use the amount of force necessary to safely apply restraints.

    (b) You may only apply the minimum number of restraints necessary to safely provide treatment and transport. (Elderly or pediatric patients may not need to be put in "4-point" restraint.)

    (c) Pain-stimulus control techniques (such as wrestling arm-locks or Koga wrist- and finger-locks) do not leave "marks" and are effective means for gaining a resistive individual's cooperation, especially when only a few restrainers are available. But EMTs should only employ them if they have been trained in the application of these techniques.

    (d) Only one EMT should talk to the patient throughout the entire restraining procedure, reassuring the patient of his safety, and encouraging the patient to understand that the restraints are for the patient's safety and care.

    (e) If an adequate number of people to ensure the safe application of restraint (a minimum of 4 persons) is not available, do not restrain the patient. Leave the patient's area, taking all others with you, and do not return until assistance arrives and safe restraint can be accomplished.

146. The restraint technique called *hobbling* or *hobble restraint* is most accurately defined as

    (a) restraining a patient's wrists together behind his back.

    (b) restraining a patient's ankles together.

    (c) connecting wrists that are restrained behind a patient's back to his restrained ankles.

    (d) Answers (a) and (b).

    (e) Answers (a), (b), and (c).

147. The restraint technique called *hog-tying* or *hog-tied* is most accurately defined as

    (a) restraining a patient's wrists together behind his back.

    (b) restraining a patient's ankles together.

    (c) connecting wrists that are restrained behind a patient's back to his restrained ankles.

    (d) Answers (a) and (b).

    (e) Answers (a), (b), and (c).

148. The medical term *positional asphyxia* is defined as when the position a person was in when his breathing and heartbeat stopped

    (a) was a position that could have obstructed his airway.

    (b) was a position that could have interfered with his mechanical means of breathing (his ability to get air in and out of his body).

    (c) is the only means of explaining his death (his autopsy reveals no natural or unnatural, medical or traumatic, chronic or acute condition that can be identified as the sole "cause" of his breathing and heartbeat initially stopping).

    (d) Answers (a) and (c).

    (e) Answers (a), (b), and (c).

149. The medical term *restraint asphyxia* is best defined as

    (a) the strangulation of a patient by a mechanical means of restraint.

    (b) the strangulation of a patient by any physical or mechanical means of restraint.

    (c) any positional asphyxia death that occurs because a form of restraint (mechanical or physical, or both) is the only thing that prevented the victim from escaping a position that was asphyxiating him.

    (d) a legal term used by family members to sue EMTs and law enforcement individuals when someone dies during application of a reasonable and safe method of restraint.

    (e) when a patient coincidentally or accidentally dies while being reasonably and safely restrained by EMS or law enforcement personnel (a death that is not the "fault" of the restrainers).

150. Which of the following statements regarding patient restraint application is true?

    (a) No patient requiring emergency medical treatment or transport should ever be hog-tied.

    (b) No patient requiring emergency medical treatment or transport should ever be restrained in a prone position (unless a posterior impalement prevents supine or lateral positioning).

    (c) Because of natural joint ranges of motion, all patients requiring full-body restraint during emergency treatment or transport should be restrained in a prone position.

    (d) Answers (a) and (b).

    (e) Answers (a) and (c).

The answer key for Test Section Five is on page 346.

6

DOT Module Five: Trauma

Subjects:

- Bleeding and Shock
- Soft-tissue Injuries
- Musculoskeletal Injuries
- Spine Injuries
- Burns

(Other Trauma Emergency subjects from DOT Module Five are addressed in Test Section Nine.)

Test Section Six consists of 120 questions and is allotted 2 hours for completion.

1.   The head is supplied with blood by the _____, producing a pulse that can be palpated on either side of the neck.
        (a) femoral arteries
        (b) radial arteries
        (c) carotid arteries
        (d) coronary arteries
        (e) brachial arteries

2.   The _____ supply the groin and both lower extremities with blood, generating a pulse that can be palpated on either side of the groin area.
        (a) femoral arteries
        (b) radial arteries
        (c) carotid arteries
        (d) coronary arteries
        (e) brachial arteries

3.   The _____ produce a pulse that can be palpated between the elbow and the shoulder on the inside of the arm.
        (a) femoral arteries
        (b) radial arteries
        (c) carotid arteries
        (d) coronary arteries
        (e) brachial arteries

4.   An artery on the posterior surface of the medial malleolus that can be palpated for a pulse is the
        (a) anterior tibial artery.
        (b) posterior tibial artery.
        (c) dorsalis pedis artery.
        (d) superior pedal artery.
        (e) posterior pedal artery.

5.   An artery on the top of the foot that can be palpated for a pulse is the
        (a) anterior tibial artery.
        (b) posterior tibial artery.
        (c) dorsalis pedis artery.
        (d) superior pedal artery.
        (e) posterior pedal artery.

6.   Capillaries are found in all parts of the body. They are tiny blood vessels that
        (a) receive blood from the smallest arteries and send it to the smallest veins.
        (b) receive blood from the smallest veins and send it to the smallest arteries.

(c) are responsible for the exchange of nutrients and waste, oxygen and carbon dioxide, at the cellular level of the body.

(d) Answers (a) and (c).

(e) Answers (b) and (c).

7. The smallest branch of an artery is called

(a) a capillary.

(b) an arteriette.

(c) an arteriole.

(d) Answers (b) or (c).

(e) None of the above.

8.   The smallest branch of a vein is called

(a) a capillary.

(b) a veinette.

(c) a venule.

(d) Answers (b) or (c).

(e) None of the above.

9. The formation of blood clots is largely dependent on the _____ found in blood.

(a) leukocytes

(b) platelets

(c) erythrocytes

(d) plasma

(e) packed cells

10. The fluid that carries blood cells and nutrients from place to place within the circulatory system is called

(a) whole blood.

(b) platelets.

(c) erythroliquid.

(d) plasma.

(e) packed cells.

11. A palpable pulse is formed when the _____ contracts, sending a wave of blood through the arteries.

(a) left atrium

(b) right atrium

(c) left ventricle

(d) right ventricle

(e) ventricular septum

12. *Peripheral* pulses include all of the following except the _____ pulse.
    (a) femoral
    (b) brachial
    (c) radial
    (d) dorsalis pedis
    (e) posterior tibial

13. *Central* pulses consist of the carotid pulse and the _____ pulse.
    (a) femoral
    (b) brachial
    (c) radial
    (d) dorsalis pedis
    (e) posterior tibial

14. The medical term *perfusion* is best defined as
    (a) the circulation of blood through an organ structure or tissues.
    (b) delivery of oxygen and other nutrients to the cells of all organ systems and tissues.
    (c) the removal of waste products from all organ systems and tissues.
    (d) Answers (a) and (b).
    (e) Answers (a), (b), and (c).

15. The medical term _____ means bleeding, or losing blood.
    (a) exsanguinary
    (b) hemorrhage
    (c) perfusion
    (d) anemia
    (e) hemoptysis

16. Three types of bleeding can occur, each having specific qualities and appearances. _____ bleeding is usually oxygen-rich and bright red in color.
    (a) Capillary
    (b) Venous
    (c) Arterial
    (d) Answers (a) and (b).
    (e) Answers (b) and (c).

17. _____ bleeding is usually oxygen-poor and dark red in color.
    (a) Capillary
    (b) Venous
    (c) Arterial
    (d) Answers (a) and (b).
    (e) Answers (b) and (c).

18. _____ bleeding is the most difficult to control.
   (a) Capillary
   (b) Venous
   (c) Arterial
   (d) Answers (a) and (b).
   (e) Answers (b) and (c).

19. _____ bleeding can be profuse; however, it is usually easy to control.
   (a) Capillary
   (b) Venous
   (c) Arterial
   (d) Answers (a) and (c).
   (e) Answers (b) and (c).

20. _____ bleeding oozes from a wound and often clots (stops bleeding) spontaneously. Bleeding control measures are usually not needed.
   (a) Capillary
   (b) Venous
   (c) Arterial
   (d) Answers (a) and (c).
   (e) Answers (b) and (c).

21. _____ bleeding may rhythmically spurt from a wound.
   (a) Capillary
   (b) Venous
   (c) Arterial
   (d) Answers (a) and (b).
   (e) Answers (b) and (c).

22. _____ bleeding usually flows from a wound in a steady stream.
   (a) Capillary
   (b) Venous
   (c) Arterial
   (d) Answers (a) and (b).
   (e) Answers (b) and (c).

23. An adult is not considered to have suffered a "serious" amount of blood loss until after _____ of blood has been lost.
   (a) 100 to 200 cc
   (b) 500 cc
   (c) 1 liter (1000 cc)
   (d) 1 ½ liters (1500 cc)
   (e) 2 liters (2000 cc)

24. A child is not considered to have suffered a "serious" amount of blood loss until after _____ of blood has been lost.

    (a) 50 cc

    (b) 100 cc

    (c) 500 cc

    (d) 750 cc

    (e) 1 liter (1000 cc)

25. An infant is not considered to have suffered a "serious" amount of blood loss until after _____ of blood has been lost.

    (a) 300 cc

    (b) 150 cc

    (c) 50 cc

    (d) 10 cc (any bleeding from an infant is considered life-threatening)

    (e) 1 liter (1000 cc)

26. Determination of blood-loss severity is based on

    (a) the patient's signs and symptoms.

    (b) an exact measurement of blood loss.

    (c) the patient's blood pressure.

    (d) Answers (a) and (b).

    (e) Answers (b) and (c).

27. Uncontrolled bleeding or significant blood loss leads to shock from _____, and possibly death.

    (a) low blood pressure

    (b) hypoperfusion

    (c) a slow pulse

    (d) hyperperfusion

    (e) Answers (a) or (c).

28. Which of the following statements regarding bleeding control methods is false?

    (a) Direct pressure to the site of bleeding is the first method of bleeding control.

    (b) Large, gaping wounds may require packing with sterile gauze and direct hand pressure.

    (c) A bleeding extremity should be kept at or below the level of the patient's heart to minimize hypoperfusion.

    (d) Pressure points may be used to control bleeding in the extremities.

    (e) Splinting may assist to control bleeding even when a fracture is not suspected.

29.   Which of the following statements regarding pressure points is true?
   (a) Pressure points are a last resort, used only when all other methods of
        bleeding control have failed.
   (b) The pressure point for upper extremities is at the brachial artery.
   (c) The pressure point for lower extremities is at the femoral artery.
   (d) Answers (b) and (c) are true.
   (e) Answers (a), (b), and (c) are true.

30.   Which of the following statements regarding the use of a tourniquet to control
      bleeding is true?
   (a) A tourniquet is a last resort, used only when all other methods of bleeding
        control have failed.
   (b) Application of a tourniquet can cause permanent damage to nerves, muscles,
        and blood vessels, resulting in the loss of the extremity.
   (c) A tourniquet should be applied only tightly enough to stop the bleeding.
   (d) Answers (b) and (c) are true.
   (e) Answers (a), (b), and (c) are true.

31.   Which of the following statements regarding the use of a tourniquet to control
      bleeding is false?
   (a) Once it has been applied, do not remove a tourniquet unless ordered to do so
        by the Medical Director.
   (b) Once it has been applied, do not loosen a tourniquet unless ordered to do so
        by the Medical Director.
   (c) The width of the tourniquet should be as thin as possible to minimize the
        amount of tissue, nerve, or blood vessel damage it may cause. A rope or the
        patient's thin belt may be used.
   (d) Do not cover a tourniquet. It should remain in open view.
   (e) Do not apply a tourniquet directly over any joint, but do apply it as close to
        the injury as possible.

32.   Bleeding from the nose may be caused by any of the following, except
   (a) internal abdominal (gastrointestinal) hemorrhage.
   (b) hypertension.
   (c) digital trauma (nose picking).
   (d) skull or facial fractures.
   (e) sinusitis or upper respiratory tract infections.

33.   The medical term for bleeding from the nose is
   (a) rhinorrhea.
   (b) epistaxis.
   (c) rhinitis.
   (d) sinusitis.
   (e) hemoptysis.

34. Which of the following statements regarding bleeding from the ears or nose is true?
   (a) Bleeding from the ears or nose may occur because of a skull fracture.
   (b) If the bleeding is the result of trauma, do not attempt to stop the blood flow.
   (c) Collect the blood with a loosely affixed sterile dressing.
   (d) All of the above are true.
   (e) None of the above is true.

35. Which of the following statements regarding emergency medical care for a nosebleed is false?
   (a) Have the patient lie flat.
   (b) Have the patient tilt his head backward.
   (c) Keep the patient calm and quiet.
   (d) Apply direct pressure by pinching the fleshy portion of the nostrils together.
   (e) If the patient becomes unconscious, place him on his side and employ suction and airway management techniques.

36. Which of the following statements regarding internal bleeding is false?
   (a) Internal bleeding can result in severe blood loss, shock, and subsequent death.
   (b) Injured or damaged internal organs commonly lead to extensive bleeding that is concealed (hidden) from emergency care providers.
   (c) Closed extremity injuries, even when painful, swollen, or deformed, are never the cause of shock from internal bleeding. Look elsewhere for sites of internal bleeding.
   (d) Suspicion of internal bleeding should be based upon the mechanism of injury.
   (e) Severity of internal bleeding should be determined by the patient's clinical signs and symptoms and the mechanism of injury.

37. Mechanisms of injury that can produce serious hypovolemia due to internal bleeding include all of the following, except
   (a) blast injuries.
   (b) any penetrating trauma to the chest, abdomen, or pelvis.
   (c) any blunt trauma to the chest, abdomen, or pelvis.
   (d) a fall from any height.
   (e) isolated penetrating trauma to the head.

38. Signs of potentially serious blood loss include all of the following, except
   (a) bright red external bleeding from the mouth, rectum, or vagina.
   (b) dark red blood flowing out of the nose.
   (c) emesis that is dark-red colored and contains coffee-ground-like material.
   (d) dark, tar-colored stools.
   (e) a tender, rigid, or distended abdomen.

39. Signs and symptoms of hypovolemic shock include all of the following, except
  (a) combativeness or altered mental status.
  (b) shallow, rapid breathing.
  (c) a slow, bounding pulse.
  (d) pale, cool, clammy skin.
  (e) complaint of extreme thirst.

40. Which of the following represents late-developing signs and symptoms of shock?
  (a) Anxiety and restlessness.
  (b) A rapid and bounding radial pulse.
  (c) Decreased blood pressure.
  (d) Answers (a) and (c).
  (e) Answers (a), (b), and (c).

41. Which of the following signs and symptoms of shock is usually the earliest to develop?
  (a) Anxiety and restlessness.
  (b) Nausea and vomiting.
  (c) Decreasing blood pressure.
  (d) Increasing pulse rate.
  (e) Increasing respiratory rate.

42. Which of the following signs and symptoms of shock is usually the last to develop?
  (a) Anxiety and restlessness.
  (b) Nausea and vomiting.
  (c) Decreasing blood pressure.
  (d) Increasing pulse rate.
  (e) Increasing respiratory rate.

43. _____ is a medical phrase indicating shock of any kind.
  (a) Hypoinfusion syndrome
  (b) Hypoperfusion syndrome
  (c) Hemorrhagic syndrome
  (d) Hyperinfusion syndrome
  (e) Hyperperfusion syndrome

44. _____ is a medical phrase specifically indicating shock from blood loss.
  (a) Hypovolemia or hypovolemic shock
  (b) Hyperperfusion syndrome or hyperinfusion syndrome
  (c) Hemorrhagic shock
  (d) Answers (a) or (b).
  (e) Answers (a) or (c).

45.   Shock is caused by
   (a) the heart failing to adequately pump blood (heart failure).
   (b) inadequate blood volume (dehydration or actual blood loss).
   (c) dilation of the body's blood vessels (a vascular container that is too large).
   (d) Answers (a) or (b).
   (e) Answers (a), (b), or (c).

46.   From the following list of activities, select all that are appropriate to the emergency medical treatment of patients in shock.
   (1) Administer high flow oxygen.
   (2) Control any external bleeding.
   (3) Elevate the lower extremities (or foot end of the backboard) by approximately 8 to 12 inches, only if the patient does not have serious injuries to the pelvis, lower extremities, head, chest, abdomen, neck, or spine.
   (4) Elevate the lower extremities (or foot end of the backboard) by approximately 8 to 12 inches, especially if the patient has serious injuries to the pelvis, lower extremities, head, chest, abdomen, neck, or spine.
   (5) If your protocol allows use of a pneumatic antishock garment (PASG), request orders to apply the garment to all abdominal-injury patients who have no chest injuries, but have shock signs and symptoms.
   (6) If your protocol allows PASG use, request orders to apply the garment to all pelvic-injury patients who have no chest injuries, but have shock signs and symptoms.
   (7) If your protocol allows PASG use, request orders to apply the garment to all chest-injury patients who have no abdominal or pelvic injuries, but have shock signs and symptoms.
   (8) Maintain the patient's airway; provide artificial ventilation or CPR if needed.
   (9) Prevent loss of body heat by covering the patient with a blanket when in cool or cold environments.
   (10) If the patient is immobilized with a long backboard, splinting of specific extremity fractures or joint injuries is optional or may be done en route to the emergency department.

      (a) 1, 2, 3, 5, 6, 7, 8, 9, and 10.
      (b) 1, 2, 4, 5, 6, 7, 8, 9, and 10.
      (c) 1, 2, 3, 7, 8, 9, and 10.
      (d) 1, 2, 4, 7, 8, 9, and 10.
      (e) 1, 2, 3, 5, 6, 8, 9, and 10.

47.   Which of the following statements regarding shock in infants or children is true?
   (a) Infants and children can maintain their blood pressure until more than 50% of their blood volume is lost.
   (b) Infants and children have less reserve blood volume than adults.

    (c) Owing to immature compensating mechanisms, the blood pressure of infants and children rapidly begins to fall ("crashes") as soon as 10% of their blood volume is lost.

    (d) Answers (a) and (b) are true.

    (e) Answers (b) and (c) are true.

48. _____ is a medical phrase specifically indicating shock from failure of the heart to adequately pump blood to the body's vital tissues.

    (a) Heart failure shock

    (b) Pump shock

    (c) Cardiogenic shock

    (d) Cardiopulmonary shock

    (e) Heterogenic shock

49. _____ is a medical phrase specifically indicating shock caused by a severe, systemic infection (infection involving all body systems).

    (a) Infectious shock

    (b) Septic shock

    (c) Vessel shock

    (d) Total body shock (TBS)

    (e) Heterogenic shock

50. Shock may be produced by a systemic infection because systemic infections release toxins that

    (a) dilate the body's blood vessels, enlarging the body's blood container, causing a "relative" hypovolemia.

    (b) constrict the body's blood vessels, enlarging the body's blood container, causing a "relative" hypovolemia.

    (c) dilate the body's blood vessels, diminishing the body's blood container, causing a "relative" hypovolemia.

    (d) constrict the body's blood vessels, diminishing the body's blood container, causing a "relative" hypovolemia.

    (e) make someone feel terribly ill, producing a relative form of "shock."

51. _____ is a medical phrase specifically indicating shock caused by spinal cord injury.

    (a) Cord shock

    (b) Spinal tap shock

    (c) Cervical shock

    (d) Neurogenic shock

    (e) CNS shock

52. Shock may be produced by spinal cord injury because
   (a) all feeling in the body becomes absent and all body functions shut down.
   (b) the heart no longer receives electrical impulses to pump the blood, so spinal cord injury causes heart failure.
   (c) the diameter of the body's blood vessels becomes constricted, and blood is no longer allowed to flow through them.
   (d) the diameter of the body's blood vessels below the level of injury becomes dilated, and there is no longer enough blood to fill them.
   (e) spinal cord injury always involves internal bleeding and immediately leads to shock from blood loss.

53. Shock usually occurs in stages. The stage called _____ is when shock is developing, but the patient's body is still able to maintain perfusion to vital organs.
   (a) decompensated shock
   (b) incomplete shock
   (c) partial shock
   (d) complete shock
   (e) compensated shock

54. The stage called _____ is when shock has fully developed, and the patient's body no longer is able to maintain perfusion to vital organs.
   (a) decompensated shock
   (b) compensated shock
   (c) partial shock
   (d) incomplete shock
   (e) complete shock

55. All of the following functions are performed by the skin, except for
   (a) protection of the body from the environment and provision of a barrier to keep out bacteria and other organisms.
   (b) prevention of body water loss and provision of a barrier to keep out environmental water.
   (c) production of white blood cells to combat infection.
   (d) regulation of body temperature.
   (e) reception and transmission of environmental information to the brain.

56. The outermost layer of skin that is composed primarily of dead cells that are constantly being rubbed or sloughed off and replaced is the
   (a) endodermis.
   (b) epidermis.
   (c) dermis.
   (d) subcutaneous layer.
   (e) sebaceous layer.

57. The layer of skin containing sweat and sebaceous glands is the
    (a) endodermis.
    (b) epidermis.
    (c) dermis.
    (d) subcutaneous layer.
    (e) sebaceous layer.

58. The layer of skin containing fat and soft tissue is largely responsible for temperature insulation and shock absorption (protection from impact injuries to the body organs). This layer is called the
    (a) endodermis.
    (b) epidermis.
    (c) dermis.
    (d) subcutaneous layer.
    (e) sebaceous layer.

59. The layer of skin containing hair follicles, blood vessels, and nerve endings is the
    (a) endodermis.
    (b) epidermis.
    (c) dermis.
    (d) subcutaneous layer.
    (e) sebaceous layer.

60. _____ is the medical term for what is commonly called a "goose egg."
    (a) Abrasion
    (b) Avulsion
    (c) Contusion
    (d) Hematoma
    (e) Laceration

61. _____ is the medical term for a bruise.
    (a) Abrasion
    (b) Avulsion
    (c) Contusion
    (d) Hematoma
    (e) Laceration

62. _____ is the medical term for a break or cut in the skin.
    (a) Abrasion
    (b) Avulsion
    (c) Contusion
    (d) Hematoma
    (e) Laceration

63. _____ is the medical term for a scraping injury.
   (a) Abrasion
   (b) Avulsion
   (c) Contusion
   (d) Hematoma
   (e) Laceration

64. _____ is the medical term for when a flap of skin or body tissue is torn loose, but remains connected to the body.
   (a) Abrasion
   (b) Avulsion
   (c) Contusion
   (d) Hematoma
   (e) Laceration

65. _____ is the medical term for when a flap of skin or body tissue is torn completely off (entirely disconnected from the body).
   (a) Abrasion
   (b) Avulsion
   (c) Contusion
   (d) Hematoma
   (e) Laceration

66. A bruise is an example of
   (a) a closed injury.
   (b) an open injury.
   (c) an open or closed injury.
   (d) an insignificant injury that never requires emergency medical attention.
   (e) None of the above.

67. A crush injury is an example of
   (a) a closed injury.
   (b) an open injury.
   (c) an open or closed injury.
   (d) an insignificant injury that never requires emergency medical attention.
   (e) None of the above.

68. A laceration is an example of
   (a) a closed injury.
   (b) an open injury.
   (c) an open or closed injury.
   (d) an insignificant injury that never requires emergency medical attention.
   (e) a serious injury that almost always results in loss of life or limb.

69. A puncture wound is an example of
  (a) a closed injury.
  (b) an open injury.
  (c) an open or closed injury.
  (d) an insignificant injury that never requires emergency medical attention.
  (e) a serious injury that almost always results in loss of life or limb.

70. An abrasion is an example of
  (a) a closed injury.
  (b) an open injury.
  (c) an open or closed injury.
  (d) an insignificant injury that never requires emergency medical attention.
  (e) a serious injury that almost always results in loss of life or limb.

71. Which of the following statements regarding amputation injuries is false?
  (a) An amputation is when a body part (usually an extremity) is completely severed from the body.
  (b) Amputations may be caused by cutting or tearing mechanisms of injury.
  (c) If properly cared for, amputated body parts may successfully be surgically reattached to the patient (resulting in few, if any, functional deficits).
  (d) Amputations most often occur in a manner that produces limited external blood loss.
  (e) Amputations always cause massive external blood loss and are accompanied by shock signs and symptoms.

72. The injury known as an *impaled object* is best defined as when
  (a) any foreign substance (such as gravel or dirt, tree leaves, twigs or branches) has become embedded in a patient's flesh.
  (b) a foreign object has punctured some part of the patient's body but was removed prior to the EMT's arrival. (The impaled object should be transported to the emergency department with the patient.)
  (c) any piece of metal has become embedded in a patient's body.
  (d) a bullet has entered the patient's body but did not exit it (as evidenced by the lack of an exit wound).
  (e) any foreign object has punctured (entered) any part of the patient's body and is still in place (in the patient's body) on the EMT's arrival.

73. A _____ is defined as any material placed on a wound to prevent further contamination or infection and/or control bleeding.
  (a) bandage
  (b) dressing
  (c) splint
  (d) Answers (a) or (c).
  (e) Answers (b) or (c).

74.   A _____ is defined as any material used to secure other material to a wound, to prevent further contamination or infection and/or control bleeding.

(a) bandage

(b) dressing

(c) splint

(d) Answers (a) or (c).

(e) Answers (b) or (c).

75.   Which of the following statements regarding open wound care is false?

(a) Remove or cut away clothing as needed, so as to expose the entire wound.

(b) Cover the entire wound with sterile material that extends at least 2 inches beyond all wound boundaries.

(c) If blood soaks through the entirety of the wound-covering material, it is imperative that all blood-soaked material be removed and replaced with fresh material.

(d) Do not apply bandages too tightly. The patient's distal pulse should remain present (unless it was absent before wound care).

(e) When caring for hands or feet, separate all the digits with gauze pads and leave the tips of all uninjured fingers or toes exposed.

76.   Which of the following statements regarding the emergency care of open chest injuries is false?

(a) Administer high flow oxygen, with positive-pressure ventilation assistance as needed.

(b) Place the patient in a position of comfort (if no spinal injury is suspected).

(c) Cover the chest wound with sterile dressings, then moisten them with sterile water or saline.

(d) Seal only three sides of the open chest wound's dressing (leaving one edge untaped).

(e) If no spinal injury is suspected, position the patient on his injured side to afford unimpeded expansion of the lung on the uninjured side.

77.   When air accumulates in the pleural space (the space between the lining of the interior chest wall and the lining of the lung) a serious condition occurs. Which of the following statements regarding this condition is true?

(a) Air may enter the pleural space via an external wound.

(b) Air may enter the pleural space via an internal lung rupture.

(c) As air accumulates in the pleural space, the lung's ability to expand becomes increasingly diminished and gas exchange becomes increasingly inadequate.

(d) Answers (a) and (c) are true.

(e) Answers (a), (b), and (c) are true.

78.   The phrase *sucking chest wound* refers to

(a) an external wound allowing air into that lung's pleural space.

(b) an internal wound leaking air into that lung's pleural space.

(c) oral trauma that causes air to be "sucked" into the pleural space via an opening in the oropharynx.

(d) Answers (a) or (c).

(e) Answers (b) or (c).

79. The condition of having air trapped in the pleural space (moderately interfering with lung function on the injured side) is called

(a) an aerothorax.

(b) a pneumothorax.

(c) a tension pneumothorax.

(d) a hemothorax.

(e) a hemopneumothorax.

80. The condition of having blood trapped in the pleural space (moderately interfering with lung function on the injured side) is called

(a) an aerothorax.

(b) a pneumothorax.

(c) a tension pneumothorax.

(d) a hemothorax.

(e) a hemopneumothorax.

81. The condition of having a large amount of air trapped in the pleural space (severely interfering with lung function on the injured side and possibly interfering with heart and opposite lung function) is called

(a) an aerothorax.

(b) a pneumothorax.

(c) a tension pneumothorax.

(d) a hemothorax.

(e) a hemopneumothorax.

82. All of the following are signs and symptoms of a condition called *traumatic asphyxia*, except

(a) a patient who is staggering about the scene, complaining of severe chest pain and difficulty breathing.

(b) obvious distention of the patient's jugular veins, with noticeably bloodshot and bulging eyes.

(c) a swollen or protruding appearance of the patient's lips or tongue.

(d) noticeable cyanosis of the patient's shoulders, neck, face, and head.

(e) possible deformity of the chest.

83. An external or internal wound to the area surrounding the heart may allow blood to accumulate between the heart and the sac that encloses it. The accumulation of blood in this area will begin to interfere with the heart's ability to expand and fully fill with blood, thus decreasing the heart's ability to pump a normal amount of blood out to the body. This condition is called

    (a) traumatic cardiac bypass.

    (b) cardiac tamponade.

    (c) cardiohemothorax.

    (d) cardiothorax.

    (e) the "bends."

84. Signs and symptoms of a heart being squeezed by the accumulation of blood in its surrounding sac include all of the following, except

    (a) distended jugular veins.

    (b) a weakening pulse.

    (c) a falling systolic blood pressure with a rising or unchanging diastolic blood pressure.

    (d) a rising systolic blood pressure with a falling or unchanging diastolic blood pressure.

    (e) a mechanism of injury that suggests blunt or penetrating chest trauma.

85. Which of the following statements regarding the emergency care of open abdominal injuries is false?

    (a) Administer high flow oxygen.

    (b) Keep the patient supine and flat (even when spine injury is not suspected). Hip or knee flexion or elevation will increase the severity of external and internal abdominal bleeding.

    (c) Cover any open abdominal wound with sterile dressings, moistened with sterile water or saline.

    (d) Consider requesting an order for application of the PASG if your protocol allows it.

    (e) Whether or not the abdominal-injury patient is immobilized to a long backboard because of suspected spine injury, as long as no hip or knee injuries are apparent, flex the patient's knees and place pillows or folded blankets beneath them to keep them flexed and elevated.

86. A dressing that does not allow air to enter or escape from a wound is called

    (a) an abusive dressing.

    (b) a hard dressing.

    (c) an occluded or "staunched" dressing.

    (d) an occlusive dressing.

    (e) a sterile dressing. (If air is allowed to enter or escape from a wound, bacteria will also enter and the dressing cannot be considered sterile.)

87.   When intestinal segments or abdominal organs are protruding from an open
      abdominal wound, the injury is called
      (a) a third-degree open abdominal injury.
      (b) an evisceration.
      (c) a visceral extrusion injury.
      (d) an external bowel herniation.
      (e) an abdominal herniation.

88.   Which of the following statements regarding emergency care for the patient with an
      open abdominal wound that has intestinal segments or abdominal organs
      protruding from it is false?
      (a) It is imperative that the protruding intestinal segments or organs be gently
           pushed back into the abdominal cavity before applying a dressing. If allowed
           to remain exposed, herniation (strangulation) or cold-exposure may result in
           tissue death of the exposed intestinal segment or organs.
      (b) Gently cover all of the abdominal wound and all exposed abdominal contents
           with a sterile dressing. Then, moisten the dressing with sterile water or saline.
      (c) Cover all of the initially applied dressing with another dressing that prevents
           air or fluid from escaping or entering the wound and that extends well beyond
           the boundaries of the first dressing.
      (d) Gently apply a clean towel or blanket on top of the dressed abdominal wound
           to preserve local body heat (in addition to covering the patient's entire body
           with a blanket to preserve total-body heat).
      (e) Whether or not the patient is immobilized to a long backboard because of
           suspected spine injury, as long as no hip or knee injuries are apparent, flex
           the patient's knees and place pillows or folded blankets beneath them to keep
           them flexed and elevated.

89.   Which of the following statements regarding emergency medical care of impaled
      objects is true?
      (a) Do not remove any impaled object from any part of the body. Only a surgeon,
           under controlled circumstances, can remove an impaled object.
      (b) All impaled objects must be removed before the wound they caused can be
           dressed and the patient can be transported. Contact the Medical Director to
           obtain specific removal instructions for each impaled object prior to removal.
      (c) An object impaled in the cheek may threaten the patient's airway. Thus, if the
           object can be removed without twisting it or increasing the size of injury, an
           object impaled in the cheek should be removed by the EMT.
      (d) Answers (b) and (c) are true.
      (e) None of the above is true.

90. Which of the following statements regarding emergency medical care of avulsions is true?
    (a) Clean the wound surface by gently rinsing with sterile saline.
    (b) Gently fold the avulsed tissue back into its normal position.
    (c) Control the bleeding and dress the wound with bulky pressure dressings.
    (d) Answers (a) and (c) are true.
    (e) Answers (a), (b), and (c) are true.

91. Which of the following statements regarding emergency medical care of full avulsions or complete amputations is true?
    (a) Immerse the part in a clean container of sterile saline for transportation with the patient. Ice should be added to the saline if transport time will be longer than 15 minutes.
    (b) Place a pressure dressing over the fully avulsed wound or the complete amputation's stump.
    (c) Do not use a tourniquet unless all other methods of bleeding control have failed.
    (d) Answers (b) and (c) are true.
    (e) Answers (a), (b), and (c) are true.

92. Which of the following statements regarding emergency medical care of large, open neck wounds is false?
    (a) Initial bleeding control of a unilateral open neck wound should consist of the EMT rapidly placing his gloved palm over the wound and applying direct pressure.
    (b) Several large blood vessels are close to the surface of the anterior neck. Thus, any open neck wound may cause life-threatening blood loss.
    (c) Never apply pressure to both sides of the patient's neck at the same time.
    (d) Any amount of direct pressure applied to a unilateral or bilateral open neck wound is likely to obstruct the airway and/or blood flow to the brain. Never apply any direct pressure to any open wound on a patient's neck.
    (e) An air embolism may enter any blood vessel exposed by an open neck wound and could easily cause the patient's death. All open neck wounds should be sealed with a dressing that does not allow air to pass through it.

93. Which of the following statements regarding bone injuries is false?
    (a) A fracture is best defined as when there is any sort of break in the bone (even just a crack).
    (b) A dislocation is best defined as when there is an alteration of the normal alignment or placement of bones, without an actual break in the bones.
    (c) It is vitally important to appropriate care provision that EMTs are able to differentiate between fractures and dislocations.
    (d) Any painful, swollen, or deformed extremity should be treated as though it were a fracture until proven otherwise.
    (e) It is not important for EMTs to be able to differentiate between a sprain and a strain injury.

94.   Correctly splinting any painful, swollen, or deformed extremity (whether a fracture or a dislocation) may accomplish which of the following effects?
   (a) Diminished pain.
   (b) Diminished blood loss.
   (c) Prevention of increased tissue, blood vessel, or nerve damage from occurring.
   (d) Answers (b) and (c).
   (e) Answers (a), (b), and (c).

95.   Which of the following statements regarding general rules of splinting is false?
   (a) Never intentionally replace protruding bone ends.
   (b) An injured extremity should always be immobilized from the joint above the injury to the joint below the injury (proximal and distal joint immobilization).
   (c) Never attempt to realign a deformed extremity. Always "splint it as it lies."
   (d) If no immediate danger or life-threats are found, splint the patient before moving the patient.
   (e) If a patient appears to be in life-threat from other injuries or conditions, disregard specific extremity immobilization. Instead, treat the life-threatening injuries or conditions while immobilizing the patient to a long backboard.

96.   Improper splinting may result in
   (a) splint compression of nerves, blood vessels, or body tissues, resulting in increased injury.
   (b) death of a patient in life-threat whose transport was delayed in order to accomplish extremity injury splinting.
   (c) reduction of circulation distal to the splinted part.
   (d) aggravation of the bone or joint injury that is being (or has been) splinted.
   (e) Any of the above.

97.   A traction splint may be applied to which of the following injuries?
   (a) A painful, swollen, and deformed midthigh injury.
   (b) A painful, swollen, and deformed knee injury.
   (c) A painful, swollen, and deformed lower leg injury.
   (d) Answers (a) and (b).
   (e) Answers (a) and (c).

98.   The use of a traction splint is contraindicated when there is a _____ injury present.
   (a) hip or pelvic
   (b) knee or ankle
   (c) partial midthigh amputation
   (d) Answers (a), (b), or (c).
   (e) None of the above injuries is a contraindication to traction splint application.

99. Mechanisms of injury that may indicate an associated spinal injury include all of the following, except

 (a) isolated, blunt trauma to the midthigh (such as the blow from a large bat) causing a fall from standing.
 (b) diving accidents where the patient lands feet first.
 (c) falls where the patient lands feet first.
 (d) soft rope hangings (soft rope stretches).
 (e) isolated, blunt trauma to the head.

100. Of the following mechanisms of injury, which is the least likely to cause spinal injury?

 (a) Penetrating trauma to the head, neck, or torso (such as a gun shot wound).
 (b) Isolated, blunt trauma to the lateral head.
 (c) A lateral fall to soft dirt from standing.
 (d) A restrained patient involved in a moderate- to high-speed motor vehicle accident.
 (e) An unrestrained patient involved in a low- to moderate-speed motor vehicle accident.

101. Which of the following statements regarding assessment of spinal injury mechanisms is true?

 (a) An elderly patient may have a spinal injury after a fall from standing.
 (b) All victims of a gunshot wound to the head, neck, chest, back, abdomen, or pelvis have a spinal injury until proven otherwise (by X ray).
 (c) All unconscious trauma victims have a spinal injury until proven otherwise (by X ray).
 (d) All lightning-strike victims have a spinal injury until proven otherwise (by X ray).
 (e) All of the above are true.

102. Which of the following statements regarding assessment of spinal injury mechanisms, signs, and symptoms is true?

 (a) The possibility of spinal injury is ruled out if the patient is already walking, is moving all extremities, and denies neurological or spinal pain complaints.
 (b) When the mechanism of injury suggests a strong potential for spinal injury, but the patient denies all possible spine-injury complaints, direct the patient to perform a variety of range-of-motion tests to be sure that a hidden spinal injury is not present.
 (c) If a victim of isolated head trauma (no direct blow to the spine area occurred) denies all neurological and spinal pain complaints the patient does not need to be treated for a spinal injury.
 (d) All of the above are true.
 (e) None of the above is true.

103. A *first-degree burn* is also known as a
   (a) superficial burn.
   (b) partial-thickness burn.
   (c) full-thickness burn.
   (d) Answers (a) or (b).
   (e) Answers (b) or (c).

104. A *third-degree burn* is also known as a
   (a) superficial burn.
   (b) partial-thickness burn.
   (c) full-thickness burn.
   (d) Answers (a) or (b).
   (e) Answers (b) or (c).

105. Reddened skin will only be present in the area of a
   (a) superficial burn.
   (b) partial-thickness burn.
   (c) full-thickness burn.
   (d) Answers (a) or (b).
   (e) Answers (b) or (c).

106. The presence of blisters indicates an area of
   (a) superficial burn.
   (b) partial-thickness burn.
   (c) full-thickness burn.
   (d) Answers (a) or (b).
   (e) Answers (b) or (c).

107. Severe pain indicates an area of
   (a) superficial burn.
   (b) partial-thickness burn.
   (c) full-thickness burn.
   (d) Answers (a) or (b).
   (e) Answers (b) or (c).

108. The loss of sensation (little to no pain) indicates an area of
   (a) superficial burn.
   (b) partial-thickness burn.
   (c) full-thickness burn.
   (d) Answers (a) or (b).
   (e) Answers (b) or (c).

109. In the real-life field situation, estimating the percentage of body surface area (BSA) that has been burned is best accomplished by using the Palmar Surface Area (or Rule of Palm) method. This method consists of recognizing that the size of _____, noting that measurement, and determining how many times that measurement can be overlaid within the entirety of the patient's burned areas.

(a) any patient's palm represents 9% of that patient's body surface area
(b) your palm represents 9% of any patient's body surface area
(c) any patient's palm represents 5% of that patient's body surface area
(d) your palm represents 1% of any patient's body surface area
(e) any patient's palm represents 1% of that patient's body surface area

110. The method most frequently addressed by written tests for determining the patient's percentage of BSA burned is the Rule of Nines. Using the Rule of Nines, if an adult patient has burned the anterior surface of his right arm, the right half of his anterior abdomen, and the anterior surface of his right leg, what is the BSA percentage of his burn?

(a) 9%.
(b) 13.5%.
(c) 18%.
(d) 22.5%.
(e) 27%.

111. Using the Rule of Nines, what is the percentage of BSA burned if an adult patient has suffered burns to his anterior chest, anterior abdomen, genital area, and anterior left leg?

(a) 23.5%.
(b) 36%.
(c) 27%.
(d) 19%.
(e) 28%.

112. Using the Rule of Nines, what is the percentage of BSA burned if an 8-year-old female has suffered burns to the front of her right arm, the right half of her anterior chest and abdomen, and the front of her right leg?

(a) 26%.
(b) 20.5%.
(c) 23%.
(d) 13.5%.
(e) 29.5%.

113. Using the Rule of Nines, what is the percentage of BSA burned if an 8-year-old male has suffered burns to his anterior chest, anterior abdomen, genital area, and anterior left leg?

(a) 26%.
(b) 20.5%.

(c) 23%.
(d) 13.5%.
(e) 29.5%.

114. Of the following burns, which one could be considered the least critical?
(a) Burns that encompass the patient's entire arm, chest, or leg.
(b) Burns accompanied by a painful, swollen, or deformed extremity.
(c) Burns associated with a respiratory injury.
(d) An adult with partial-thickness burns over 10% of his BSA (not involving his hands, feet, face, or genitalia).
(e) A pediatric or geriatric patient with partial-thickness burns over 5% of his BSA (not involving his hands, feet, face, or genitalia).

115. Of the following burns, which should be considered the most critical?
(a) Any patient with partial-thickness burns involving the hands, feet, face, or genitalia.
(b) An adult with partial-thickness burns of 15 to 30% of his BSA (not involving his hands, feet, face, or genitalia).
(c) An adult with full thickness burns of 2 to 10% of his BSA (not involving his hands, feet, face, or genitalia).
(d) All of the above are equally critical burns.
(e) None of the above is considered critical burns.

116. A burn that encircles an entire body part (such as an arm, the chest, or a leg) is called
(a) a circumoral burn.
(b) a full-thickness burn.
(c) a full-surface burn.
(d) a circumferential burn.
(e) an amputating burn.

117. Which of the following statements regarding emergency care measures for thermal burns is false?
(a) Do not break any blisters.
(b) Request orders from the Medical Director to apply a topical burn antiseptic (available in ointment or lotion form).
(c) Remove all smoldering clothing (even after any flames are extinguished).
(d) Remove all jewelry from burned extremities as soon as possible.
(e) Do not bandage burned hands and feet until you have separated burned digits with sterile gauze pads.

118. Place the following emergency care measures for thermal burns in the order in which they are performed (from first performed to last performed).

    (1) Assess the airway.
    (2) Assess the patient's breathing.
    (3) Assess the patient's circulation.
    (4) Assure personal safety.
    (5) Manage any airway problems.
    (6) Stop the burning process, initially with water or saline.
    (7) Take body substance isolation precautions.
    (8) Manage any breathing problems.
    (9) Treat the patient for shock signs and symptoms.
  (10) Determine an estimated percentage of BSA burned, additionally assessing for burn depth and severity.

        (a) 1, 2, 3, 4, 5, 6, 7, 8, 9, and 10.
        (b) 4, 6, 1, 2, 3, 7, 5, 8, 10 and 9.
        (c) 4, 7, 6, 1, 5, 2, 8, 3, 9, and 10.
        (d) 4, 7, 1, 2, 3, 10, 5, 8, and 10.
        (e) Any of the above orders of performing these emergency care measures are acceptable. Different patients may require vastly different care approaches.

119. Which of the following statements regarding emergency care measures for chemical burns is false?

    (a) Dry powders should be brushed off before any flushing with water or sterile saline is performed.
    (b) Flushing of any chemical burn area should be continued for at least 20 minutes (if not longer) and can be done en route to the emergency department.
    (c) Do not contaminate unexposed areas when flushing.
    (d) Remove all clothing, shoes, socks, belts, and jewelry before beginning any decontamination measures (including flushing).
    (e) Treat the patient for shock.

120. Which of the following statements regarding emergency care measures for electrical burns is false?

    (a) A doubled pair of latex gloves, or a dry tree branch, will protect the EMT from electrical shock while removing a patient from contact with an active electrical source.
    (b) All electrocution victims have a spine injury until proven otherwise.
    (c) Monitor the patient closely for cardiac arrest (consider the need for AED).
    (d) Electrical burns usually are much more severe than their outward appearance.
    (e) Look for both an electrical injury entrance and exit wound.

The answer key for Test Section Six is on page 351.

7

OB/GYN, Pediatric and Geriatric Patients

From DOT Module Four and DOT Module Six

Subjects:

- Obstetrics and Gynecology
- Pediatric Age and Developmental Differences
- Pediatric Airway Differences
- Pediatric Assessment Considerations
- Pediatric Emergency Care Considerations
- Pediatric Seizures, Poisoning, Fevers, and Drowning
- Sudden Infant Death Syndrome
- Pediatric Trauma, Child Abuse, and Neglect
- Geriatric Patient Considerations
- Cerebral Vascular Accidents

Test Section Seven consists of 105 questions and is allotted 1 hour and 45 minutes for completion.

1.   The medical term for a developing, unborn baby is
        (a) a zygote.
        (b) a fetus.
        (c) an ovum.
        (d) a spermatozoa.
        (e) a uterus.

2.   The medical term for the organ in which the developing unborn baby grows is
        _____. This organ is also responsible for labor and expulsion of the infant.
        (a) the placenta
        (b) the vagina
        (c) the cervix
        (d) the abdomen
        (e) the uterus

3.   The actual *birth canal* consists of the lower part of the uterus and
        (a) the vagina.
        (b) the cervix.
        (c) the placenta.
        (d) Answers (b) and (c).
        (e) None of the above (the birth canal is a completely separate organ).

4.   The *placenta* is best defined as
        (a) the organ in which the developing unborn baby grows.
        (b) the bag of waters in which a baby develops.
        (c) the organ through which the unborn baby exchanges nourishment and waste
             products during pregnancy.
        (d) the cushion that protects the unborn baby from harm.
        (e) the organ that seals the bottom of the womb, to prevent premature expulsion
             of the developing baby.

5.   The *umbilical cord* is best defined as
        (a) the "anchor" that attaches the developing baby to the mother's abdomen
             (preventing premature expulsion).
        (b) the "anchor" that attaches the developing baby to the placenta (preventing
             premature expulsion).
        (c) an organ that creates its own oxygenated blood cells to "ventilate" the
             developing baby until its lungs are functional.
        (d) a cord that acts as an extension of the placenta, through which the
             developing baby receives nourishment while in the womb.
        (e) None of the above.

6. The _____ is the medical term for a container, within the womb, that surrounds the developing baby. This container floats the baby in about one to two quarts of fluid; thus the common term for this container is the "bag of waters."
    (a) amniotic sac
    (b) placental sac
    (c) vaginal sack
    (d) uterine sack
    (e) cervical sac

7. The lower part of the birth canal is called the
    (a) uterus.
    (b) placenta.
    (c) hymen.
    (d) fallopian tube.
    (e) vagina.

8. The area of skin between the vaginal opening and the anus is often torn during delivery. This area of skin is called the
    (a) hymen.
    (b) perineum.
    (c) cervix.
    (d) genitalia.
    (e) "no man's land" (because the EMT is not to touch it).

9. The medical term _____ refers to when the vaginal opening appears to "bulge out," because the first portion of the infant is pressing against it.
    (a) breech presentation
    (b) pushing phase
    (c) bloody show
    (d) crowning
    (e) caudal presentation

10. Technically, *labor* is divided into three (sometimes four) stages. As a whole, however, the entire process of labor is best defined as beginning when
    (a) contractions are 3 minutes apart.
    (b) the first uterine contraction is felt.
    (c) the vagina begins to bulge out.
    (d) the "bloody show" occurs.
    (e) the uterus begins to bulge out.

11. The entire process of labor is best defined as ending when the
    (a) baby is delivered.
    (b) amniotic sac is broken.
    (c) placenta is delivered.
    (d) hymen is perforated or torn.
    (e) postpartum bleeding has been controlled.

12.   The medical phrase *presenting part* is best defined as
  (a) the delivery of the placenta.
  (b) the appearance of the infant's head in the vaginal opening.
  (c) the part of the infant that first appears at the vaginal opening.
  (d) Answers (a) or (b).
  (e) Answers (a) or (c).

13.   The medical term *crowning* is best defined as
  (a) the breaking of the bag of waters.
  (b) the bulging caused at the vaginal opening by the infant's presenting part.
  (c) the stage of labor when the mother needs to push.
  (d) Answers (a) or (b).
  (e) Answers (a) or (c).

14.   The phrase *bloody show* refers to
  (a) the excessive amount of bleeding that accompanies even normal childbirth (up to 4 L of blood may be lost).
  (b) the breaking of the bag of waters.
  (c) the stage of labor when the mother needs to push and begins to bleed heavily.
  (d) a small vaginal discharge of blood-tinged, watery mucus that may occur as labor begins.
  (e) the delivery of the placenta.

15.   The medical term *miscarriage* is best defined as
  (a) the delivery of products of conception early in a pregnancy.
  (b) the spontaneous termination of a pregnancy.
  (c) the induced termination of a pregnancy.
  (d) Answers (a) or (b).
  (e) Answers (a), (b), or (c).

16.   The medical term *abortion* is best defined as
  (a) the delivery of products of conception early in a pregnancy.
  (b) the spontaneous termination of a pregnancy.
  (c) the induced termination of a pregnancy.
  (d) Answers (a) or (b).
  (e) Answers (a), (b), or (c).

17.   Emergency care for a miscarriage includes all of the following, except
  (a) obtaining baseline vital signs.
  (b) providing treatment based upon signs and symptoms.
  (c) application of an external vaginal pad (the EMT must not actually pack the internal vagina).
  (d) close inspection of conception or fetal tissues passed into the toilet prior to flushing them (the EMT must be able to clearly describe the tissues observed).
  (e) emotional support to the mother.

18. Which of the following statements regarding seizures in pregnancy are true?

  (a) Pregnancy does not cause seizures. If a pregnant patient has a seizure, she either already has a seizure disorder, or she has recently been the victim of head trauma.

  (b) Low blood pressure is associated with seizures caused by pregnancy.

  (c) Pregnancy-related seizures only cause a serious life threat to the unborn baby.

  (d) Answers (b) and (c) are true.

  (e) None of the above is true.

19. Emergency care for a seizing pregnant patient includes

  (a) providing high flow oxygen, aggressive airway maintenance, rapid transport to the emergency department, and requesting an ALS intercept.

  (b) positioning the patient on her right side for transport (to improve the unborn baby's oxygenation).

  (c) obtaining an order from the Medical Director to assist the patient with taking her prescribed seizure medication.

  (d) Answers (a) and (b).

  (e) Answers (a), (b), and (c).

20. Vaginal bleeding

  (a) may occur early or late in pregnancy.

  (b) will only occur early in pregnancy if the patient is a trauma victim (consider spousal abuse to be possible if the first- or second-trimester patient neglects to report trauma; this is a mandatory reporting situation).

  (c) may or may not be accompanied by abdominal pain.

  (d) Answers (a) and (b).

  (e) Answers (a) and (c).

21. Emergency care for vaginal bleeding includes

  (a) performing a complete (but discreet) physical examination, obtaining baseline vital signs, and obtaining the patient's medical and gynecological history.

  (b) high flow oxygen administration, and providing treatment based upon vital signs and symptoms.

  (c) obtaining an order to "pack" the vagina with sterile pads to occlude excessive and serious bleeding. (Packing is almost always required to stop excessive and serious vaginal bleeding, because "direct" pressure cannot be externally accomplished.)

  (d) Answers (a) and (b).

  (e) Answers (a), (b), and (c).

AUTHOR'S NOTE: *Take a deep breath, then let it out and relax. Read the next question and its numbered factors carefully and calmly. Using your scratch paper, simply make a list of your selections for question 22. Do the same for questions 23 and 24. By now, you should be comfortable enough with these kinds of questions that you'll NOT need to stop timing your performance to answer them.*

22. When assessing a patient in labor, it is important to be able to determine the likelihood of imminent delivery (delivery within the next 10 minutes), so as to decide whether to stay on scene and deliver the baby, or to transport the patient to the hospital for delivery. Which of the following patient history factors, signs and symptoms, represents information that might be associated with an imminent OR a delayed delivery and thus is of very little value to making a transport decision?

    (1) The patient has previously delivered three children.
    (2) The patient is quite anxious and insists, "This baby is coming NOW!"
    (3) The patient reports no previous pregnancies or deliveries.
    (4) Contractions are lasting between 30 seconds and 1 minute in duration, and are occurring every 2 to 3 minutes.
    (5) Contractions have just started, lasting no more than 10 to 20 seconds in duration, and are occurring 5 to 10 minutes apart.
    (6) The "bag of waters" has already broken.
    (7) The "bag of waters" has not yet broken.
    (8) The infant is crowning.
    (9) The infant is not crowning.
   (10) The patient strongly complains of needing to move her bowels.
   (11) The patient describes having had a small, blood-tinged, vaginal discharge immediately prior to your arrival.
   (12) The patient strongly feels the need to push the baby out.
   (13) During each contraction, the patient is screaming and insisting that her pain is excruciating.

        (a) 3, 6, 7, 9, 11, and 13.
        (b) 1, 2, 4, 8, 10, and 12.
        (c) 5.
        (d) 1, 4, 6, 10, 11, and 13.
        (e) 1, 5, 7, and 13.

23. Which of question number 22's patient history factors, signs and symptoms, strongly indicate a patient who is unlikely to be delivering her baby within the next 10 minutes (and should immediately be transported to the emergency department for delivery)?

    (a) 3, 6, 7, 9, 11, and 13.
    (b) 1, 2, 4, 8, 10, and 12.
    (c) 5.
    (d) 1, 4, 6, 10, 11, and 13.
    (e) 1, 5, 7, and 13.

24. Which of question number 22's patient history factors, signs and symptoms, strongly indicate a patient who is highly likely to be delivering her baby within the next 10 minutes?

   (a) 3, 6, 7, 9, 11, and 13.
   (b) 1, 2, 4, 8, 10, and 12.
   (c) 5.
   (d) 1, 4, 6, 10, 11, and 13.
   (e) 1, 5, 7, and 13.

25. Once the Medical Director has agreed with the EMT's reasons for deciding to remain on scene for delivery, which of the following statements regarding on-scene delivery assistance is true?

   (a) If delivery fails to occur within 10 minutes after prepping the patient for an on-scene delivery, contact the Medical Director for permission to alter the plan, and transport the patient to the emergency department.
   (b) Advise your dispatcher of the situation, and be prepared for a long stay on scene. To deliver a newborn on scene (even without any birth complications), you may have to remain there for 40 to 60 minutes—sometimes even longer. Birth is not an exact science.
   (c) The pregnant patient in labor is "always right." If delivery seems imminent, but the mother absolutely insists on going to the bathroom first, assist her to do so before prepping her for delivery. (Prehospital delivery is embarrassing enough without also causing the patient to suffer embarrassment about becoming incontinent of urine or feces. Even new moms know when they just have to "void"!)
   (d) If delivery fails to occur within 30 minutes after prepping the patient for an on-scene delivery, have the patient move to her left side and hold her legs together. Then, contact the Medical Director for permission to alter the plan, and transport the patient to the emergency department.
   (e) Answers (b) and (c) are true.

26. Timing the frequency of contractions and the duration of each contraction are both very important labor and delivery assessment steps. Contraction duration is measured by timing from

   (a) the beginning of each contraction to its end (from start to finish).
   (b) the end of one contraction to the beginning of the next contraction (from end to start).
   (c) the beginning of one contraction to the beginning of the next contraction (from start to start).
   (d) the beginning of one contraction to the end of the next contraction (from start to next-finished).
   (e) the end of one contraction to the end of the next contraction (from end to end).

27.   The frequency (or interval) of contractions is measured by timing from
  (a) beginning of each contraction to its end (from start to finish).
  (b) the end of one contraction to the beginning of the next contraction (from end to start).
  (c) the beginning of one contraction to the beginning of the next contraction (from start to start).
  (d) the beginning of one contraction to the end of the next contraction (from start to next-finished).
  (e) the end of one contraction to the end of the next contraction (from end to end).

28.   When the infant's head begins to emerge, place your fingers
  (a) within the vaginal opening on either side of the infant's head so that you may gently grasp the infant's jaws (as in the jaw-thrust airway maneuver). Apply gentle traction to speed up the delivery in a controlled manner.
  (b) around the bony parts of the infant's exposed skull (avoiding the face and the skull's soft spot) and apply evenly distributed, gentle traction to speed the delivery in a controlled manner.
  (c) at a distance from the infant's skull and the mother's vaginal area, forming a "cup" with which to "catch" the infant's head and prevent trauma.
  (d) on the bony parts of the infant's exposed skull (avoiding the skull's soft spot), applying evenly distributed, gentle pressure to prevent an explosive delivery.
  (e) and your hands at your sides! Mothers have been delivering babies without assistance since time began. Occupy yourself by recording this moment as the official time of birth.

29.   If the "bag of waters" has not already broken by the time the infant's head is being delivered,
  (a) instruct the mother to stop pushing, place her on her left side, and have her hold her legs together. Immediately remove her to the ambulance for rapid transport to the emergency department.
  (b) use a sterile scalpel to carefully puncture the sac and pull all of the sac tissues away from the baby's head.
  (c) use your fingers to pinch and puncture the sac, pulling the sac tissues away from the emerging skull or face.
  (d) do not attempt to break it. The membrane will break on its own, at the appropriate time. Simply continue with your assistance of the delivery.
  (e) have the mother reach down and break the sac. (EMTs who break membranes are often charged with negligence).

30.   As the infant's head completes its delivery, determine if the umbilical cord is around the infant's neck. If the cord is around the infant's neck,
  (a) gently loosen it before sliding it over the infant's upper shoulder and head. If the cord will not loosen, securely clamp it in two places, carefully cut the cord between the clamps, and then gently remove the cord from around the infant's neck.
  (b) instruct the mother to stop pushing, place her on her left side, and have her hold her legs together. Immediately remove her to the ambulance for rapid transport to the emergency department.

(c) immediately sever the cord using a sterile scalpel; then continue with the delivery. At this late point, blood loss from a severed cord will not affect the mother or the infant.

(d) leave the cord in place and continue the delivery without deviation from protocol.

(e) immediately clamp the cord (without severing it) and then continue the delivery without deviation from protocol.

31. After the infant's head is born, support the head and suction the infant's
   (a) nose, once or twice in each nostril. Then suction the mouth two or three times.
   (b) nose, once in each nostril, before suctioning the mouth once. Repeat this process, in this order, as needed until the infant's airway seems clear.
   (c) mouth first, then each of its nostrils.
   (d) nose only (infants are "nose breathers").
   (e) mouth only (infants are "mouth breathers").

32. After the infant is completely delivered,
   (a) perform the time-honored "smack on the bottom" to initiate breathing. Invert the baby, holding it firmly by the feet (infants are slippery; be careful), and slap the baby's buttocks at least once or twice.
   (b) wrap the infant in a warm blanket and place it on its side with the head slightly lower than the trunk to allow for drainage.
   (c) if the umbilical cord has not been cut, keep the baby level with the vagina.
   (d) Answers (b) and (c).
   (e) Answers (a), (b), and (c).

33. To sever the umbilical cord of a normally delivered baby, you should
   (a) wait until the baby is breathing on its own and the cord no longer has a pulse before clamping and cutting.
   (b) place one clamp approximately 10 inches away from the baby, and another clamp approximately 7 inches away from the baby, then cut the cord between these two clamps.
   (c) place one clamp approximately 4 inches away from the baby, and another clamp approximately 7 inches away from the baby, then cut the cord between these two clamps.
   (d) Answers (a) and (b).
   (e) Answers (a) and (c).

34. The umbilical cord should normally be severed
   (a) beyond the farthest clamp (neonatal blood samples will be obtained from the section of cord retained between the clamps).
   (b) in between the two clamps (thus, the closest clamp must be far enough away from the baby to allow for blood sample work or IV access to be performed on the section that remains with the baby).
   (c) in the emergency department. Do not cut the cord in the field.
   (d) before the baby is wrapped in a blanket (bleeding from the cut end may soil the blanket).
   (e) by the mother (EMTs who cut cords are often charged with negligence).

35. Bleeding from the clamp at the end of the umbilical cord segment that remains attached to the baby
   (a) is a normal occurrence and may continue for 15 to 30 minutes.
   (b) is a serious emergency and is also the reason why EMTs are not allowed to cut the umbilical cord in the field.
   (c) should be controlled by immediately removing the clamp (or umbilical tape tie) and reapplying it closer to the baby, in a slightly tighter manner.
   (d) should be controlled by immediately applying an additional clamp (or umbilical tape tie) as close to the first one as possible, in a slightly tighter manner.
   (e) should be controlled by removing the clamp, squeezing the excess blood out of the cord (beginning at the baby's end) and reapplying the clamp at the cord end.

36. Which of the following statements is true?
   (a) Delivery of the placenta is not an EMT assisted-field-delivery function. Transport the patient to the emergency department prior to placenta delivery, having the mother keep her legs together, and using "lights and sirens" if placental delivery appears imminent (Mom keeps wanting to "push").
   (b) If the mother and the baby are doing well (there is no suggestion of any life threat), EMTs may wait on scene for up to 20 minutes for placental delivery. If placental delivery doesn't occur by then, initiate transport of the patient. Placental delivery may or may not occur en route to the emergency department.
   (c) Delivery of the placenta must occur within 5 minutes after delivery, and prior to transporting the mother and baby. If it doesn't deliver spontaneously, the EMT should apply and maintain aggressive downward pressure to the uterus (over the abdomen) until the placenta is delivered.
   (d) Delivery of the placenta is a natural occurrence that always immediately follows childbirth, but is rather messy and embarrassing for both the patient and the EMT. Closely observe the delivered placenta before discretely disposing of it (using the nearest toilet), and then transport the mother and child to the emergency department.
   (e) Until the placenta delivers, do not, for any reason, move the mother. Doing so may increase maternal blood loss and pose a significant risk of maternal death. If the placenta does not deliver within 5 minutes after the infant is born, summon another vehicle to separately transport the newborn, and remain on scene until the mother delivers the placenta.

37.   Once the placenta is delivered,

   (a) place it in a container or towel, put both in a plastic bag, and transport it to the hospital with the mother and child. All placental tissues must accompany the mother to the hospital.

   (b) the patient may finally be transported to the emergency department. Closely observe the delivered placenta before discretely disposing of it (using the nearest toilet), and record your observations prior to leaving the scene.

   (c) the patient may finally be transported. If the infant was not transported earlier than the mother, have the mother begin breast-feeding the baby while you closely observe the delivered placenta before discretely disposing of it (using the nearest toilet). Then transport the mother and baby to the emergency department.

   (d) closely observe it before discretely disposing of it (using the nearest toilet). Avoid allowing the mother to observe the placenta, as this sight is often emotionally disturbing.

   (e) the patient may finally be transported to the emergency department without the EMT risking charges of negligence for premature transport.

38.   After delivery of the baby and/or the placenta, emergency care for the mother includes all of the following, except

   (a) vigorous soap and water cleansing of the vaginal opening to prevent infection (especially if any tearing of the mother's genitalia occurred during delivery).

   (b) placing a sterile pad over the vaginal opening.

   (c) lowering the mother's legs and supporting her knees with towels or pillows to help her keep her legs together (advise her that "squeezing" them together is not necessary).

   (d) assisting with control of postdelivery bleeding by massaging the mother's uterus (massaging the mother's abdomen).

   (e) assisting control of postdelivery bleeding by allowing the mother to nurse the baby (only if she desires to do so).

39.   Which of the following statements regarding vaginal bleeding following delivery is false?

   (a) Blood loss after delivery is common and does not threaten the mother's well-being. Up to 500 cc of blood loss is well tolerated and thus should not cause undue psychological stress to the EMT or the mother.

   (b) Blood loss after delivery is common and does not threaten the mother's well-being. Up to 2,000 cc (2 L) of blood loss is well tolerated and thus should not cause undue psychological stress to the EMT or the mother.

   (c) If blood loss seems excessive, the EMT should massage the uterus (massage the abdomen).

   (d) Regardless of the EMT's estimation of blood loss, if the mother appears to be in shock (hypoperfusion), treat her for shock and transport her prior to uterine massage. Massage may occur en route.

   (e) If bleeding continues despite uterine massage, check the massage technique and transport the patient immediately, providing oxygen and treatment for shock, in addition to ongoing assessments.

40. Initial care of the newborn includes all of the following, except

(a) wrapping in a warm, dry blanket and covering the infant's head to conserve heat.

(b) positioning the infant on its side, level with the vagina, until the umbilical cord is cut.

(c) airway suctioning.

(d) the traditional inverted buttocks-spanking (tactile stimulation) to encourage the baby to breathe.

(e) assessing the infant's breathing, skin color, and muscle tone.

41. If a new born has not begun breathing by _____ after delivery, the EMT should begin artificial ventilation.

(a) one minute

(b) 10 seconds

(c) 15 seconds

(d) 30 seconds

(e) 5 seconds

42. A newborn infant's heart rate is considered to be "slower than normal" when it falls below _____ beats per minute (bpm).

(a) 60

(b) 80

(c) 100

(d) 110

(e) 120

43. One minute after birth, you are caring for a breathing newborn who has a heart rate of 100 bpm, pink central skin color, and cyanotic hands and feet. You should

(a) administer chest compressions.

(b) provide positive-pressure ventilation with oxygen at 15 1pm.

(c) provide supplemental oxygen at 15 1pm, free-flowing near the infant's face.

(d) continue to ensure warmth and observe the baby. These findings are normal.

(e) Answers (a) and (b).

44. One minute after birth, you are caring for a breathing newborn who has a heart rate of 110 bpm with cyanotic hands, feet, and trunk. You should

(a) administer chest compressions.

(b) provide positive-pressure ventilation with oxygen at 15 1pm.

(c) provide supplemental oxygen at 15 1pm, free-flowing near the infant's face.

(d) continue to provide warmth and observe the baby. These findings are normal.

(e) Answers (a) and (b).

45.   One minute after birth, you are caring for a breathing newborn who has a heart rate of 80 bpm. You should
    (a) administer chest compressions.
    (b) provide positive-pressure ventilation with oxygen at 15 1pm.
    (c) provide supplemental oxygen at 15 1pm, free-flowing near the infant's face.
    (d) continue to provide warmth and observe the baby. These findings are normal.
    (e) Answers (a) and (b).

46.   One minute after birth, you are caring for an apneic newborn who has a heart rate of 50 bpm. You should
    (a) administer chest compressions.
    (b) provide positive-pressure ventilation with oxygen at 15 1pm.
    (c) provide supplemental oxygen at 15 1pm, free-flowing near the infant's face.
    (d) continue to provide warmth and observe the baby. These findings are normal.
    (e) Answer (a) and (b).

47.   Two minutes after birth, you are caring for a breathing newborn with a heart rate of 110 bpm who still has cyanotic hands, feet, and trunk. You should
    (a) administer chest compressions.
    (b) provide positive-pressure ventilation with oxygen at 15 1pm.
    (c) provide supplemental oxygen at 15 1pm, free-flowing near the infant's face.
    (d) continue to provide warmth and observe the baby. These findings are still normal.
    (e) Answers (a) and (b).

48.   If a newborn infant requires artificial ventilation, the EMT should provide ventilations at a rate of _____ times per minute (_____).
    (a) 12 to 20 / one ventilation every 5 or 3 seconds.
    (b) 20 to 30 / one ventilation every 3 or 2 seconds.
    (c) 40 to 60 / one ventilation every $1\frac{1}{2}$ seconds, or each second.
    (d) 60 to 80 / one ventilation each second, or 3 ventilations every 2 seconds.
    (e) 80 / 3 ventilations every 2 seconds.

49.   The newborn's APGAR assessment and scoring should be performed
    (a) only on the way to the hospital (after all critical care has been performed).
    (b) at 1 and 5 minutes after the infant's birth (two scores).
    (c) at 1 and 5 minutes after the placenta delivers (two scores).
    (d) every minute during the first 5 minutes after the infant's birth (five scores).
    (e) by the emergency department staff, immediately upon arrival.

50.   The G of the APGAR score's mnemonic stands for
   (a) Gasping (poor respiratory effort).
   (b) Gurgling (indication of aspiration).
   (c) Gross deformity (presence of obvious congenital anomalies).
   (d) Groaning (poor crying ability).
   (e) Grimace (irritable facial expression, sneezing, coughing, or crying in response to stimulus).

51.   For the majority of births, the baby's head is the first part to emerge from the birth canal. This head-first presentation is called a
   (a) dorsal presentation.
   (b) ventral presentation.
   (c) cephalic presentation.
   (d) caudal presentation.
   (e) cranial presentation.

52.   If the umbilical cord is visible, protruding from the vaginal opening prior to the infant's delivery, this condition is called
   (a) umbilical crowning.
   (b) cord crowning.
   (c) a prolapsed cord.
   (d) a presenting cord.
   (e) a prelooped cord.

53.   Which of the following statements about when the umbilical cord is protruding from the vaginal opening prior to the infant's delivery is true?
   (a) This condition presents a serious emergency that endangers the life of the unborn fetus; delivery absolutely cannot be accomplished in the field. Transport the patient immediately, using lights and sirens.
   (b) This condition is not unusual and not a concern; proceed with delivery as normal.
   (c) Although unusual, this condition is easily rectified in the field. Contact your Medical Director for special delivery orders.
   (d) If the umbilical cord is the crowning part, clamp the cord in two places, sever the cord between the clamps, and proceed with delivery as normal.
   (e) None of the above is true.

54.   When the umbilical cord is protruding from the vaginal opening prior to the infant's delivery, emergency care includes all of the following, except
   (a) high flow oxygen administration.
   (b) positioning the mother on her left side with her legs tightly squeezed together until special delivery orders can be obtained and implemented.

(c) insertion of the EMT's sterile-gloved hand into the mother's vagina, to push the infant's presenting part away from the umbilical cord.

(d) assessment of the mother's baseline vital signs.

(e) gentle, but rapid transport to the emergency department.

55. A *breech presentation* is best defined as
(a) when the infant's face is crowning.
(b) when one of the infant's limbs protrudes from the vaginal opening.
(c) when both lower extremities or the buttocks of the infant are the first portions to present at the vaginal opening.
(d) when the buttocks of the infant (and no limbs) appear as the first presenting part at the vaginal opening.
(e) when the infant explosively delivers, head first, from the vaginal opening (something usually accompanied by tearing or "breeching" of the mother's vaginal tissues).

56. A *single limb presentation* birth
(a) is most commonly a foot presentation, with the infant in a breech position within the womb.
(b) cannot be delivered in the field. Position the patient supine with her head down and her pelvis (buttocks) elevated, and rapidly transport her to the emergency department.
(c) can be delivered in the field with the assistance of on-line medical direction.
(d) Answers (a) and (b).
(e) Answers (a) and (c).

57. Which of the following statements regarding multiple births (twins, triplets) is true?
(a) A multiple-birth delivery cannot be accomplished in the field. If the mother knows that there is more than one fetus to be delivered, position her on her left side with her legs tightly squeezed together and transport her with lights and sirens to the emergency department.
(b) Multiple-birth deliveries may require more than one infant resuscitation. Call for additional assistance as soon as you become aware that more than one fetus may be delivered and be prepared to transport the patient if the second (or third) infant has not delivered within 10 minutes of the previous one.
(c) Multiple-birth deliveries, although more time-consuming (commonly generating on-scene times well over an hour), are no different than single-birth deliveries. Simply coach the mother through each birth and proceed normally.
(d) All multiple-birth deliveries in the field will involve the death of at least one of the infants. Do not be upset by this and be prepared to counsel and support the mother when one (or more) of the infants is born dead.
(e) None of the above is true.

58. Amniotic fluid should be clear. If it is greenish or brownish-yellow, this indicates that

    (a) the fetus has expelled stool into the fluid prior to birth.

    (b) fetal distress (or maternal distress) may have occurred during labor.

    (c) the mother and the infant have an infectious disease. The EMT should employ full-body BSI precautions and notify the emergency department to prepare an isolation room.

    (d) Answers (a) or (b).

    (e) Answers (a), (b), or (c).

59. The medical term for amniotic fluid that is greenish or brownish-yellow is

    (a) mercromium or mercromium staining.

    (b) bile or bile staining.

    (c) meconium or meconium staining.

    (d) lymph or lymph staining.

    (e) micromium or micromium staining.

60. A premature birth is defined as any infant that weighs less than $5\frac{1}{2}$ pounds at birth or any infant born before the 37th week of pregnancy. Which of the following statements regarding premature newborns is false?

    (a) Premature newborns are always at risk for profound hypothermia; if the environment does not feel "too hot" to the EMT, it probably is not warm enough for the infant.

    (b) Suctioning of the premature infant's airway is particularly important. Keep the airway clear.

    (c) If supplemental oxygen should be administered via oxygen tubing, run at 10 to 15 lpm and directed across ("blow by"), not directly "at," the premature newborn's face.

    (d) Resuscitation is often required for premature infants and may be unsuccessful.

    (e) Premature infants require chest compressions at a rate twice as fast as full-term newborns but delivered at only half the depth to prevent injury.

61. Which of the following statements appropriately describe aspects of the condition called *placenta previa*?

    (1) This is caused by the placenta separating (partially or fully) from the wall of the uterus.

    (2) This is caused by the placenta developing abnormally low in the uterus, partially or completely covering the opening to the uterus.

    (3) This occurs when the placenta is undeveloped and unable to perform its functions (the mother's body is naturally ridding itself of a "defective" organ).

    (4) S/Sx often include vaginal bleeding without complaints of abdominal pain.

(5) S/Sx often include complaints of abdominal pain without vaginal bleeding.

(6) This is a life-threatening emergency for the unborn infant.

(7) This is a life-threatening emergency for the pregnant patient.

(a) 1, 5, 6, and 7.

(b) 2, 4, 6, and 7.

(c) 3, 4 or 5, 6, and 7.

(d) 1 or 2, 4 or 5, and 6.

(e) 1 or 2, 4 or 5, and 7.

62. Which of question number 61's numbered statements describe aspects of the condition called *abruptio placentae?*

(a) 1, 5, 6, and 7.

(b) 2, 4, 6, and 7.

(c) 3, 4 or 5, 6, and 7.

(d) 1 or 2, 4 or 5, and 6.

(e) 1 or 2, 4 or 5, and 7.

63. When a pregnant woman is transported on her back, the weight of her enlarged uterus (containing the developing baby, the placenta, and the amniotic fluid) may compress the inferior vena cava and obstruct blood return to her heart. This obstruction causes classic signs and symptoms that include

(a) a severe headache.

(b) low blood pressure.

(c) the sensation of dizziness or lightheadedness.

(d) Answers (a) and (b).

(e) Answers (b) and (c).

64. Because the inferior vena cava lies behind the uterus, on the _____ side of midline, pregnant women should always be transported with the weight of the uterus shifted to the _____ side.

(a) right / left

(b) left / right

(c) right / right

(d) left / left

(e) right or left / left or right (blood vessel location differs in some women)

65. The condition caused by a uterus enlarged because of pregnancy obstructing the return of blood to the heart when the patient is transported flat on her back is called

(a) migraine positioning disorder.

(b) supine hypotensive syndrome.

(c) supine positioning disorder.

(d) migraine position syndrome.

(e) prebirth position syndrome.

66. Which of the following activities are appropriate to the EMT's care of a patient who reports having been sexually assaulted?

(1) Question the patient extensively about the assailant's physical description and appearance, documenting all nonmedically related information (information that may assist law enforcement in their crime investigation) in the first or last paragraph of your patient care report.

(2) Closely examine every sexual assault victim's genitals to determine if any trauma or bleeding is present or requires treatment.

(3) Do not handle the patient's clothing, and provide basic medical interventions only if the patient appears to be in serious physical shock.

(4) To provide the patient as much privacy as possible, avoid making conversation or engaging in eye contact while transporting the patient to the closest emergency department.

(5) Allow the patient time to bathe and use the toilet before transportation to the emergency department for a rape examination (this is the least you can do to provide support for an emotionally traumatized patient).

(6) Provide all standard medical assessments and treatments; however, you do not need to examine the genitalia of a patient with stable vital signs and no obvious indication of severe genital bleeding.

(7) Provide a gentle, but honest explanation for why you cannot allow the patient to wash, bathe, urinate, or change clothing prior to transportation.

    (a) 1, 2, and 4.
    (b) 1, 3, and 4.
    (c) 1, 4, 5, and 6.
    (d) 2, 4, 5, and 6.
    (e) 6 and 7.

67. A *stillborn* infant is best defined as a baby that
    (a) is delivered alive but dies within 24 hours of birth.
    (b) dies within the mother's womb several hours before delivery.
    (c) dies within the mother's womb several weeks before delivery.
    (d) Answers (a) or (b).
    (e) Answers (b) or (c).

68. A child is considered an *infant* until he has reached _____ of age.
    (a) 4 months
    (b) 6 months
    (c) 12 months
    (d) 18 months
    (e) 24 months

69.   A *toddler* is best defined as a child from the age of

    (a) 6 months to 2 years.

    (b) 1 to 3 years.

    (c) 18 months to 3 years.

    (d) 24 months to 2 years.

    (e) 2 to 5 years.

70.   A *preschooler* is best defined as a child from the age of

    (a) 3 to 6 years.

    (b) 2 to 8 years.

    (c) 5 to 9 years.

    (d) birth to 5 years (or 4 years, if born in the fall months).

    (e) 2 to 5 years.

71.   A *school-age child* is best defined as a child from the age of

    (a) 6 to 18 years.

    (b) 8 to 18 years.

    (c) 9 to 12 years.

    (d) 4 or 5 to 18 years.

    (e) 6 to 12 years.

72.   An *adolescent* is best defined as a child from the age of

    (a) 6 to 18 years.

    (b) 8 to 18 years.

    (c) 13 to 15 years.

    (d) 12 to 18 years.

    (e) 13 to 20 years.

73.   Respiratory assessment of the infant or child includes

    (a) noting chest expansion, symmetry, and effort of breathing.

    (b) observing for nasal flaring, stridor, crowing, or retractions.

    (c) listening for any noisy breathing, especially grunting.

    (d) Answers (a) and (b).

    (e) Answers (a), (b), and (c).

74.   The respiratory rate considered normal for an infant (not a newborn) at rest is
_____ breaths per minute.

    (a) 10 to 12

    (b) 12 to 20

    (c) 15 to 30

    (d) 20 to 30

    (e) 25 to 40

75. The respiratory rate considered normal for a 13-year-old adolescent at rest is
     _____ breaths per minute.
     (a) 10 to 12
     (b) 12 to 20
     (c) 15 to 30
     (d) 20 to 30
     (e) 25 to 40

76. The respiratory rate considered normal for a 6-year-old child at rest is _____
     breaths per minute.
     (a) 10 to 12
     (b) 12 to 20
     (c) 15 to 30
     (d) 20 to 30
     (e) 25 to 40

77. A child who requires artificial ventilation should be ventilated at a minimum rate of
     (a) 12 times per minute (one ventilation every 5 seconds).
     (b) 60 times per minute (one ventilation every second).
     (c) 15 times per minute (one ventilation every 4 seconds).
     (d) 30 times per minute (one ventilation every 2 seconds).
     (e) 20 times per minute (one ventilation every 3 seconds).

78. The pulse rate considered normal for an infant (not a newborn) at rest is
     _____ beats per minute.
     (a) 120 to 150
     (b) 100 to 120
     (c) 60 to 105
     (d) 70 to 110
     (e) 80 to 140

79. The pulse rate considered normal for a 13-year-old adolescent at rest is _____
     beats per minute.
     (a) 120 to 150
     (b) 100 to 120
     (c) 60 to 105
     (d) 70 to 110
     (e) 80 to 140

80. The pulse rate considered normal for a 6-year-old child at rest is _____ beats per minute.

  (a) 120 to 150
  (b) 100 to 120
  (c) 60 to 105
  (d) 70 to 110
  (e) 80 to 140

81. Obtaining the pediatric patient's blood pressure requires the availability and use of an appropriately sized blood pressure cuff. To accurately measure blood pressure, the blood pressure cuff must go all the way around the patient's arm (securely attaching to the available Velcro), and be wide enough to cover _____ length of the patient's upper arm (from shoulder to elbow).

  (a) one-fourth of the
  (b) two-thirds of the
  (c) one-half of the
  (d) three-fourths of the
  (e) the entire

82. According to National Standards, the EMT is required to obtain at least one prehospital blood pressure measurement for all patients who are

  (a) 12 years and older.
  (b) 8 years and older.
  (c) 3 years and older.
  (d) 1 year and older.
  (e) of any age (including infants).

83. There are special considerations to remember when assessing and treating the pediatric patient in respiratory distress. Which of the following special considerations is false?

  (a) Respiratory failure is the most frequent cause of cardiac arrest in infants and children.
  (b) Cyanosis is a late finding in children and indicates a critically ill patient.
  (c) Respiratory failure in pediatric patients is almost always due to a foreign body airway obstruction. Thus, EMT-Basics are not allowed to assist pediatric patients with inhaler use.
  (d) Indications and contraindications for EMT-assisted metered-dose inhaler usage are exactly the same for a pediatric patient as for an adult patient.
  (e) "Grunting" while breathing indicates a critically ill pediatric patient.

84. Which of the following statements indicates the correct protocol and dosage for EMT-assisted infant or child epinephrine auto-injector use?

(a) Assist with only one infant/child auto-injector use (0.15 mg of medication).

(b) If the patient has both respiratory distress and signs and symptoms of shock, assist with two simultaneous infant/child auto-injector uses (0.3 mg of medication, total).

(c) Assist with one infant/child auto-injector use (0.15 mg of medication), followed by another assisted injection (if ordered) every 5 minutes until the patient's injectors are all used or you arrive at the emergency department.

(d) If the patient has both respiratory distress and signs and symptoms of shock, assist with two simultaneous infant/child auto-injector uses (0.6 mg of medication) every 5 minutes until the patient's injectors are all used or you arrive at the emergency department.

(e) None of the above. Infants and children are not prescribed epinephrine auto-injectors.

85. The most common cause of seizure in an infant or child (especially between the ages of 6 months and 3 years) is

(a) hypoxia.

(b) high fever.

(c) poisoning.

(d) failure to take prescribed anticonvulsant (antiseizure) medication.

(e) excessive oxygen administration (most often caused by using a nonrebreather mask to treat children who don't need the extra oxygen).

86. Which of the following statements regarding pediatric seizures is true?

(a) Seizures in children who have a chronic seizure disorder and have been taking their medication as they are supposed to are rarely ever life-threatening. If no injury occurred during the "break through" seizure, emergency treatment and ambulance transportation are not needed. Reassure the parents and instruct them to call the child's pediatrician during regular office hours.

(b) All infants and children, no matter what their medical history, who have any kind of seizure (even a "febrile seizure") should be treated by the EMT as if the seizure indicates a life-threatening illness or hidden injury.

(c) Children with chronic seizure disorders may have very brief seizures (10 seconds to 3 minutes) or prolonged seizures (5 to 10 minutes), depending upon their individual history. If no injury occurred during the seizure, and a parent reports that the child's seizure was not of an unusual length, emergency treatment and ambulance transportation are not needed. Reassure the parents and instruct them to call the child's pediatrician during regular office hours.

(d) All of the above are true.

(e) Answers (a) and (c) are true.

87. Which of the following statements regarding treatment of the conscious pediatric patient who has been poisoned is true?
    (a) Administer oxygen and monitor vital signs closely.
    (b) Contact the Medical Director and report the poisoning substance.
    (c) Depending upon the poisoning substance, request orders to administer activated charcoal.
    (d) Answers (a) and (b) are true.
    (e) Answers (a), (b), and (c) are true.

88. Which of the following statements regarding treatment of the unconscious pediatric patient who has been poisoned is true?
    (a) Administer oxygen, artificial ventilations, and monitor vital signs closely.
    (b) Contact the Medical Director and report the poisoning substance.
    (c) Depending upon the poisoning substance, request orders to administer activated charcoal.
    (d) Answers (a) and (b) are true.
    (e) Answers (a), (b), and (c) are true.

89. Which of the following statements regarding pediatric fevers is false?
    (a) Fevers often accompany ear infections and common childhood diseases such as measles or chicken pox.
    (b) Fevers often accompany life-threatening diseases such as meningitis or epiglottitis.
    (c) A fever accompanied by a rash indicates a potentially life-threatening illness.
    (d) Fevers frequently cause pediatric dehydration and hypoglycemia.
    (e) It is normal for a fever to cause infants or children to have a seizure (in fact, this indicates that their body's defense mechanism against hyperthermia is functioning properly). If no injury occurred during the "febrile seizure," emergency treatment and ambulance transportation are not needed. Reassure the parents and instruct them to call the child's pediatrician during regular office hours.

90. Which of the following statements regarding pediatric patients in shock is false?
    (a) Pediatric shock most often occurs because of cardiac failure (children will successfully compensate for all other shock causes until their heart "gives out").
    (b) It takes very little blood or fluid loss to produce shock in a pediatric patient.
    (c) Vomiting or diarrhea may quickly dehydrate the pediatric patient and result in shock.
    (d) Because children have strong, resilient bodies and can compensate for shock far longer than adults can, they may appear "fine," even when they are in the initial stage of shock.
    (e) Once pediatric patients reach the point where they are no longer able to compensate for a cause of shock, they deteriorate much more rapidly than an adult (they "crash").

91. *Sudden infant death syndrome* (SIDS) is caused by
  (a) child abuse (often due to hidden injuries without external signs of abuse).
  (b) external suffocation, either purposefully (by parents) or accidentally (by bed covers).
  (c) aspiration of vomitus and subsequent suffocation during sleep.
  (d) Answers (b) or (c).
  (e) None of the above.

92. Emergency care for the SIDS patient includes all of the following, except
  (a) performing all resuscitation methods for suspected SIDS babies, unless the child has rigor mortis (a stiff, cold body in a warm environment).
  (b) avoiding any comments that might suggest blame to the parents.
  (c) reassuring the parents that SIDS occurs to apparently healthy babies, without any warning.
  (d) ensuring that the parents will receive emotional support and counseling.
  (e) the mandatory completion of a "suspected child abuse" report.

93. Which of the following statements regarding pediatric trauma is false?
  (a) Trauma is the second leading cause of death in infants and children (idiopathic respiratory failure being the most common cause of pediatric death).
  (b) Blunt trauma is the most common lethal pediatric trauma mechanism.
  (c) Pediatric respiratory arrest is common secondary to head injuries and may occur during transport.
  (d) The most common cause of hypoxia in the unconscious pediatric head injury patient is obstruction of the airway by the tongue.
  (e) Sand bags should never be used to stabilize a pediatric trauma patient's head.

94. Which of the following statements regarding pediatric trauma is false?
  (a) Because children have very soft, pliable ribs, they may have significant internal chest injuries without any external signs.
  (b) The abdomen is a more common site of injury in children than in adults.
  (c) Always consider hidden abdominal injury in the pediatric trauma patient who is deteriorating without external signs of serious injury.
  (d) Children have very flexible bones and are often frightened by splinting techniques. Therefore, only apply splints to extremities with obvious deformities (simple pain and swelling is not an indication for splinting in the pediatric patient).
  (e) Pneumatic antishock garments (PASGs) should only be used if they fit the pediatric patient. Never place both legs of a child inside an adult PASG leg section.

95. Possible child abuse signs and symptoms include all of the following, except
  (a) multiple bruises in various stages of healing.
  (b) an injury that doesn't seem to fit the mechanism described by the parent or caretaker.

    (c) repeated calls to the same address.

    (d) a parent or caretaker who acts unusually concerned about a seemingly innocent injury.

    (e) a parent or caretaker who appears angry that the child is "always falling down or getting hurt!"

96.   Possible child neglect signs and symptoms include

    (a) the absence of adult supervision.

    (b) a child who appears malnourished.

    (c) a living environment that appears unsafe.

    (d) Answers (b) and (c).

    (e) Answers (a), (b), and (c).

97.   Which of the following statements regarding EMT actions, when suspicious of child abuse or neglect, is false?

    (a) Report your suspicions that abuse or neglect is involved to the emergency department staff.

    (b) Clearly document your suspicion that the child was abused or neglected on the patient care report. In this way, more attention will be paid to your assessment of the child's situation, and you will not be accused of "missing" the signs of abuse or neglect.

    (c) Avoid accusing or confronting any parties you suspect of child abuse or neglect.

    (d) Document only your objective findings (what you saw, heard, and so on) on the patient care report. Do not officially document your suspicion of child abuse or neglect.

    (e) If you have any suspicion of child abuse or neglect, transport the child to the emergency department (even when the injuries do not warrant ambulance transport).

98.   When communicating with any-aged patient who has suffered a hearing loss (or is completely deaf) in one ear, the EMT should

    (a) shout all questions as loudly as possible, to ensure that the patient hears them and feels less embarrassed about having a hearing deficit.

    (b) assume a position where the patient can see the EMT while she or he speaks; patients with hearing deficits often rely upon watching lip movement in order to "hear" better.

    (c) determine which ear has suffered a hearing loss, and assume a position closest to the patient's "good" ear, so that the patient is better able to hear the EMT's questions.

    (d) Answers (b) and (c).

    (e) Answers (a), (b), and (c).

99.   Which of the following statements regarding geriatric (elderly) patient special considerations is false?

   (a) The EMT's index of medical- or trauma-suspicion when assessing a geriatric patient should be exactly the same when assessing a young adult patient. Suspecting someone of having a greater potential for illness or injury simply by virtue of their age is a form of discrimination and is illegal (in addition to being medically inappropriate).

   (b) Because even "healthy" adults over the age of 65 naturally have a greater risk of suffering from heart disease and hypertension, the EMT's index of suspicion for these emergencies should be increased when assessing an elderly individual.

   (c) Elderly patients are more prone to falls and suffer greater injury from minor falls than do younger adults.

   (d) Elderly patients are more prone than younger adults to suffering hypo- or hyperthermia emergencies due to small changes in environmental temperatures.

   (e) Elderly individuals are more prone to suffering from accidental prescription medication overdose (because they get confused or forgetful), or serious side effects from adverse prescription medication interactions (because they have so many medications), than are younger adults.

100. Which of the following statements regarding geriatric trauma patient assessment considerations is false?

   (a) All geriatric patients are acutely sensitive to pain. Thus, when an elderly trauma patient denies pain in an area that does not appear injured, the EMT can reasonably be sure that no injury exists there, in spite of what the MOI may indicate.

   (b) Elderly persons may suffer falls caused by a spontaneous fracture of one or more brittle bones. Thus, they may be suffering from a fall-causing fracture, as well as one or more fall-caused fractures.

   (c) Because of brittle bones, geriatric patients are more prone to incurring fractures from lesser MOIs than are younger adults.

   (d) Geriatric patients may suffer traumatic injuries due to falls caused by a medical problem. Thus, all geriatric trauma patients must also be thoroughly assessed for acute medical problems.

   (e) Although geriatric patients are prone to complaining of being cold when the environment they are in is warm, always consider hypothermia as an additional factor when assessing any geriatric trauma patient who has been "down" in a warm environment for a prolonged period of time.

101. An altered level of consciousness (altered mental status) may be caused by a "stroke." The medical term for a stroke is abbreviated CVA, which stands for

   (a) cardiovascular accident.
   (b) cerebral vascular accident.
   (c) cardiovertebral accident.
   (d) cerebro-volume accident.
   (e) cranial vault accident.

102. A CVA may be caused by
  (a) brain tissue bleeding due to head trauma.
  (b) a blocked artery in the brain (from a fat or plaque emboli, or a blood clot).
  (c) a ruptured artery in the brain.
  (d) Answers (b) or (c).
  (e) Answers (a), (b), or (c).

103. Which of the following are possible signs and symptoms of a CVA?

  (1) Headache
  (2) Seizure activity
  (3) Slurred speech
  (4) Hemiparesis
  (5) Hypertension
  (6) Loss of consciousness
  (7) Nausea or vomiting
  (8) Bowel or bladder incontinence
  (9) Numbness or weakness on one side of the body

  (10) Dyspnea
  (11) Dizziness
  (12) Confusion
  (13) Paraplegia
  (14) Unequal pupils
  (15) Unilateral vision loss

  (a) 1, 2, 3, 4, 5, 6, 7, 8, 9, 10, 11, 12, 14, and 15.
  (b) 2, 3, 4, 5, 9, 11, 12, 14, and 15.
  (c) 3, 4, 5, 9, 11, 12, 14, and 15.
  (d) 3, 6, 8, 9, 10, 11, 12, 14, and 15.
  (e) 1, 2, 5, 9, 11, 12, 13, and 14.

104. Patients of any age may have a spinal column alignment abnormality. (For instance, a condition called *scoliosis* is when the spinal column curves left and/or right from midline, and may be present at birth.) Any patient with a spinal column alignment abnormality must be spinally immobilized with padding provided to avoid stressing the patient's "normal" spinal alignment. Geriatric patients with osteoporosis (or after a lifetime of poor posture) may have a spinal column curvature abnormality commonly referred to as a "hump back" or "hunch back." The medical term for this kind of spinal curvature is
  (a) thoracic hypertrophy.
  (b) humphosis.
  (c) kyphosis.
  (d) lordosis.
  (e) a sacral spine curvature.

105. The medical term for the spinal column curvature abnormality commonly referred to as a "sway back" is
  (a) thoracic hypertrophy.
  (b) inverted humphosis.
  (c) kyphosis.
  (d) lordosis.
  (e) a sacral spine curvature.

The answer key for Test Section Seven is on page 355.

8

DOT Module Seven: Operations

Subjects:

- Ambulance Operation
- Scene Operations
- Rescue Operations
- Hazardous Materials Incident Management
- Multiple-Casualty Incident Management
- Infectious Diseases

Test Section Eight consists of 60 questions and is allotted 1 hour for completion.

1. When operating an emergency vehicle with lights and sirens engaged,
    (a) the emergency vehicle driver is just as liable as any other motorist for the occurrence of accidents due to negligent driving practices.
    (b) if an accident occurs because another motorist failed to yield the right-of-way to the emergency vehicle, the motorist will be found at fault.
    (c) flashing red signals may be ignored.
    (d) red stop signals may be ignored.
    (e) stop signs may be ignored.

2. When operating with lights and sirens engaged, the emergency vehicle
    (a) may exceed the posted speed limit without any liability.
    (b) does not need to signal turns.
    (c) may pass other vehicles without signaling or "clearing" the passing lane.
    (d) may pass an off-loading school bus even when its red warning lights are blinking.
    (e) may disregard regulations governing direction of travel (may drive east-bound in a west-bound lane of traffic), but only if using proper caution and a regard for the safety of others.

3. When operating without lights and sirens engaged, the emergency vehicle
    (a) may exceed the posted speed limit without any liability.
    (b) does not need to signal turns.
    (c) may park anywhere, including in a lane of traffic, as long as personal property or lives are not threatened.
    (d) must follow every traffic rule and regulation that any other vehicle is subject to.
    (e) must follow only the traffic rules and regulations that apply to vehicles equipped with lights and sirens.

4. Which of the following statements regarding the use of sirens is false?
    (a) Some states require the use of sirens anytime an emergency vehicle is traveling with its emergency lights engaged.
    (b) Studies have shown that the longer a siren is sounded (especially in one sound pattern) the more likely it is that motorists will hear it and yield the right-of-way.
    (c) An ill or injured patient may experience increased anxiety and discomfort when transported with lights and sirens in continuous use.
    (d) Use of sirens may cause hearing loss for the unprotected emergency vehicle operator.
    (e) Emergency vehicle operators may be unaware that they tend to increase their speed of travel the longer their siren is sounded.

5. Which of the following statements regarding the use of lights and sirens is false?

(a) Some states require that an emergency vehicle must come to a complete stop at a red stop light or stop sign before proceeding through the intersection, even when using lights and sirens.

(b) After determining that all other motorists are yielding the right-of-way, some states allow an emergency vehicle, using lights and sirens, to proceed through the intersection without coming to a full stop (having only slowed for a red stop light or stop sign).

(c) Most states require that lights and sirens only be used for situations that threaten life or limb, and then only with due regard for public safety.

(d) In any state, if an emergency vehicle operator does not drive with due regard for the safety of others, the operator may be ticketed, sued, or even incarcerated.

(e) Even if not required by law, it is best to always have the siren engaged when traveling with emergency lights engaged, and to avoid altering siren-sound patterns.

6. Which of the following statements regarding the use of sirens is false?

(a) Modern-day sirens are specifically designed to penetrate buildings, dense shrubbery, and civilian vehicle soundproofing.

(b) Even when they can hear them, motorists may ignore emergency vehicle sirens.

(c) Motorists listening to loud radios or car stereos may not hear a siren.

(d) Be prepared for motorists to panic when they hear the siren.

(e) If the siren must constantly be used when traveling with emergency lights engaged, it is best to periodically alter the siren-sound pattern.

7. The faster an emergency vehicle travels,

(a) the more likely it is to be involved in a collision.

(b) the greater the distance required to stop.

(c) the more lives will be saved.

(d) Answers (a) and (b).

(e) Answers (a), (b), and (c).

8. When responding to an emergency through city streets, a police escort should be used

(a) during rush hours, when traffic is most congested.

(b) when responding to a call where CPR is in progress.

(c) only when absolutely necessary (such as when you are unfamiliar with the area where the call is located).

(d) Answers (a) and (b).

(e) Answers (a), (b), and (c).

9.   When following an emergency police escort through city streets, you should
   (a) turn off the ambulance siren, so that motorists are not confused by two different sirens.
   (b) keep the ambulance siren exactly the same as that used by the police escort, so that motorists are not confused by two different sirens.
   (c) stay at least one block behind the escort vehicle so that motorists realize there are two emergency vehicles approaching.
   (d) follow the escort as closely as possible, so that motorists cannot pull in between your vehicle and the police vehicle.
   (e) be aware that following an escort vehicle is an extremely hazardous endeavor, and be even more cautious than you normally would be before you follow the escort vehicle through any intersection.

10.   Collisions involving emergency vehicles most commonly occur
   (a) within 5 blocks of quarters.
   (b) in a parking lot.
   (c) at an intersection.
   (d) when traveling a busy, grid-locked city street.
   (e) when traveling a busy, grid-locked interstate highway.

11.   Duties of the EMT who is not trained in rescue or extrication techniques include all of the following, except
   (a) assessment and administration of necessary care to the patient before and during extrication, only if the patient can be safely accessed.
   (b) assuring that the patient is removed in a manner that will not unnecessarily cause further injury.
   (c) directing the efforts of all rescue and extrication personnel.
   (d) cooperation with the activities of the rescue or extrication personnel.
   (e) assuring that the activities of rescue or extrication personnel do not interfere with patient safety and care.

12.   Duties of the EMT who is also trained in rescue or extrication techniques include
   (a) first assuring that at least one EMS-provider will be focusing on the patient's needs prior to beginning rescue or extrication (establishing assigned duties).
   (b) assuring that patient care precedes extrication unless delayed movement would endanger the life of the patient or other rescuers.
   (c) assuring that the activities of rescue or extrication personnel do not interfere with patient safety and care.
   (d) Answers (a) and (b).
   (e) Answers (a), (b), and (c).

13.   The first priority for all EMS, rescue, and extrication personnel is
   (a) patient safety and appropriate care.
   (b) personal protection and safety of other team members.

    (c) implementing cervical spine precautions for the patient.

    (d) gaining access at any cost.

    (e) representing the service well when being filmed by news crews.

14. The second priority for all EMS, rescue, and extrication personnel is

    (a) patient safety and appropriate care.

    (b) personal protection and safety of other team members.

    (c) implementing cervical spine precautions for the patient.

    (d) gaining access at any cost.

    (e) representing the service well when being filmed by news crews.

15. The EMT who is untrained in rescue or extrication operation may

    (a) engage in simple access rescue techniques (ones that do not pose a danger to the EMT and do not require special training or equipment to accomplish).

    (b) engage in complex access rescue techniques if the patient is in life threat and the required special equipment is available (like public AEDs, almost all rescue devices have directions printed on them).

    (c) direct the activities of the other rescue/extrication personnel (as "medical officer," the EMT is in command of any scene that involves injury or illness).

    (d) Answers (a) and (b).

    (e) Answers (a), (b), and (c).

16. You are dispatched to a vehicle collision that is blocking one lane of the roadway. Your ambulance is equipped with 7 reflective, orange emergency cones. On your arrival you see that a law enforcement vehicle has already strategically parked and set up emergency cones between the collided vehicles and the flow of oncoming traffic in that lane. You should park your vehicle

    (a) inside the law enforcement emergency cones already placed across the accident-blocked lane and engage your vehicle's rear warning flashers (you will not need to use your cones).

    (b) beyond the accident site, in the accident-blocked lane or on the shoulder adjacent to the blocked lane, so that the law enforcement and collided vehicles are between the flow of that lane's oncoming traffic and the back of your vehicle, and engage your vehicle's rear warning flashers (you will not need to use your cones).

    (c) in the lane immediately next to the law-enforcement and accident-blocked lane, so that two lanes are closed and scene operation safety is fully ensured; then, set up all 7 of your emergency cones across the second lane, between oncoming traffic and the back of your vehicle.

    (d) Answers (a) or (c), depending upon personal preference.

    (e) Answers (b) or (c), depending upon personal preference.

17. You are dispatched to a vehicle collision that is blocking one lane of the roadway. Your ambulance is equipped with 7 reflective, orange emergency cones. If yours is the first emergency vehicle to arrive on scene, you should park your vehicle

   (a) in the accident-blocked lane, between the collided vehicles and the flow of oncoming traffic; then, engage your vehicle's rear warning flashers and set up all 7 emergency cones between oncoming traffic and the back of your vehicle.

   (b) beyond the accident site, in the accident-blocked lane or on the shoulder adjacent to the blocked lane, so that the collided vehicles are between the flow of that lane's oncoming traffic and the back of your vehicle; then, set up all 7 emergency cones between oncoming traffic and the collided vehicles.

   (c) in the lane immediately next to the accident-blocked lane, so that two lanes are blocked and scene operation safety is fully ensured; then, set up all 7 emergency cones across both lanes, between oncoming traffic in the accident-blocked lane and the lane your vehicle is blocking.

   (d) Answers (a) or (c), depending upon personal preference.

   (e) Answers (b) or (c), depending upon personal preference.

18. When parking at the site of a vehicle collision that is blocking one lane of a roadway, you should

   (a) turn off your vehicle's headlights, unless your headlights are required to illuminate the accident scene.

   (b) engage your vehicle's warning flashers, in addition to keeping your vehicle's revolving beacon lights on.

   (c) engage your vehicle's warning flashers and turn your vehicle's revolving beacon lights off.

   (d) Answers (a) and (b).

   (e) Answers (a) and (c).

19. Which of the following statements about emergency removal of a patient to a safer location is false?

   (a) If danger of rescuer injury exists (in addition to risk of increased patient injury), and the danger cannot be alleviated, patient stabilization and spinal immobilization may be delayed until after removal to a safe area.

   (b) If the MOI suggests possible C-spine injury, the patient cannot be moved, under any circumstances, until after appropriately immobilized.

   (c) Patients in rising, swift-running water will require extrication before they can be spinally immobilized.

   (d) Patients being assessed in a vehicle that suddenly catches fire may be rapidly removed before they are spinally immobilized.

   (e) Patients being assessed in a building that begins to collapse may be rapidly removed before they are spinally immobilized.

20.   You arrive on the scene where a small passenger car has struck a utility pole. Your scene size-up reveals that there is a sparking electrical line lying across the hood of the car. The vehicle's driver is visibly unconscious, and gurgling respirations are audible. You should immediately
   (a) access the patient, provide C-spine control, perform a jaw-thrust airway maneuver, and assess his airway.
   (b) use rapid extrication techniques to carefully remove the patient from the car without touching any metal surfaces.
   (c) summon the utility company to immediately respond to the scene and wait for their arrival before accessing the patient.
   (d) attempt to rouse the patient without touching any metal.
   (e) use rubber gloves to gain access to the gear shift (avoiding body contact with any metal surfaces), place the vehicle in neutral, and roll it away from the live electrical line.

21.   Which of the following statements regarding the establishment of a helicopter landing zone (LZ) is false?
   (a) A 100-foot-square area (approximately 30 large steps on each side) is preferred for a safe LZ, but, during the daytime, a 60-foot-square LZ (19 or 20 large steps) is usually considered safe.
   (b) If one side of a divided highway (a highway with a median separating one or more lanes of common traffic-flow direction) will be used for the LZ, traffic only needs to be stopped in the lane(s) on the LZ-side of the median. (That's why an LZ should not be established in a median. If it was, you'd have to stop all lanes of traffic, on both sides.)
   (c) The LZ should be a minimum of 150 feet (50 yards) away from the collision site, so that noise and rotor wash will minimally affect those who are still in it.
   (d) A flat LZ is always preferred; however, a helicopter can land on a moderate slope or incline.
   (e) Even when landing on a perfectly flat LZ, a helicopter's main rotor blades can dip down to as low as 4 feet from the ground.

22.   Which of the following statements regarding LZ establishment is false?
   (a) Direct all unoccupied individuals to clear the LZ of all lightweight debris (paper, tree branches, garbage, folding chairs—whatever the rotor wash might cause to become airborne).
   (b) Mark at least the four corners of a daytime LZ with a highly visible device, such as an emergency cone, or a flag, or the like.
   (c) Mark at least the four corners of a nighttime LZ with a rotating beacon, or a flare (if there is no fire danger), or by positioning four vehicles just beyond each corner with their headlights on and directed into the center of the LZ.
   (d) A fifth marker should be placed on the up-wind side of either a daytime or a nighttime LZ, so that the pilot will be advised of the wind direction at the LZ.
   (e) Helicopter pilots do not want to be guided by ground personnel. Even if someone on scene is familiar with aeronautical guidance techniques, keep everyone at least 100 yards away from the LZ—otherwise, the pilot will not be able to safely land the helicopter.

23.   Which of the following statements regarding safe operational practices associated with helicopters is false?

(a) If an LZ's terrain is extremely dry or dusty, and a fire department vehicle is available, have the entire LZ's area lightly wetted down to prevent a huge dust cloud being created by the landing helicopter's rotor wash. (Be sure that the area is not turned into a mud wallow, however!)

(b) Never approach a helicopter until the pilot has signaled you to do so, and never go anywhere near the helicopter's tail rotor.

(c) After it lands, if the LZ area has a slight incline or slope, approach the helicopter from the uphill side, not the downhill side. (The main rotor blades of all helicopters remain horizontally stationary, and will be striking closest to the downhill side of a slope.)

(d) If you can't see the pilot as you approach the helicopter, the pilot can't see you, and you are approaching from the wrong place.

(e) Be sure that all loose clothing articles (blankets, hats, or the like) worn by the patient (and by all the care providers) are removed or secured prior to approaching the helicopter.

24.   The first emergency response team to arrive at a hazardous materials (HAZMAT) scene should establish zones of operation. The most dangerous HAZMAT zone is the one that includes the immediate area of the HAZMAT incident. This zone is called the _____ and is usually associated with the color _____.

(a) "hot" zone / black

(b) "hot" zone / red

(c) "cold" zone / black

(d) "cold" zone / red

(e) "cold" zone / blue

The following four questions pertain to the same scenario.

You and your crew have been dispatched to a "truck accident" on a north-/south-bound interstate highway. You are approaching from the south and the wind is blowing from the south. As you near the scene, you see some kind of a tanker truck on its side, in a grassy area about 10 or 15 feet east of the highway. Something that looks like smoke is seeping from the crumpled part of the tank.

25.   You should park your vehicle on the highway's shoulder, well out of traffic lanes

(a) and approximately 100 feet before reaching the highway area that is even with the accident site.

(b) and approximately 100 feet beyond the highway area that is even with the accident site.

(c) and no more than approximately 50 feet before reaching the highway area that is even with the accident site (you don't want to have to carry equipment farther than that).

(d) and no more than approximately 50 feet beyond the highway area that is even with the accident site (you don't want to have to carry equipment farther than that).

(e) at the highway area even with the accident site (the truck is far enough off the road for this parking area to be safe).

26. You and your crew are not trained in (or equipped for) HAZMAT handling. After parking your vehicle, your initial tasks include all of the following, except

(a) establishing a "safe zone," a "control zone," and a "danger zone."

(b) removing as many patients from the danger zone as possible, using rapid extrication techniques.

(c) attempting to identify the tanker contents from a safe distance.

(d) directing all bystanders away from the site (politely asking them to leave the area if they weren't involved in the accident).

(e) staying in the safe zone and radioing for appropriate support resources.

27. To identify the contents of the tanker truck, you should

(a) use binoculars to search for and read any hazardous material placard that is posted on the tank.

(b) interview the conscious driver in the safe zone (while another EMT is assessing and caring for him).

(c) search the overturned truck for the bill of lading or shipping papers, being careful to avoid the spill area.

(d) Answers (a) and (b).

(e) Answers (a), (b), and (c).

28. Although some studies show that vehicles are correctly placarded only 50 to 75% of the time, if you see a hazardous material placard, you may identify the indicated material by

(a) looking up the placard's numbers, shape, and/or colors in *Hazardous Materials, The Emergency Response Handbook*, if it is carried in your vehicle.

(b) having your dispatcher look up the placard's numbers, shape, and/or colors in *Hazardous Materials, The Emergency Response Handbook*, if the book is kept at dispatch.

(c) having your dispatcher call CHEMTREC, a 24-hour hotline number (800-424-9300), to report the placard's numbers, shape, and/or colors.

(d) Answers (a) or (b).

(e) Answers (a), (b), or (c).

29. A critical incident stress debriefing (CISD) is designed to assist EMS providers in dealing with stress following a critical incident. Critical incidents include calls that involve

(1) 3 or more casualties.   (4) the injury or suicide of an EMS worker.
(2) 5 or more casualties.   (5) an EMS worker causing civilian injury or death.
(3) 25 or more casualties.   (6) the injury or death of an infant or child.

(a) 1, 2, and 3.
(b) 2 and 3.
(c) 3.
(d) 2, 3, and 6.
(e) 1, 2, 3, 4, 5, and 6.

30. A multiple-casualty incident (MCI), sometimes called a multiple-casualty situation (MCS), is best defined as any incident, event, or situation

(a) that places a great demand on EMS equipment or personnel resources.
(b) involving 3 or more patients.
(c) involving 10 or more patients.
(d) involving 25 or more patients.
(e) involving 50 or more patients.

31. An incident management system is a system developed by local jurisdictions for planned and coordinated response to MCIs. This system should provide for

(a) orderly means of communication between other agencies and resources.
(b) a central means of coordinating multiple agencies and resources.
(c) the predetermined identification of one agency (usually the Sheriff's Department or State Patrol) to be considered "in command" of every MCI, regardless of its nature.
(d) Answers (a) and (b).
(e) Answers (a), (b), and (c).

32. You and your EMT partner are the first emergency responders to arrive on the scene of an obvious MCI. Your first duty is to

(a) begin counting the number of patients, so that the total number of victims is known, and a "false alarm" is not sounded.
(b) activate the MCI incident management system.
(c) begin clearing uninjured and uninvolved persons away from the scene so that an accurate count can be made.
(d) begin treating patients.
(e) establish a danger zone and a safe zone.

33. The process called *triage* comes from the French word that means,

(a) "to select."
(b) "determine the first."

    (c) "to sort."

    (d) "determine the worst."

    (e) "determine the best."

34. During an MCI, initial triage should be done in a manner that will

    (a) save the greatest number of lives possible, given the available resources.

    (b) quickly identify which patients require rapid treatment and transportation and which patients can wait.

    (c) rapidly determine the name, age, and address of each patient before confusion (or unconsciousness) prevents patient identification.

    (d) Answers (a) and (b).

    (e) Answers (a), (b), and (c).

35. The most widely recognized and utilized system of MCI triage is the START system. START is an acronym for

    (a) Safety Triage Assessment Removal Treatment.

    (b) Simple Treatment Assessment Removal Tag.

    (c) Safety Treatment Assessment Reporting Termination.

    (d) Simple Triage And Rapid Transport.

    (e) Scene Treatment And Rapid Transportation.

To answer the following four questions, consider this MCI scenario: A suspended second story walkway within a busy shopping mall has entirely collapsed, apparently because of structural instability. No other sections of the walkway remain suspended, so there is no danger of further collapse. At the time of its collapse, an unknown number of people were on or below the walkway.

36. The first step of the START triage system is to announce (using a bullhorn),

    (a) "If you can walk, get up and come to the ambulance behind me now, please." (If another landmark or location will be used as a "walking-wounded" collection point, order them to that point instead of "the ambulance behind me.")

    (b) "Everyone who is injured should hold up an arm or call for help, now!"

    (c) "If you are not injured, please leave the area now!"

    (d) "Everyone who is injured should stay where you are. We will come to you!"

    (e) None of the above. You should never order a group of injured people to do something. It would cause a mass panic and create more injuries.

37. As you begin your systematic MCI triage, the first patient you encounter is unconscious and apneic. Using the START triage system, you should immediately

    (a) tag the patient red (dead) and move on to search for viable patients.

    (b) tag the patient red (critical) and move on to find more viable patients.

    (c) tag the patient green (a "pass over," nonviable patient) and move on to search for viable patients.

    (d) check for a pulse before tagging the patient critical or dead.

    (e) open the patient's airway and assess for spontaneous return of breathing.

38.   The next patient you assess is unconscious, has an open airway with a respiratory rate of 30, with a weak and rapid pulse. You should immediately

   (a) remove the patient to the nearest ambulance and initiate definitive treatment.

   (b) initiate and maintain spinal immobilization, waiting until others can assume spinal immobilization and treatment before resuming your triage process.

   (c) tag the patient green (he's breathing, has a pulse, and can wait for additional treatment) and move on to the next victim.

   (d) initiate and provide all appropriate treatment for that victim, avoiding patient abandonment charges by forgoing further patient triage duties, and continue to provide treatment for that patient until his care is assumed by another EMT.

   (e) tag the patient red (critical), and move on to the next patient.

39.   You assess the next patient and determine that she is awake, has a respiratory rate of 28, with a rapid and bounding radial pulse. Your next START triage system step is to

   (a) ask her if her neck hurts.

   (b) ask her if her chest hurts.

   (c) tag her with a "black" tag (she is "critical" but "viable"), then move on to the next patient.

   (d) ask her to tell her name and write it on her forehead, then move on to the next patient.

   (e) assess her mental status before tagging her. ("Who is the president of the United States?")

40.   According to the START triage system, patients designated as being those of the highest priority for rapid treatment and ambulance transport are identified by a tag with _____ as the bottom color.

   (a) red

   (b) blue

   (c) yellow

   (d) green

   (e) black

41.   According to the START triage system, patients designated as being those who require treatment but do not require ambulance transportation (minor injury victims) are identified by a tag with _____ as the bottom color.

   (a) red

   (b) blue

   (c) yellow

   (d) green

   (e) black

42. Which of the following are *communicable* diseases?
(1) AIDS (acquired immune deficiency syndrome)
(2) Bacterial meningitis
(3) Chickenpox (varicella)
(4) German measles (rubella)
(5) Hepatitis
(6) Measles (rubeola)
(7) Mumps
(8) Pneumonia (bacterial)
(9) Pneumonia (viral)
(10) Staphylococcal skin infections ("staff" infections)
(11) Tuberculosis (TB)
(12) Whooping cough (pertussis)
(13) SARS (severe acute respiratory syndrome)

   (a) 1, 2, 3, 4, 5, 6, 7, 8, 9, 10, 11, 12, and 13.
   (b) 1, 4, 5, 7, 8, 10, 11, 12, and 13.
   (c) 1, 3, 4, 5, 8, 9, 11, and 13.
   (d) 1, 2, 4, 5, 9, 10, and 11.
   (e) 1, 5, and 11.

43. Body substance isolation (BSI) infection control precautions consist of
   (a) wearing protective equipment (contact barriers).
   (b) following mandated procedures for infection control.
   (c) obtaining vaccinations for specific diseases.
   (d) Answers (a) and (b).
   (e) Answers (a), (b), and (c).

44. Which of the following statements regarding BSI infection control precautions is true?
   (a) For every single patient an EMT encounters, every available BSI infection control precaution should be utilized.
   (b) Only moist (undried) body fluids present an infection risk. Once infectious fluids have dried, they no longer retain any form of infectious pathogen.
   (c) Any body fluid, whether dried or moist, should be considered to be "infectious" until proven otherwise.
   (d) Answers (a) and (b) are true.
   (e) Answers (a) and (c) are true.

45. _____ is an infectious disease that causes an inflammation of the liver.
   (a) AIDS
   (b) Bacterial Meningitis
   (c) Hepatitis
   (d) Staphylococcal skin infection ("Staff" infection)
   (e) Tuberculosis (TB)

46. AIDS can be transmitted by
   (a) blood transfusions of AIDS-infected blood.
   (b) blood contact (via open wounds or IV drug use) and unprotected sexual contact with an AIDS-infected person.
   (c) having any contact with the body surface or clothing of an AIDS-infected person.
   (d) Answers (a) and (b).
   (e) Answers (a), (b), and (c).

47. AIDS is caused by the
   (a) homosexual infected virus (HIV).
   (b) human immunodeficiency virus (HIV).
   (c) heroin intravenous virus (HIV).
   (d) homosexual intravenous virus (HIV).
   (e) human intravenous virus (HIV).

48. Which of the following statements regarding hepatitis is true?
   (a) Hepatitis can be contracted via any contact with the body surface or clothing of an infected person.
   (b) Hepatitis can be contracted via blood, stool, or other body fluids (both dried and moist).
   (c) Hepatitis can be contracted via moist blood, stool, or other body fluids. Once dried, the hepatitis virus is rendered inactive.
   (d) Answers (a) and (b) are true.
   (e) Answers (a) and (c) are true.

49. Which of the following statements regarding AIDS is true?
   (a) AIDS can be contracted via any contact with the body surface or clothing of an infected person.
   (b) AIDS is contracted via unprotected sexual contact or contact with AIDS-infected blood (both dried and moist).
   (c) AIDS is contracted via unprotected sexual contact or contact with AIDS-infected blood (moist blood only). Once dried, the AIDS virus is rendered inactive.
   (d) Answers (a) and (b) are true.
   (e) Answers (a) and (c) are true.

50. Which of the following statements regarding staphylococcal skin infections ("staff" infections) is true?
   (a) An EMT who has direct, unprotected contact with infected wounds may become infected with "staff."
   (b) An EMT who has direct, unprotected contact with infected sores may become infected with "staff."

(c) Any direct, unprotected contact with "staff"-contaminated objects may infect an EMT.

(d) Answers (a) and (b).

(e) Answers (a), (b), and (c).

51. Which of the following statements regarding tuberculosis (TB) is true?

(a) TB was eradicated in the late 1950s. Health care provider contraction of TB (from patients) is virtually unheard of in today's society.

(b) TB contraction by health care providers from patients is a rare event, especially since health care providers are routinely tested for the disease.

(c) TB is highly contagious, and TB cases have become more and more frequent since the late 1980s. Any patient with a cough should be suspected of having TB, until proven otherwise.

(d) Answers (a) and (b) are true.

(e) None of the above is true.

52. Human skin is

(a) a highly effective barrier against pathogen-caused infections, unless it is broken by a cut or opening.

(b) a very poor barrier against pathogen-caused infections. Any lethal pathogen can be absorbed though unbroken skin.

(c) only an effective barrier to viral pathogens (such as AIDS and hepatitis).

(d) Any of the above.

(e) None of the above.

53. Cross-infection caused by an EMT (or other health care provider) transferring one patient's pathogens to another patient is

(a) a complication that is virtually impossible, unless the contaminating pathogen remains moist.

(b) a serious concern that is best avoided by vigorous hand washing between every patient contact. BSI precautions, alone, will not always protect a health care provider's next patient from cross-infection.

(c) something that will happen, no matter what kind of precautions a health care provider takes. It is a risk that all patients must face when seeking emergency care.

(d) something that often occurs but is so easily remedied by administration of IV antibiotics that it is not a concern for health care providers in the emergency setting.

(e) something that is a serious concern for in-hospital care providers but does not apply to prehospital care providers.

54. Which of the following statements regarding mucous membranes is true?

    (a) Mucous membranes are present only in the mouth.

    (b) Mucous membranes are present only in the nose.

    (c) Mucous membranes cannot be crossed by infectious pathogens (they are the most effective barrier a person has, by virtue of the thickness of their secretions).

    (d) Mucous membranes are present in the mouth, the nose, and the eyes. They present an easy access for any sort of infectious pathogen.

    (e) Answers (a) and (c) are true.

55. Which of the following statements regarding direct (unprotected) mouth-to-mouth artificial respiration performance is true?

    (a) No EMT should ever have to perform direct mouth-to-mouth artificial respirations while on duty.

    (b) Every EMT, no matter what his certification level, must be prepared to perform direct mouth-to-mouth artificial respirations, whether on or off duty.

    (c) Only basic EMTs must be prepared to perform direct mouth-to-mouth artificial respirations while on duty. (Intermediate EMTs and paramedics may perform orotracheal intubation; thus they can always avoid performing mouth-to-mouth artificial respirations.)

    (d) All of the above are true.

    (e) None of the above is true.

56. Equipment and supplies that have been exposed to infectious pathogens

    (a) do not present a cross-contamination (or EMT-contamination) threat once their surface has dried.

    (b) should not be disposed of at the scene, whether they are moist or dry.

    (c) should not be reintroduced to the ambulance until after their surface has dried.

    (d) Answers (a) and (b).

    (e) Answers (a) and (c).

57. According to federal law, every employer of emergency health care providers must provide, free of charge to the employee,

    (a) personal protective equipment that does not allow blood or other infectious body fluid to pass through it.

    (b) the hepatitis B series of vaccinations.

    (c) education and training in the avoidance of infectious contact and procedures for infection control.

    (d) Answers (a) and (c). (Obtaining vaccinations is the responsibility of each individual employee.)

    (e) Answers (a), (b), and (c).

58. Immunizations are available against which of the following diseases?

    (a) Tetanus

    (b) Hepatitis-B

    (c) Tuberculosis

    (d) Answers (a) and (b).

    (e) Answers (a), (b), and (c).

59. Immunizations are available against which of the following diseases?

    (a) Chickenpox

    (b) Measles

    (c) Hepatitis-C

    (d) Answers (a) and (b).

    (e) Answers (a), (b), and (c).

60. Within one day of returning from overseas travel, your patient has developed a fever, a persistent dry cough, and serious difficulty breathing. Which of the following is a patient care practice that represents the best way to protect others from contracting what may be an airborne-droplet-transmitted infectious disease?

    (a) Immediately ensuring that you and your partner(s) each don a paper face mask and wear it during the entirety of your contact with the patient.

    (b) Immediately placing a paper face mask on the patient, so as to prevent him from ejecting airborne droplets into the environment, and being sure to advise the care providers to whom you deliver the patient of the potential for an airborne-droplet-transmitted illness.

    (c) Immediately giving each family member a paper face mask and ensuring that they are worn during all further contact with the patient.

    (d) Immediately administering high flow oxygen to the patient via a snugly fitted nonrebreather mask, and being sure to advise the care providers to whom you deliver the patient of the potential for an airborne-droplet-transmitted illness.

    (e) Answers (a), (b), and (c).

The answer key for Test Section Eight is on page 359.

9

Random-Ordered Questions

Questions from a Variety of DOT Modules

(A Nonelective Section)

AUTHOR'S NOTE: This section contains questions that are based upon DOT requirements but are not covered elsewhere in this text. Additionally, all previous test sections contained questions grouped together by subject relationship. However, actual tests often do not offer subject-associated groups of questions. Thus, this section offers you an opportunity to practice answering randomly ordered questions.

Subjects:

- Acute Abdomen
- Basic Life Support
- Drug and Alcohol Abuse
- Dual Lumen Airways
- Eye Injuries
- Glasgow Coma Scale, Revised Trauma Score, APGAR Score
- Head and Spine Injuries
- Inhaled and Injected Poisonings
- Medical Terminology

Test Section Nine consists of 135 questions and is allotted 2 hours and 15 minutes for completion.

1.   Anatomy is the study of
        (a) body structure.
        (b) body function.
        (c) body strength.
        (d) Answers (a), (b), or (c).
        (e) None of the above.

2.   The tough outer coat of the eye's globe is called the
        (a) epidermis.
        (b) cornea.
        (c) vitreous body.
        (d) orbit.
        (e) sclera.

3.   The compression-to-ventilation ratio 2 trained rescuers should perform for cardiopulmonary arrest victims aged 1 to 13 years old (puberty) is
        (a) 5:1 (1 ventilation for every 5 chest compressions).
        (b) 15:2 (2 ventilations for every 15 chest compressions).
        (c) 30:2 (2 ventilations for every 30 chest compressions).
        (d) 15:1 (1 ventilation for every 15 chest compressions).
        (e) 30:1 (1 ventilation for every 30 chest compressions).

4.   CPR chest compressions for an adult should be performed at a depth of
        (a) $\frac{1}{2}$ to 1 inch.
        (b) 1 to $1\frac{1}{2}$ inches.
        (c) $1\frac{1}{2}$ inches to 2 inches.
        (d) at least 2 inches.
        (e) $2\frac{1}{2}$ to 3 inches.

5.   A finding noted on only one side of the body (or only one side of a particular body region or part) may be called _____ finding.
        (a) a unilateral
        (b) a bilateral
        (c) a trilateral
        (d) a quadrilateral
        (e) an unusual

6.   You have been called by worried friends to assess a 25 y/o chronic alcoholic. He
        smells strongly of alcohol, has slurred speech, and staggers when he tries to walk.
        You notice a small abrasion on his upper left forehead. There is no swelling,
        deformity, or instability in that area, and you don't find any other obvious signs or
        symptoms of illness or injury. Although verbally abusive of everyone, he is not
        threatening himself or others. He knows who he is, where he is, and accurately
        identifies the day/date. He is refusing treatment and transport (Tx/Trans). Which
        of the following statements regarding this scenario is true?
        (a) Chronic alcoholics may suffer a serious subdural hematoma from even a
            relatively "minor" head injury. Although he is grossly AAOx3, you should not
            allow this adult to refuse Tx/Trans. You should summon police assistance
            and call your Medical Director to obtain orders for implementing involuntary
            Tx/Trans measures (including restraint application).
        (b) It is not illegal for an adult to drink or become intoxicated. Because this
            person has not committed a crime, does not demonstrate a clearly life-
            threatening injury or illness, and is grossly AAOx3, you cannot perform
            involuntary Tx/Trans measures.
        (c) Because his friends generated a 911 call, you have a contractual obligation to
            perform involuntary Tx/Trans measures, even though the patient does not
            appear seriously injured or ill and is technically competent to refuse
            Tx/Trans.
        (d) Until this person loses consciousness, you cannot perform involuntary
            Tx/Trans measures. Before leaving the scene, instruct his friends to call 911
            again when he passes out.
        (e) Before leaving the scene, instruct his friends to call the police and report this
            person as "disturbing the peace" (or the like). After he is arrested, the police can
            call you back and you'll then be able to perform involuntary Tx/Trans measures.

7.   Which position of the human body is referred to as the *anatomical position*?
        (a) Standing upright with arms outstretched above the head (thumbs out).
        (b) Lying prone with arms along the side of the body (thumbs pointing up).
        (c) Lying supine with arms outstretched above the head (thumbs in).
        (d) Any of the above.
        (e) None of the above.

8.   Which of the following statements regarding infant, child, or adult CPR
        performance by 2 rescuers after an advanced airway is in place, is false?
        (a) Chest compressions are no longer performed in cycles with interruptions to
            allow for ventilation.
        (b) The compressing rescuer should deliver compressions at a rate of at least 100
            per minute.
        (c) The ventilating rescuer should provide at least 8 to 10 breaths per minute.
        (d) The compressing rescuer should be replaced approximately every 2 minutes
            to prevent compressor fatigue and deterioration in quality and rate of
            compressions.
        (e) Having an advanced airway in place does not negate the need to provide
            periodic pauses in compressions to allow for effective ventilation.

9. Which of the following statements regarding the advantages of using a Pharyngeo-tracheal Lumen (PtL®) airway is false?

   (a) Because it can function whether its tube enters the esophagus or the trachea, the PtL® cannot be improperly placed.

   (b) Because the upper airway is sealed by the large pharyngeal cuff, a mask seal (to the face) is not required.

   (c) Unlike the Combitube®, once inserted into an unconscious patient and secured, the PtL® may remain in place even after the patient begins to regain consciousness.

   (d) The PtL® is especially helpful for airway control and ventilation of trauma patients because the head and neck do not need to be moved during insertion.

   (e) The large pharyngeal cuff helps prevent secretions or blood from the nasopharynx or mouth from entering the lower airway.

10. Any MOI that causes the head to be abruptly thrust backward will probably produce a _____ injury of the spine.

    (a) compression

    (b) hyperflexion

    (c) hyperextension

    (d) distraction

    (e) rotation

11. The *semi-Fowler's* position is best defined as when the patient

    (a) has his legs straight out or bent, with his upper body (torso and head) elevated at a 50 to 60 degree angle to his buttocks.

    (b) has his legs straight out or bent, with his upper body (torso and head) elevated at less than a 45 degree angle to his buttocks.

    (c) is lying prone with his feet elevated higher than his head.

    (d) is lying supine with his feet elevated higher than his head.

    (e) is lying on either his right or left side with his feet elevated higher than his head.

12. Which of the following statements regarding carbon monoxide (CO) inhalation poisoning is true?

    (a) CO is one of the most common causes of inhalation poisoning.

    (b) CO poisoning often produces flu-like symptoms and (like the flu) often causes multiple-patient situations.

    (c) CO has a distinctive odor (much like natural gas). Do not enter an area when you smell CO on approach.

    (d) Answers (a) and (b) are true.

    (e) Answers (a), (b), and (c) are true.

13. A person in the *prone* position is lying

(a) on his stomach.

(b) on his side.

(c) on the floor.

(d) on a bed with his head elevated 40 degrees.

(e) on his back.

14. Which of the following statements regarding the irrigation of a chemical burn to the eyes is true?

(a) You will probably have to hold the eye(s) open during irrigation unless the patient is able to do so and you have provided the patient with protective gloves.

(b) Especially when only one eye is contaminated, always irrigate from the medial aspect of the eye to the lateral aspect of the eye, being sure not to contaminate the other eye with water run-off.

(c) Especially when only one eye is contaminated, always irrigate from the lateral aspect of the eye to the medial aspect of the eye, being sure not to contaminate the other eye with water run-off.

(d) Answers (a) and (b) are true.

(e) Answers (a) and (c) are true.

15. The function of the _____ is to store bile, which aids in the digestion of fats.

(a) gallbladder

(b) liver

(c) kidneys

(d) pancreas

(e) duodenum

16. Which of the following best defines *lateral rotation*?

(a) Standing in an upright position and bending forward.

(b) To straighten a joint.

(c) To bend a joint.

(d) To turn a joint or limb away from the body's midline.

(e) To turn a joint or limb toward the body's midline.

17. Which of the following statements regarding use of a flow-restricted, oxygen-powered ventilation device (FROPVD) to deliver ventilations to a pediatric patient is false?

(a) Use of a standard FROPVD model for ventilation of pediatric patients is absolutely contraindicated.

(b) Pediatric FROPVD models are available but may only be used on pediatric patients if the EMT has been given special training in their use.

(c) Gastric distention is a common side effect of FROPVD use and may lead to regurgitation and aspiration of stomach contents.

(d) Simultaneous spinal immobilization is still required when ventilating a trauma patient with a FROPVD.

(e) FROPVDs are especially helpful for treating pediatric (or adult) chest trauma victims because positive-pressure ventilation always improves oxygen delivery.

18. When withdrawing from a substance the addicted abuser may suffer a condition called the *DTs*. "DTs" stands for
    (a) drunk tremors.
    (b) drug tremors.
    (c) delirium tremens.
    (d) drink and drug taker syndrome.
    (e) drug taker syndrome.

19. Which of the following statements regarding insertion steps for Combitube® and PtL® airways is false?
    (a) The distal end of the tube must be lubricated with a petroleum jelly product prior to insertion.
    (b) The patient should be hyperventilated for at least 2 minutes (at a rate of 24 ventilations per minute) prior to and following insertion.
    (c) Both cuffs should be inflated and checked for leaks prior to insertion.
    (d) Both cuffs must be inflated prior to determining where the tube has lodged (the esophagus or the trachea).
    (e) During the first ventilation, auscultate over the epigastrium first; if gurgling sounds are heard, immediately discontinue ventilating that tube.

20. Which of the following statements regarding the Revised Trauma Score (RTS) is true?
    (a) Use of the RTS assists in determining whether a patient should be transported to the closest emergency department, or to a trauma center.
    (b) Use of the RTS assists trauma centers in evaluating and improving the quality of care they provide to trauma patients.
    (c) Calculation of the RTS is a mandatory emergency care assessment step for every trauma patient who has an altered level of consciousness or an airway control problem, and care provision may need to be paused to accomplish RTS calculation prior to contacting the Medical Director or the receiving facility.
    (d) Answers (a) and (b) are true.
    (e) Answers (a), (b), and (c) are true.

21. Another term for the posterior surface of the body is the _____ surface.
    (a) dorsal
    (b) ventral
    (c) plantar
    (d) palmar
    (e) inguinal

TEST SECTION NINE   263

22.   Which of the following statements regarding situations in which a head trauma
       patient is wearing a helmet is false?
       (a) Effective spinal immobilization cannot be accomplished without removing the
            helmet.
       (b) If there are no indications of dyspnea or airway problems in an alert patient,
            and the helmet fits well (snugly), it is better to leave it on.
       (c) Even when using controlled and careful techniques, helmet removal may
            cause further cervical spine injury.
       (d) If the helmet has an unusual shape and interferes with effective spinal
            immobilization, it must be removed.
       (e) When a patient in cardiac arrest is wearing a helmet, it must be removed.

23.   Which of the following statements regarding injected poisons is true?
       (a) Bites from deer flies, horseflies, or gnats can be painful, but they do not
            transmit venom or poison, and will not cause allergic reactions or
            anaphylaxis.
       (b) Although they don't have stingers, spiders and ticks can bite and inject
            poison under the skin, which may cause allergic reactions or anaphylaxis.
       (c) Because they keep their stinger, individual bees can sting repeatedly. But
            individual yellow jackets, wasps, and hornets are able to sting someone only
            once. Unless a swarm is present, repeat injury (multiple stings) will not occur.
       (d) Answers (a) and (b) are true.
       (e) Answers (a) and (c) are true.

24.   The medical term *adduction* refers to
       (a) movement toward the body.
       (b) movement toward the head.
       (c) movement away from the body.
       (d) movement toward the feet.
       (e) movement toward the back.

25.   The white area of the eye is called the
       (a) iris.
       (b) cornea.
       (c) sclera.
       (d) pupil.
       (e) conjunctiva.

26.   Which of the following best defines *extension*?
       (a) Standing in an upright position and bending forward.
       (b) To straighten a joint.
       (c) To bend a joint.
       (d) To turn a joint or limb away from the body's midline.
       (e) To turn a joint or limb toward the body's midline.

27. Common signs and symptoms of *appendicitis* (inflammation of the appendix) include all of the following, except
    (a) abnormally increased appetite (polyphagia).
    (b) pain or cramping around the umbilicus.
    (c) low-grade fever and chills.
    (d) a rigid abdomen.
    (e) pain or cramping in the right lower quadrant of the abdomen.

28. For infant CPR, the chest should be compressed to a depth of at least
    (a) one third of the anterior-posterior diameter of the chest (1 $\frac{1}{2}$ inches).
    (b) two thirds of the anterior-posterior diameter of the chest (2 inches).
    (c) $\frac{1}{2}$ inch.
    (d) 1 inch.
    (e) Answer (b) or (d), depending upon local protocol.

29. Which of the following statements regarding the signs and symptoms commonly associated with substance abuse is true?
    (a) The "acetone breath" that accompanies hyperglycemic emergencies may be mistaken as an odor of alcohol on a person's breath or clothing and may be detected before the adult patient develops a demonstrably altered LOC.
    (b) When there are no apparent signs or symptoms of injury or illness, an adult with slurred speech and an unsteady gait, who clearly smells of alcohol, has simply had too much to drink. As long as the person is "AAOx3," you cannot treat or transport him against his will.
    (c) Any person demonstrating visual or auditory hallucinations has an altered LOC and can be treated and transported involuntarily, even if he knows who he is, where he is, and what the day/date is.
    (d) Answers (a) and (c) are true.
    (e) Answers (b) and (c) are true.

30. The use of a Combitube® is contraindicated for all of the following patients, except
    (a) a patient with a gag reflex prior to Combitube® ventilation (and if a gag reflex is regained after Combitube® ventilation, the tube must be removed).
    (b) a patient less than 5 feet tall.
    (c) a patient who has swallowed a caustic substance.
    (d) a patient with esophageal disease.
    (e) trauma patients (because Combitube® insertion requires slight hyperextension of the neck).

31. Another term for the anterior surface of the hand is the _____ surface.
    (a) dorsal
    (b) ventral
    (c) plantar
    (d) palmar
    (e) inguinal

32.   A trauma patient who is apneic and pulseless will have a Glasgow Coma Scale valuation of

(a) 9 points.
(b) 6 points.
(c) 3 points.
(d) 1 point.
(e) 0 points.

33.   Which of the following statements regarding situations when a trauma patient is wearing a helmet is false?

(a) If the patient complains of new or increased pain as you are removing the helmet, stop the removal and consider other options of immobilization with the helmet remaining in place.
(b) If the patient's head can move about within it, the helmet should be removed.
(c) If the patient complains of increased pain during removal of a loosely fitting helmet, discontinue removal and place padding between the patient's head and the helmet interior.
(d) If a helmet interferes with your ability to assess or manage an airway, it must be removed.
(e) When an alert football player without airway or breathing problems is wearing a helmet and full shoulder pads, and the helmet fits well (snugly), the shoulder pads must come off, but the helmet should be left in place.

34.   Which of the following signs and symptoms are common to most poisonous bites or stings?

(a) Pain, redness, and/or swelling at the site.
(b) Chills and/or fever.
(c) Nausea or vomiting, weakness and/or dizziness.
(d) Answers (a) and (c).
(e) Answers (a), (b), and (c).

35.   A patient should be considered to have a seriously high blood pressure when the _____ reading is greater than _____ mmHg (millimeters of mercury).

(a) systolic / 150
(b) diastolic / 90
(c) systolic / 120
(d) Answers (a) or (b).
(e) Answers (b) or (c).

36.   Which of the following best defines *medial rotation*?

(a) Standing in an upright position and bending backward.
(b) To straighten a joint.
(c) To bend a joint.
(d) To turn a joint or limb away from the body's midline.
(e) To turn a joint or limb toward the body's midline.

37. Which of the following statements regarding treatment of an eye with an object impaled in it is true?

    (a) If the patient is wearing contact lenses (soft or hard), the impaled eye's lens must be removed to avoid further injury.

    (b) Pad around the impaled object to stabilize it in place, being sure to allow the patient's unaffected eye to remain open and unimpaired (this is an important psychological comfort measure).

    (c) Pad around the impaled object to stabilize it in place, then be sure to bandage the uninjured eye closed.

    (d) Answers (a) and (b) are true.

    (e) Answers (a) and (c) are true.

38. The major functions of the _____ are to secrete hormones that regulate blood sugar levels and to release enzymes that assist in breaking down food in the small intestine.

    (a) gallbladder

    (b) liver

    (c) kidneys

    (d) pancreas

    (e) duodenum

39. You are off-duty and alone, without a cell phone, when you discover an 8-year-old in cardiopulmonary arrest. You'll have to leave to find a phone and summon assistance. You should

    (a) immediately leave to activate the EMS system, then return and begin CPR.

    (b) perform CPR for about two minutes before leaving to activate the EMS system.

    (c) perform CPR for at least five minutes before leaving to activate the EMS system.

    (d) immediately leave to activate the EMS system, and then wait until you've obtained at least one CPR assistant before returning to the patient.

    (e) immediately begin CPR and continue until someone else arrives or you are too exhausted to continue.

40. The standard "*shock position*" is best defined as when the patient

    (a) has his legs straight out or bent, with his upper body (torso and head) elevated at a 45 to 60 degree angle to his buttocks.

    (b) has his legs straight out or bent, with his upper body (torso and head) elevated at less than a 45 degree angle to his buttocks.

(c) is lying prone with his feet elevated higher than his head.

(d) is lying supine with his feet elevated higher than his head.

(e) is lying on either his right or left side with his feet elevated higher than his head.

41. Which of the following signs and symptoms may be exhibited by someone suffering from alcohol withdrawal?

(1) Seizures

(2) Extremity tremors

(3) Restlessness or anxiety

(4) Profuse diaphoresis

(5) Confusion

(6) Altered LOC

(7) Seriously unusual and agitated behaviors or comments

(8) Profound elation (extremely "happy" behavior or comments)

(9) Auditory or visual hallucinations

(10) Tactile hallucinations

    (a) 2, 3, 4, 5, 6, 7, 8, 9.

    (b) 1, 2, 3, 4, 5, 6, 7, 8, 9, 10.

    (c) 1, 2, 3, 4, 5, 6, 7, 9, 10.

    (d) 2, 3, 5, 6, 7, 8, 9, 10.

    (e) 2, 3, 6, 7, 8, 9, 10.

42. Which of the following statements regarding inflation of the various Combitube® and PtL® cuffs is false?

(a) Simultaneously inflate both of the PtL's cuffs by blowing a sustained breath into the main inflation valve (#1) until the pilot balloon inflates or resistance is met.

(b) Inflate the Combitube's large pharyngeal cuff by injecting approximately 100 cc of air into the #1 inflation valve.

(c) Inflate the PtL's large pharyngeal cuff first, by injecting approximately 250 cc of air, then inflate the tube's cuff with approximately 10 to 15 cc of air.

(d) Inflate the Combitube's distal (tube) cuff by injecting approximately 10 to 15 cc of air into the #2 inflation valve.

(e) If cuff-inflation resistance is met, but the inflation valve's pilot balloon has not inflated, the cuff may have a leak. Withdraw the air from both cuffs and remove the device.

43. The two "A"s of the APGAR mnemonic stand for

(a) Appearance (skin color) and Apnea (absent respirations).

(b) Activity (extremity movement) and Altered level of consciousness.

(c) Appearance (skin color) and Activity (extremity movement, muscle tone).

(d) Appearance (skin color) and Activity (heart rate).

(e) Activity (extremity movement, muscle tone) and Abnormality (presence of obvious congenital anomalies).

44. Which of the following statements regarding spinal immobilization using a child safety seat is true?

    (a) If the child has an altered level of consciousness, he must be removed from the safety seat and immobilized to a long backboard.

    (b) If your assessment reveals no need for immediate resuscitation measures, leave the child in the safety seat and secure pads around his body as needed, to ensure that movement within the seat is prevented.

    (c) To secure the seat-immobilized child to your stretcher, tip the seat backward so that the child is in a supine position. (This also puts the child in the "shock position" because his feet will be elevated.)

    (d) Answers (a) and (b) are true.

    (e) Answers (a), (b), and (c) are true.

45. Which of the following statements regarding emergency care of an insect sting when the stinger is still present is true?

    (a) Use tweezers or forceps (not your fingers) to pluck the stinger free as soon as possible (before additional poison is injected).

    (b) With gloves on and without touching the stinger, use your thumb and forefinger to squeeze the site from either side and expel the stinger. Wipe the loosened stinger from the site with a sterile 4 × 4. (Do not pick the stinger up with your fingers because it may penetrate your glove!)

    (c) Scrape the stinger from the site as soon as possible, using the edge of something like a credit card, ATM card, matchbook, or pocket knife.

    (d) Answers (a) and (b) are true.

    (e) None of the above is true. The stinger should be left in place (and the site dressed) until a physician can determine the appropriate removal technique.

46. Which of the following best defines *flexion*?

    (a) Standing in an upright position and bending backward.

    (b) To straighten a joint.

    (c) To bend a joint.

    (d) To turn a joint or limb away from the body's midline.

    (e) To turn a joint or limb toward the body's midline.

47. The _____ is the largest organ in the human body.

    (a) liver

    (b) right lung

    (c) small intestine

    (d) large intestine

    (e) skin

48. Assessment of the pupils with a penlight is performed to determine all of the following, except

(a) visual acuity.

(b) reactivity to light.

(c) pupil shape.

(d) pupil size.

(e) pupil equality.

49. Common signs and symptoms of an abdominal aortic aneurysm include all of the following, except

(a) severe, constant abdominal pain.

(b) complaint of a "ripping," "tearing," or "burning" pain in the lower back.

(c) periodic "sharp" or "stabbing" abdominal pain relieved by flexing the knees.

(d) an absent or decreased femoral pulse.

(e) a soft abdomen with a centralized, pulsating mass palpable.

50. Which of the following statements regarding anatomical and physiological pediatric airway considerations is false?

(a) Because infants and children have smaller respiratory system airway passages than adults, it takes less swelling to obstruct pediatric airways.

(b) Because the tongues of infants and children take up more space in the mouth than do adult tongues, it is easier for the pediatric airway to become obstructed by the tongue.

(c) An infant's or child's chest wall is softer, more pliant and elastic than an adult's. Thus infants and children rely upon their diaphragm to accomplish breathing less than adults do.

(d) Because the trachea is softer and narrower in infants and children, positioning for an open pediatric airway is different than positioning for an open adult airway.

(e) Because infants and children have smaller respiratory system airway passages than adults, it takes less secretions or bleeding to obstruct pediatric airways.

51. The best definition of the midclavicular line is an imaginary line drawn from the middle of either clavicle,

(a) down to the great toe on either side.

(b) down to the lowest margin of the anterior torso on the same side.

(c) diagonally across the chest to the umbilicus.

(d) Answers (a) or (b).

(e) Answers (a) or (c).

52.   Which of the following statements regarding withdrawal from alcohol addiction is false?

   (a) An alcoholic who is too sick to drink alcohol may go into withdrawal.

   (b) An alcoholic may go into withdrawal as soon as 12 to 24 hours after his last drink.

   (c) An alcoholic who elects to suddenly stop drinking should expect to suffer withdrawal.

   (d) Although it is an extremely painful, profoundly frightening, and psychologically debilitating experience, alcohol withdrawal is not a life-threatening condition.

   (e) Anyone who suffers a seizure suspected to be caused by alcohol withdrawal may have a seriously life-threatening condition.

53.   The use of a PtL® is contraindicated for all of the following patients, except

   (a) a patient with a gag reflex prior to PtL® ventilation (if a gag reflex is regained after PtL® ventilation, the tube must be removed).

   (b) a patient less than 5 feet tall.

   (c) a patient who has swallowed a caustic substance.

   (d) a patient with esophageal disease.

   (e) trauma patients (because PtL® insertion requires slight hyperextension of the neck).

54.   The maximum number of points available when evaluating a trauma patient's Revised Trauma Score (the best possible score) is

   (a) 15 points.

   (b) 13 points.

   (c) 12 points.

   (d) 10 points.

   (e) 9 points.

55.   When a patient's head receives a direct blow that causes brain injury at the site of the blow and also causes brain injury at the site opposite to the blow (from his brain rebounding and impacting his skull interior), this kind of injury is called

   (a) an acceleration–deceleration injury.

   (b) a coup-contrecoup injury.

   (c) a classic French concussion pattern.

   (d) a bilateral hematoma.

   (e) a contralateral hematoma.

56.   The best definition of the midaxillary line is an imaginary line drawn

   (a) horizontally, from armpit to armpit, across the chest.

   (b) diagonally, from one armpit to the opposite hip.

   (c) vertically, from the middle of one armpit to the lateral aspect of the ankle on
        the same side.
   (d) horizontally, from hip to hip, across the lower abdomen.
   (e) vertically, from the chin to the pubic bone.

57.   Which of the following statements describe appropriate emergency care measures
      for the treatment of stings or bites?
      (1) Apply constricting bands above and below any extremity bite or sting site
           that involves a joint.
      (2) Apply one constricting band between the extremity bite or sting site and the
           body.
      (3) Consult medical direction regarding the use of constricting bands for
           extremity injury sites.
      (4) Apply a cold pack to any insect sting or snakebite site (especially if it is a
           rattlesnake bite).
      (5) A cold pack should not be applied to marine animal stings.
      (6) Splint and elevate the injured extremity (above the level of the patient's
           heart) to diminish swelling and minimize spread of the venom into
           surrounding tissues.
         (a) 1, 3, 4, 5, and 6.
         (b) 2, 3, 4, 5, and 6.
         (c) 3, 4, 5, and 6.
         (d) 3 and 5.
         (e) 3 and 6.

58.   The medical term for the small, odd-looking, soft structure that hangs down from
      the roof of the posterior oropharynx is
         (a) the epiglottis.
         (b) an idiosyncratic anomaly (not everyone has one).
         (c) that "hangy-down-thingie."
         (d) the gag organ.
         (e) the uvula.

59.   Which of the following situations requires removal of the patient's contact lenses in
      the prehospital setting?
         (a) A chemical burn to the eye.
         (b) Blunt injury to the globe of the eye.
         (c) The eye is impaled with an object.
         (d) Answers (a) and (b).
         (e) Answers (a), (b), and (c).

60. Functions of the _____ include hydration regulation (retention or excretion of water), as well as regulation and maintenance of the body's electrolyte and acid-base balance.

    (a) gallbladder

    (b) liver

    (c) kidneys

    (d) pancreas

    (e) duodenum

61. The *apex* of an organ is best defined as it's

    (a) pointed portion.

    (b) superior portion.

    (c) inferior portion.

    (d) flat portion.

    (e) largest (usually rounded) portion.

62. Which of the following conditions may also cause the signs, symptoms, and unusual behaviors frequently associated with individuals who are intoxicated because of alcohol and/or drug abuse?

(1) Hypoglycemia	(9) Electrolyte imbalance
(2) Hyperglycemia	(10) Gastrointestinal bleeding
(3) Hyperthermia	(11) Communicable diseases
(4) Hypothermia	(12) Infections
(5) Seizure disorders	(13) Poisoning
(6) Stroke	(14) Head injury
(7) Fever	(15) Hypoxia
(8) Overdose	(16) Brain tumor

    (a) 1, 2, 3, 4, 5, 6, 7, 8, 9, 10, 11, 12, 13, 14, 15, and 16.

    (b) 1, 4, 5, 7, 8, 9, 12, 13, 14, 15, and 16.

    (c) 1, 2, 4, 5, 6, 8, 9, 10, 13, 14, 15, and 16.

    (d) 2, 3, 4, 5, 6, 8, 9, 10, 13, 14, 15, and 16.

    (e) 1, 3, 4, 5, 6, 7, 8, 13, 14, 15, and 16.

63. Once begun, BLS CPR must be continued until the patient spontaneously resumes circulation and breathing, or

    (a) ALS arrives and ALS CPR measures are performed.

    (b) until rigor mortis develops.

    (c) a physician orders that life support be discontinued.

    (d) Answers (a) or (c).

    (e) Answers (a), (b), or (c).

64. When 2 or more trained rescuers are available to perform CPR, the chest-compressor should switch roles with the ventilator, or be replaced by another chest-compressor, after performing

    (a) 1 minute of chest compression (approximately 5 cycles of CPR).

    (b) 2 minutes of chest compression (approximately 5 cycles of CPR).

    (c) 5 minutes of chest compression (approximately 15 cycles of CPR).

    (d) 10 minutes of chest compression.

    (e) 15 minutes of chest compression.

65. Which of the following statements regarding the advantages of using a Combitube® airway is false?

    (a) Because it can function whether its tube enters the esophagus or the trachea, the Combitube® cannot be improperly placed.

    (b) Because its pharyngeal cuff is self-adjusting and self-positioning (an advantage over the PtL®), a mask seal is not required.

    (c) Unlike the PtL®, once inserted into an unconscious patient and secured, the Combitube® may remain in place even after the patient begins to regain consciousness.

    (d) The Combitube® is especially helpful for airway control and ventilation of trauma patients because the head and neck do not need to be moved during insertion.

    (e) There is no stylet in the distal lumen of the Combitube's #2 tube, which allows for gastric content suctioning when esophageal placement occurs (another advantage over the PtL®).

66. The "P" of the APGAR mnemonic stands for

    (a) Pulse (heart rate).

    (b) Pupils (equal or unequal).

    (c) Pink (skin color).

    (d) Pallor (skin color).

    (e) Purple (cyanosis).

67. The tibia is _____ to the femur.

    (a) superior

    (b) medial

    (c) midline

    (d) inferior

    (e) lateral

68. _____ typically occurs in auto accidents (especially rear-impacts), when the patient's head comes to a sudden stop, but his brain continues to travel within the skull. The brain impacts the halted skull interior, then rebounds to also impact the opposite side of his skull interior, causing injury at two sites.

    (a) An acceleration–deceleration brain injury

    (b) A coup-contrecoup brain injury

    (c) A classic French concussion pattern

    (d) A bilateral cranial hematoma

    (e) A contralateral cranial hematoma

69. Which of the following statements describe appropriate emergency care measures for the treatment of stings or bites?

    (1) Gently cleanse the snakebite area with soap and water.

    (2) Do not stimulate a bite or sting site by cleansing it.

    (3) Contact the Medical Director to obtain an order for the application of an antidote salve or rinse to a bite or sting site.

    (4) Observe for signs and symptoms of allergic reaction (or anaphylaxis) and treat as directed.

    (5) Oxygen should be administered only if the patient is complaining of shortness of breath. (Altered vital signs may be present, but oxygen administration will not alleviate the effects of an extremity sting/bite, and will only increase patient anxiety or agitation.)

    (6) Splint a stung or bitten extremity and keep it positioned below the level of the patient's heart.

    (7) Remove all jewelry from beyond the injured area.

        (a) 1, 4, 6, and 7.

        (b) 2, 4, and 5.

        (c) 1, 3, 4, and 5.

        (d) 2, 3, 4, 5, and 7.

        (e) 2, 3, 4, 5, 6, and 7.

70. The best definition of the midscapular line is an imaginary line drawn from the middle of either scapula,

    (a) down to the heel on either side.

    (b) down to the lowest margin of the posterior torso on the same side.

    (c) across to the other scapula.

    (d) Answers (a) or (b).

    (e) Answers (a) or (c).

71. Which of the following statements regarding effective adult chest-compression performance is false?

    (a) For chest compression to achieve effective artificial blood flow, the chest must be depressed at least 2 inches (5 cm).

    (b) If EMS providers fail to compress the chest deep enough, effective artificial blood flow will not be achieved.

(c) The AHA recommendation for effective chest compression is "Push Hard and Push Fast."

(d) Allowing the chest to completely "recoil" (return to its original position) after each compression is contraindicated because it causes lower intrathoracic pressures and decreases coronary perfusion.

(e) Chest compressions should be delivered at a rate of at least 100 per minute.

72. The cranium is _____ to the spine.
   (a) superior
   (b) medial
   (c) midline
   (d) inferior
   (e) lateral

73. Among several other functions, the _____ filters and detoxifies the blood, is a major site of glucose (sugar) storage, and aids in the production of bile for fat digestion.
   (a) gallbladder
   (b) liver
   (c) kidneys
   (d) pancreas
   (e) duodenum

74. CPR chest compressions for children 1 to 8 years old should be performed with enough force to cause the child's sternum to descend a distance of
   (a) only $\frac{1}{2}$ to 1 inch ("less is more" when it comes to compressing pediatric chests).
   (b) at least $\frac{1}{3}$ of the child's anterior-posterior chest diameter (2 inches).
   (c) approximately $\frac{1}{2}$ of the child's anterior-posterior chest diameter (7 centimeters).
   (d) Answers (a) or (b), depending upon local protocol.
   (e) Answers (a) or (c), depending upon local protocol.

75. The maximum number of points available when evaluating a trauma patient's Glasgow Coma Scale (the best possible score) is
   (a) 25 points.
   (b) 15 points.
   (c) 13 points.
   (d) 12 points.
   (e) 10 points.

76. Which of the following statements regarding brain injuries that occur due to circumstances unrelated to trauma is false?

 (a) Nontraumatic brain injuries rarely produce the same symptoms as traumatic brain injuries.

 (b) Brain injuries may occur because of blood clots becoming lodged within the brain.

 (c) Brain injuries may occur because of blood vessels becoming weakened, breaking and hemorrhaging within the brain.

 (d) Nontraumatic brain injuries can cause an altered level of consciousness.

 (e) Lack of oxygen (hypoxia) can cause symptomatic brain injury.

77. The great toe is on the _____ side of the foot.

 (a) superior

 (b) medial

 (c) midline

 (d) inferior

 (e) lateral

78. Which of the following statements regarding CO inhalation poisoning is false?

 (a) Cherry red lips or skin and complaint of a headache are the earliest signs and symptoms exhibited by a CO poisoning victim.

 (b) Blue lips or skin color (cyanosis) can be a sign of CO poisoning.

 (c) CO poisoning will cause falsely high pulse oximeter readings.

 (d) An altered level of consciousness is a very early sign of CO poisoning, but it may go unnoticed by the victim or other persons present (who are also probably suffering from CO poisoning).

 (e) Early signs of CO poisoning include isolated or combined complaints of dizziness, weakness, dyspnea, nausea, or vomiting.

79. Another term for the inferior surface of the foot is the _____ surface.

 (a) dorsal

 (b) ventral

 (c) plantar

 (d) palmar

 (e) inguinal

80. A child who has a pulse but is in respiratory arrest should be ventilated at a rate of

 (a) 12 to 20 times per minute (ventilate once every 3 seconds).

 (b) 60 times per minute (ventilate once per second).

 (c) 10 times per minute (ventilate once every 6 seconds).

 (d) 30 times per minute (ventilate once every 2 seconds).

 (e) 120 times per minute (ventilate twice per second).

81.   A _____ injury of the spine is often produced by a hanging mechanism of injury.

    (a) compression

    (b) hyperflexion

    (c) hyperextension

    (d) distraction

    (e) rotation

82.   Which of the following statements regarding basic rules for the care of any eye injury is true?

    (a) If an injured eye is swollen shut, do not force the lid open unless irrigation for the removal of chemicals is required.

    (b) Every patient with an eye injury requires emergency department evaluation.

    (c) When only one eye is injured, it is important to the patient's psychological well-being to allow the uninjured eye to remain open after bandaging the injured eye (you should never "blind" an eye-injured patient).

    (d) Answers (a) and (b) are true.

    (e) Answers (a), (b), and (c) are true.

83.   Under which of the following circumstances should CPR not be initiated?

    (a) The presence of obvious mortal wounds such as decapitation or incineration.

    (b) The presence of rigor mortis or lines of lividity.

    (c) When an infant is born apneic and pulseless, with blistered skin and a strong, disagreeable odor.

    (d) Answers (a) or (b).

    (e) Answers (a), (b), or (c).

84.   In the anatomical position, the ulna is _____ to the humerus.

    (a) proximal

    (b) anterior

    (c) superior

    (d) posterior

    (e) distal

85.   Your patient is a 28-year-old male who opens his eyes only when physically stimulated, has severely slurred speech, and withdraws from pain without appearing to localize the painful site. What is his Glasgow Coma Scale point total?

    (a) 10 points.

    (b) 8 points.

    (c) 15 points.

    (d) 3 points.

    (e) 0 points.

86. After delivering a newborn infant, it is important to _____. Suctioning in an opposite order may cause the baby to gasp and begin breathing, aspirating the fluids or mucus that haven't already been suctioned away.

(a) suction the mouth before suctioning the nostrils

(b) suction the nostrils before suctioning the mouth

(c) suction or remove the drool that is outside the mouth before suctioning the interior airway

(d) Answers (a) or (b), depending upon local protocol

(e) None of the above. Concern for the order of newborn airway suctioning is an "old wives' tale." It does not make a difference

87. Your patient is an unconscious 23-year-old male who was struck once in the head with a wooden baseball bat. Which of the following vital sign patterns suggests that your patient has a head injury serious enough to cause increased intracranial pressure (excess pressure inside his skull, also called the "Cushing's reflex" or "Cushing's Triad")?

(a) Increasing blood pressure; increasing pulse rate; slow, deep, irregular respirations.

(b) Decreasing blood pressure; decreasing pulse rate; slow, shallow, irregular respirations.

(c) Increasing blood pressure; decreasing pulse rate; slow, deep, irregular respirations.

(d) Decreasing blood pressure; increasing pulse rate; rapid, shallow respirations.

(e) Decreasing systolic blood pressure, increasing diastolic blood pressure; rapid, thready pulse; slow, shallow respirations.

88. The *Trendelenburg* position is best defined as when the patient

(a) has his legs straight out or bent, with his upper body (torso and head) elevated at a 45 to 60 degree angle to his buttocks.

(b) has his legs straight out or bent, with his upper body (torso and head) elevated at less than a 45 degree angle to his buttocks.

(c) is lying prone with his feet elevated higher than his head.

(d) is lying supine with his feet elevated higher than his head.

(e) is lying on either his right or left side with his feet elevated higher than his head.

89. Which of the following statements regarding the irrigation of a chemical burn to the eyes is false?

(a) Sterile saline may be used to irrigate the eyes.

(b) Sterile water may be used to irrigate the eyes.

(c) If the chemical is an acid, irrigate the eyes with a diluted sodium bicarbonate solution to neutralize the acid and stop the burning process.

(d) Clean tap water may be used to irrigate the eyes.

(e) Never use any kind of chemical antidote, diluted vinegar solutions, or the like to irrigate the eyes.

90. Which of the following statements regarding emergency medical care for the pregnant trauma patient is true?
  (a) Trauma assessment and treatment is exactly the same for pregnant patients as for any other patient.
  (b) Perform a standard initial trauma assessment and physical examination, obtain the same vital signs, but be sure to obtain the patient's gynecological history when obtaining the patient's medical history.
  (c) Transport the patient on her right side. If the patient requires spinal immobilization, secure her to a long backboard as you would secure any other patient, then elevate the left side of the board to cause the patient's abdomen to shift its weight to the right side.
  (d) Answers (b) and (c) are true.
  (e) None of the above are true.

91. The sternum is _____ to the thoracic spine.
  (a) proximal
  (b) anterior
  (c) superior
  (d) posterior
  (e) distal

92. Use back blows and chest thrusts to clear a complete airway obstruction in patients
  (a) less than 1 year old.
  (b) aged 1 to 8 years old.
  (c) over 8 years old.
  (d) from birth to 8 years old.
  (e) None of the above (these techniques are no longer used).

93. The R of the APGAR mnemonic stands for
  (a) Rigor (stillborn infant).
  (b) Rapid (heart rate or respiratory rate).
  (c) Rate (heart rate or pulse).
  (d) Respiratory effort (rate and effort of respirations).
  (e) Robust (healthy, crying infant).

94. If a newborn infant has a pulse but its breathing is absent or inadequate, ventilate at a rate of
  (a) 12 to 20 times per minute (one ventilation every 3 to 5 seconds).
  (b) 20 to 30 times per minute (one ventilation every 5 to 6 seconds).
  (c) 40 to 60 times per minute (one ventilation every $1\frac{1}{2}$ seconds, or each second).
  (d) 60 to 80 times per minute (one ventilation each second, or 3 ventilations every 2 seconds).
  (e) 80 times per minute (3 ventilations every 2 seconds).

95.   The only injury on the body of your unconscious adult patient is a large hematoma on his right temple. His blood pressure is 100/80, his pulse is 140 per minute, and his respiratory rate is 32 per minute. Which of the following statements regarding this patient is true?

   (a) He is developing increased intracranial pressure (pressure inside his skull).
   (b) He has probably overdosed on drugs or alcohol.
   (c) He is developing neurogenic shock.
   (d) He is developing cardiogenic shock.
   (e) He is in danger of shock from hidden hemorrhage elsewhere in his body.

96.   *Physiology* is the study of

   (a) body structure.
   (b) body function.
   (c) body strength.
   (d) Answers (a), (b), or (c).
   (e) None of the above.

97.   The metatarsals are _____ to the tarsals.

   (a) proximal
   (b) anterior
   (c) superior
   (d) posterior
   (e) distal

98.   The colored area of the eye is called the

   (a) iris.
   (b) cornea.
   (c) sclera.
   (d) pupil.
   (e) conjunctiva.

99.   Which of the following statements regarding interruption of CPR is false?

   (a) CPR may be briefly interrupted for defibrillation or other ALS treatment measures.
   (b) If chest compressions produce vomiting, immediately discontinue CPR until all of the stomach contents have been evacuated or suctioned away, so that additional CPR pauses will not have to occur.
   (c) CPR may be briefly interrupted to move a patient down (or up) a flight of stairs.
   (d) When resuming CPR after an interruption, begin with chest compressions rather than with ventilations.
   (e) Interrupt CPR for no longer than 10 seconds to perform return-of-pulse checks.

100. Your patient is a 37-year-old female who is awake. She obeys commands to perform physical activities appropriately, but she doesn't know the day, date, or where she is. What is her Glasgow Coma Scale point total?

(a) 15 points.

(b) 14 points.

(c) 10 points.

(d) 8 points.

(e) 3 points.

101. Any MOI that causes the head to be abruptly thrust forward will probably produce a _____ injury of the spine.

(a) compression

(b) hyperflexion

(c) hyperextension

(d) distraction

(e) rotation

102. The cervical spine is _____ to the esophagus.

(a) proximal

(b) anterior

(c) superior

(d) posterior

(e) distal

103. Which of the following statements regarding the irrigation of a chemical burn to the eyes is true?

(a) Irrigate a contaminated eye for no more than 10 minutes (transportation should not be delayed longer than that); then bandage both eyes and transport the patient to the emergency department.

(b) Initiate eye irrigation as soon as you discover the MOI, beginning on scene while you prepare a method for irrigation to use en route to the emergency department, and continuing irrigation until you reach the emergency department (the minimum amount of eye-irrigation time is 20 minutes unless you arrive at the emergency department before then).

(c) There is no maximum amount of eye-irrigation time (an alkali burn to the eyes should be irrigated for at least an hour).

(d) Answers (b) and (c) are true.

(e) None of the above is true; irrigation times are specific to each chemical substance and vary widely. Call the Medical Director for instructions prior to beginning irrigation.

104. When artificially ventilating an infant or child, the duration of each ventilation should be

   (a) $\frac{1}{2}$ to 1 second.
   (b) no less than 1 second.
   (c) $1\frac{1}{2}$ to 2 seconds.
   (d) 2 to $2\frac{1}{2}$ seconds.
   (e) $2\frac{1}{2}$ to 3 seconds.

105. Your patient is a 50-year-old female who makes no response to verbal or painful stimuli. She has agonal respirations and no palpable pulses. What is her Glasgow Coma Scale point total?

   (a) 10 points.
   (b) 8 points.
   (c) 5 points.
   (d) 3 points.
   (e) 0 points.

106. In the anatomical position, the palm of the hand is considered to be the _____ surface.

   (a) proximal
   (b) superior
   (c) anterior
   (d) inferior
   (e) posterior

107. Your patient is a 15-year-old female who suffered penetrating trauma to her skull, producing unconsciousness. When you apply physical stimuli, she extends and straightens both her arms and legs. Your patient is exhibiting _____ posturing.

   (a) decerebrate
   (b) coma-position
   (c) concussion
   (d) declinicate
   (e) decorticate

108. The *Fowler's* position is best defined as when the patient

   (a) has his legs straight out or bent, with his upper body (torso and head) elevated at a 45 to 60 degree angle to his buttocks.
   (b) has his legs straight out or bent, with his upper body (torso and head) elevated at less than a 45 degree angle to his buttocks.
   (c) is lying prone with his feet elevated higher than his head.
   (d) is lying supine with his feet elevated higher than his head.
   (e) is lying on either his right or left side with his feet elevated higher than his head.

109. You are off-duty and alone, without a cell phone, when you discover an unresponsive 45-year-old male who occasionally seems to be "gasping" for breath but has no carotid pulse. You should
   (a) begin CPR by performing 30 chest compressions, followed by ventilating the victim twice.
   (b) provide 2 ventilations, followed by performance of 30 chest compressions.
   (c) perform CPR for at least 2 minutes before leaving to find a phone and activate the EMS system.
   (d) immediately leave to find a phone and activate the EMS system. (He's breathing and doesn't require CPR, but he's *unconscious* and requires EMS assistance!)
   (e) Answers (a) and (c).

110. The approximate rate suggested for newborn CPR chest compression performance is _____ times per minute.
   (a) no faster than 50
   (b) approximately 60
   (c) no less than 80
   (d) at least 100
   (e) at least 150

111. A person in the *supine* position is lying
   (a) on his stomach.
   (b) on his side.
   (c) on the floor.
   (d) on a bed with his head elevated 40 degrees.
   (e) on his back.

112. When an MOI such as a direct blow to the top of the head causes the weight of the head to be driven downward into the spine (along a direct line of force), a _____ injury of the spine will probably occur.
   (a) compression
   (b) hyperflexion
   (c) hyperextension
   (d) distraction
   (e) rotation

113. Another term for the anterior surface of the body is the _____ surface.
   (a) dorsal
   (b) ventral
   (c) plantar
   (d) palmar
   (e) inguinal

114. Use the Heimlich maneuver (abdominal thrusts) to clear a complete airway obstruction in patients
    (a) less than 1 year old.
    (b) aged 1 to 8 years old.
    (c) over 8 years old.
    (d) 1 year old and older.
    (e) of all ages (including infants).

115. A trauma patient who is apneic and pulseless will have a Revised Trauma Score of
    (a) 5 points.
    (b) 3 points.
    (c) 2 points.
    (d) 1 point.
    (e) 0 points.

116. When used as a medical term, *abduction* refers to
    (a) movement toward the body.
    (b) movement toward the head.
    (c) movement away from the body.
    (d) movement toward the feet.
    (e) movement toward the back.

117. Your adult patient is unconscious after being struck in the head by a baseball while she was sitting in the grass watching the game. Her signs and symptoms indicate increasing intracranial pressure. Which of the following treatment measures or considerations is false?
    (a) To elevate her head and prevent further intracranial pressure increase, secure her to a long backboard in a "semi-seated" position by creating a wedge of firm blankets between the board and her head, neck, and torso.
    (b) Hyperventilate her with 100 percent oxygen at a rate of at least 20 breaths per minute.
    (c) Perform vital sign checks every 5 minutes.
    (d) Do not attempt to stop the blood flow if she is bleeding from her ears, nose, or mouth.
    (e) Anticipate emesis and be prepared to provide aggressive suctioning.

118. In the anatomical position, the thumb is on the _____ side of the hand.
    (a) superior
    (b) medial
    (c) midline
    (d) inferior
    (e) lateral

119. Which of the following statements regarding incidents of "lay rescuers" (citizens without any medical background) performing CPR on a patient prior to your arrival is true?

   (a) Lay rescuers are trained to begin chest compressions immediately after determining that someone is unconscious, without bothering to check for a pulse.

   (b) Citizens should never be criticized for failing to perform mouth-to-mouth ventilation on a stranger. Providing chest compressions without ventilations is far better than providing no CPR at all.

   (c) If you discover that a lay rescuer initiated chest compressions without first checking for the presence of a pulse, be sure to obtain that individual's name and phone number. It is good "PR" to contact the citizen after the call and explain the correct CPR protocol.

   (d) Answers (a) and (b) are true.

   (e) Answers (b) and (c) are true.

120. When performing two-rescuer CPR on a newborn, the compression/ventilation ratio is

   (a) 5 chest compressions to each ventilation (5:1).

   (b) 15 chest compressions to 2 ventilations (15:2).

   (c) 5 chest compressions to 2 ventilations (5:2).

   (d) 3 chest compressions to each ventilation (3:1).

   (e) 3 chest compressions to 2 ventilations (3:2).

121. A finding noted on both sides of the body (or on both sides of a particular body region or part) may be called _____ finding.

   (a) a unilateral

   (b) a bilateral

   (c) a trilateral

   (d) a quadrilateral

   (e) an unusual

122. Signs and symptoms of an orbital fracture include

   (a) double vision or suddenly decreased visual acuity.

   (b) paralysis of upward gaze.

   (c) numbness above the eye, over the cheek, or in the upper lip.

   (d) Answers (a) and (c).

   (e) Answers (a), (b), and (c).

123. The umbilicus is considered to be in the _____ area of the abdomen.

   (a) superior

   (b) circumflex

   (c) midline

   (d) inferior

   (e) lateral

124. To provide the best possible open airway for infants and children, place a folded towel under the patient's
    (a) head to aid in hyperextension, and to align and maintain the airway in an open, neutral position.
    (b) neck to align and maintain the airway in an open, neutral position.
    (c) torso to align and maintain the airway in an open, neutral position.
    (d) Answers (a) or (b).
    (e) Answers (a) or (c).

125. Which of the following elements is assessed in order to calculate the patient's Revised Trauma Score?
    (1) The patient's systolic blood pressure.
    (2) The patient's diastolic blood pressure.
    (3) The difference between the patient's systolic and diastolic blood pressure (his pulse pressure).
    (4) The patient's respiratory rate.
    (5) The patient's Glasgow Coma Scale.

        (a) 1, 2, 3, 4, and 5.
        (b) 1, 2, 3, and 4.
        (c) 1, 4, and 5.
        (d) 3, 4, and 5.
        (e) 1 and 4.

126. Your patient is a 42-year-old female who suffered blunt trauma to her skull, producing unconsciousness. When you apply physical stimuli, she flexes both wrists, bringing her arms into her chest, and straightens her legs. Your patient is exhibiting _____ posturing.
    (a) decerebrate
    (b) coma-position
    (c) concussion
    (d) declinicate
    (e) decorticate

127. The small toe is on the _____ side of the foot
    (a) superior
    (b) medial
    (c) midline
    (d) inferior
    (e) lateral

128. When using an oral airway adjunct for an infant or child, the EMT should employ

    (a) an entirely different method of airway adjunct sizing than the one used for adults.

    (b) a tongue depressor to push and lift the tongue out of the way, then inserting the adjunct into the airway without rotation.

    (c) the same method of airway adjunct insertion as used for an adult.

    (d) Answers (a) and (b).

    (e) Answers (a) and (c).

129. The maximum (best) APGAR score possible is

    (a) 5.

    (b) 10.

    (c) 15.

    (d) 25.

    (e) 50.

130. The universal single-rescuer CPR compression-to-ventilation ratio for cardiopulmonary arrest victims of all ages (except infants) is

    (a) 5:1 (1 ventilation for every 5 chest compressions).

    (b) 15:2 (2 ventilations for every 15 chest compressions).

    (c) 30:2 (2 ventilations for every 30 chest compressions).

    (d) 15:1 (1 ventilation for every 15 chest compressions).

    (e) 30:1 (1 ventilation for every 30 chest compressions)

131. A patient should be considered to have seriously low blood pressure when the _____ reading is less than _____ mmHg (millimeters of mercury).

    (a) systolic / 150

    (b) diastolic / 90

    (c) systolic / 120

    (d) systolic / 90

    (e) Answers (b) or (c).

132. Rescuer fatigue has been shown to result in inadequate performance of chest compression rates and/or depth. When 2 or more rescuers are available to perform adult CPR, the chest-compressor should switch roles with the ventilator, or be replaced by another chest-compressor, after performing

    (a) 5 cycles of chest compression (approximately 2 minutes).

    (b) 5 minutes of chest compression (approximately 20 cycles).

    (c) 10 cycles of cheste compression (approximately 3 minutes).

    (d) 10 minutes of chest compression (approximately 20 cycles).

    (e) 15 minutes of chest compression (approximately 30 cycles).

133. Which of the following statements regarding trauma and pregnancy is false?
   (a) A pregnant woman normally has a pulse rate that is 10 to 15 beats per minute slower than a nonpregnant woman.
   (b) In the late stages of pregnancy, a woman may have a blood volume that is up to 48% greater than a nonpregnant woman. Thus, a greater blood loss may be required before a pregnant woman shows signs of blood loss.
   (c) Because pregnant women have a slower digestive tract and delayed gastric emptying, they are at a greater risk for vomiting and aspiration of emesis.
   (d) In the late stages of pregnancy, a woman requires 10 to 20% more oxygen than a nonpregnant woman.
   (e) Transport the patient on her left side. If the patient requires spinal immobilization, secure her to a long backboard as you would secure any other patient, then elevate the right side of the board to cause the patient's abdomen to shift its weight to the left side.

134. A person in a *lateral recumbent* position is lying
   (a) on his stomach.
   (b) on his side.
   (c) on the floor.
   (d) on a bed with his head elevated 40 degrees.
   (e) on his back.

135. Which of the following statements regarding the EMT's assessment and treatment of an individual adamantly identified (by family, friends, or police) as being under the influence of alcohol and/or drugs is false?
   (a) No one is ever "just drunk," until after they've been cleared by a thorough emergency department evaluation.
   (b) No one is ever "just high on drugs," until after they've been cleared by a thorough emergency department evaluation.
   (c) Anyone with an altered LOC requires high-flow oxygen administration, thorough prehospital medical assessment and care measures (including a blood sugar measurement and/or glucose administration), and transportation to the emergency department.
   (d) Anyone who battles with the police to the extent that the police employ maximum forms of restraint has an altered LOC until proven otherwise (by an emergency department evaluation), should be supinely restrained on the EMT's wheeled stretcher, thoroughly evaluated and appropriately treated en route to the emergency department.
   (e) Confusion due to intoxication (from drugs or alcohol use, or both) is not the same thing as an altered LOC and does not require emergency care.

The answer key for Test Section Nine is on page 361.

10

Advanced Airway Management (An Elective Section)

Subjects:

- Airway Anatomy Review (repeated per DOT emphasis)
- Adult Orotracheal Intubation
- Pediatric Orotracheal Intubation
- Endotracheal Tube Suctioning
- Nasogastric Tube Insertion

Test Section Ten consists of 75 questions and is allotted 1 hour and 15 minutes for completion.

1.   When breathing through the mouth, the first area that air enters is the
      (a) pharynx.
      (b) nasopharynx.
      (c) larynx.
      (d) hypopharynx.
      (e) oropharynx.

2.   When breathing through the nose, the first area that air enters is the
      (a) pharynx.
      (b) nasopharynx.
      (c) larynx.
      (d) hypopharynx.
      (e) oropharynx.

3.   The area that lies directly above the openings of the windpipe and the tube leading to the stomach is called the
      (a) pharynx.
      (b) nasopharynx.
      (c) larynx.
      (d) hypopharynx.
      (e) oropharynx.

4.   A leaf-shaped valve that prevents food and liquid from entering the wind pipe is called the
      (a) cricoid cartilage.
      (b) larynx.
      (c) valecula.
      (d) epiglottis.
      (e) trachea.

5.   A groovelike space (sometimes considered a structure) that is immediately anterior to the leaf-shaped valve that prevents food and liquid from entering the wind pipe is called the
      (a) cricoid cartilage.
      (b) larynx.
      (c) valecula.
      (d) epiglottis.
      (e) trachea.

6.   The medical term for the "wind pipe" is the
         (a) cricoid cartilage.
         (b) larynx.
         (c) valecula.
         (d) epiglottis.
         (e) trachea.

7.   The firm ring that forms the lower portion of the voice box is the
         (a) cricoid cartilage.
         (b) larynx.
         (c) valecula.
         (d) epiglottis.
         (e) trachea.

8.   The medical term for the "voice box" is the
         (a) cricoid cartilage.
         (b) larynx.
         (c) valecula.
         (d) epiglottis.
         (e) trachea.

9.   The windpipe divides into two large air tubes at a junction called the *carina*.
         The medical term for these air tubes is the
         (a) right and left rhonchi.
         (b) right and left bronchi.
         (c) right and left alveoli.
         (d) anterior and posterior rhonchi.
         (e) anterior and posterior bronchi.

10.   At the end of the respiratory "tree" are groups of tiny sacs. These sacs are called the
         (a) rhonchi.
         (b) bronchi.
         (c) alveoli.
         (d) petechia.
         (e) cilia.

11.   The narrowest area of an infant or child's airway is at the level of the
         (a) cricoid cartilage.
         (b) larynx.
         (c) valecula.
         (d) epiglottis.
         (e) trachea.

12. An ET tube is designed to be inserted through the _____ and into the _____
     (a) cricoid cartilage / larynx
     (b) larynx / trachea
     (c) valecula / larynx
     (d) epiglottis / valecula
     (e) trachea / larynx

13. The medical term *intubation* is best defined as
     (a) an airway maneuver that is too advanced for EMT-Basics.
     (b) the insertion of a tube into the mouth.
     (c) the insertion of a tube.
     (d) the insertion of a tube into the esophagus.
     (e) the insertion of a tube through the nose.

14. The medical phrase *orotracheal intubation* is best defined as
     (a) the insertion of a tube into the trachea via the nose.
     (b) the insertion of a tube into the trachea via the mouth.
     (c) the insertion of a tube into the esophagus via the mouth.
     (d) the insertion of a tube into the esophagus via the nose.
     (e) the insertion of any tube through the nose or mouth.

15. A *laryngoscope* is best defined as an illuminating tool that is inserted into the
     pharynx, and used to visualize the pharynx and
     (a) larynx (vocal cords).
     (b) cricoid cartilage (vocal cords).
     (c) vocal cords (cricoid cartilage).
     (d) trachea (cricoid cartilage).
     (e) nasopharynx.

16. All of the following advantages accompany successful orotracheal intubation, except
     (a) provision of complete control of the patient's airway.
     (b) minimized risk of aspiration.
     (c) better access for suctioning the esophagus.
     (d) better oxygen delivery to the lungs.
     (e) allowance of deeper suctioning of the airways.

17. Complications of orotracheal intubation include all of the following, except
     (a) physical stimulation of the airway may produce a dangerously rapid heart
          rate.
     (b) trauma to lips, teeth, tongue, gums, or airway structures.
     (c) inadequate oxygenation due to prolonged intubation attempts.
     (d) right main-stem intubation.
     (e) esophageal intubation.

18.   Complications of orotracheal intubation include all of the following, except
        (a) stimulation of vomiting.
        (b) self-extubation by the patient who regains consciousness.
        (c) physical stimulation of the airway may produce a dangerously slow heart rate.
        (d) unrecognized accidental extubation during moving or transporting the
             patient.
        (e) self-extubation by the unconscious patient.

19.   The most serious potential complication of orotracheal intubation is
        (a) airway stimulation that produces a rapid heart rate.
        (b) right main stem intubation.
        (c) esophageal intubation.
        (d) stimulation of vomiting.
        (e) patient self-extubation.

20.   Laryngoscope blades come in two general types, curved and straight. Each type of
        blade comes in a variety of sizes, from the smallest size (_____) to the largest size
        (_____).
        (a) 6 / 0
        (b) 3 / 0
        (c) 0 / 6
        (d) 0 / 4
        (e) 4 / 1

21.   The straight laryngoscope blade (a "Miller," "Wisconsin," or "Flagg" blade) is
        designed to be inserted so that the tip of the blade
        (a) enters the valecula and lifts it, indirectly lifting the epiglottis, so that the lower
             airway opening can be visualized.
        (b) is placed under the epiglottis, directly lifting it, to visualize the lower airway
             opening.
        (c) enters the epiglottis, just above the cricoid cartilage, to indirectly lift the
             valecula, so that the lower airway opening can be visualized.
        (d) is placed into the valecula, sliding it to the right side, to visualize the cricoid
             cartilage opening to the airway.
        (e) enters the cricoid cartilage, just above the valecula, to indirectly lift the cricoid
             cartilage and visualize the lower airway opening.

22.   The endotracheal (ET) tube size commonly considered appropriate for the average
        adult male is _____ millimeters in diameter.
        (a) 9.5 to 10.0
        (b) 8.5 to 9.5
        (c) 8.0 to 8.5
        (d) 7.5 to 8.5
        (e) 7.0 to 8.0

23. The curved laryngoscope blade (a "MacIntosh" blade) is designed to be inserted so that the tip of the blade

    (a) enters the valecula and lifts it, indirectly lifting the epiglottis, so that the lower airway opening can be visualized.

    (b) is placed under the epiglottis, directly lifting it, to visualize the lower airway opening.

    (c) enters the epiglottis, just above the cricoid cartilage, to indirectly lift the valecula, so that the lower airway opening can be visualized.

    (d) is placed into the valecula, sliding it to the right side, to visualize the cricoid cartilage opening to the airway.

    (e) enters the cricoid cartilage, just above the valecula, to indirectly lift the cricoid cartilage and visualize the lower airway opening.

24. The ET tube size commonly considered appropriate for the average adult female is _____ millimeters in diameter.

    (a) 9.5 to 10.0

    (b) 8.5 to 9.5

    (c) 8.0 to 8.5

    (d) 7.5 to 8.5

    (e) 7.0 to 8.0

25. In an emergency, an ET tube that is _____ millimeters in diameter may be used for an average adult male or female.

    (a) 9.5

    (b) 8.5

    (c) 7.5

    (d) 6.0

    (e) 5.0

26. At the top of the ET tube is an adapter that is designed to connect the tube with a bag-valve for ventilation. Because there are many manufacturers of both bag-valve-mask devices and ET tubes, this adapter (and the port of the bag-valve) must be of a standard size on all brands. The standard size of the adapter at the top end of an ET tube is

    (a) 5 millimeters.

    (b) 10 millimeters.

    (c) 15 millimeters.

    (d) 20 millimeters.

    (e) 25 millimeters.

27. Many ET tubes have a small hole opposite to the beveled, bottom end of the ET tube. This hole is called "Murphy's eye" and is designed to

    (a) be a port through which an endotracheal suctioning device is passed.

    (b) decrease the chance of ET tube obstruction.

    (c) allow for extra ventilation, in case the selected ET tube is too small for the patient.

    (d) Answers (a) and (b).

    (e) Answers (a), (b), and (c).

28.   At the far end of adult ET tubes is an inflatable cuff. The purpose of this cuff is to

    (a) anchor the tube in place (the inflated cuff is larger than the cricoid cartilage). Thus, if tape or tube-tying material is not immediately available, you do not need to use such devices.

    (b) keep vomitus from entering the ET tube.

    (c) keep air from leaking around the tube (escaping, rather than ventilating the patient).

    (d) Answers (a) and (b).

    (e) Answers (b) and (c).

29.   The ET tube's inflatable cuff holds _____ of air.

    (a) 5 cc

    (b) 10 cc

    (c) 15 cc

    (d) 20 cc

    (e) 30 cc

30.   The ET tube's cuff is inflated by injecting air into the inflation valve at the top of the ET tube. Just beyond the inflation valve is a pilot balloon. The pilot balloon is designed to

    (a) verify that the cuff has inflated and is maintaining its inflation.

    (b) prevent air from escaping the cuff.

    (c) provide an injection site for medications that can be administered through the ET tube.

    (d) Answers (a) and (b).

    (e) Answers (a) and (c).

31.   The length of a standard, adult ET tube is

    (a) 15 centimeters.

    (b) 20 centimeters.

    (c) 25 centimeters.

    (d) 33 centimeters.

    (e) 47 centimeters.

32.   In the average adult, the distance between the teeth and the carina is

    (a) 15 centimeters.

    (b) 20 centimeters.

    (c) 25 centimeters.

    (d) 33 centimeters.

    (e) 47 centimeters.

33. In the average adult, the distance between the teeth and the vocal cords is
   (a) 15 centimeters.
   (b) 20 centimeters.
   (c) 25 centimeters.
   (d) 33 centimeters.
   (e) 47 centimeters.

34. A malleable metal stylet is often used to provide extra stiffness and shape to the ET tube during intubation. Prior to intubation, this stylet should be inserted until the tip of the stylet is
   (a) visible just beyond the ET tube's distal opening.
   (b) between the Murphy's eye and the ET tube's distal opening.
   (c) protruding from the Murphy's eye.
   (d) at the distal end of the inflatable cuff, approximately $1/4$ inch before reaching Murphy's eye.
   (e) Any of the above is acceptable.

35. Which of the following statements regarding use of lubricants for intubation is false?
   (a) Only water-soluble lubricants should be used.
   (b) The stylet may be lubricated to allow for easy removal after intubation.
   (c) A lubricant should be applied to the ET tube prior to intubation.
   (d) Lubrication is mandatory when performing intubation. If a water-soluble lubricant is not available, Vaseline® jelly (or the like) may be used.
   (e) Only sterile lubricants should be used.

36. Indications for the performance of orotracheal intubation include all of the following, except
   (a) the inability to ventilate an apneic patient.
   (b) to protect the airway of a patient who is unresponsive to any painful stimuli.
   (c) to protect the airway of any unconscious patient with no gag reflex.
   (d) to provide the best possible ventilation and airway protection for a cardiac arrest patient.
   (e) to secure the airway of an unconscious patient who coughs when attempts to insert an oropharyngeal airway are made.

37. Prior to an intubation attempt, the adult patient should be hyperventilated with 100% oxygen, using the bag-valve-mask with an oropharyngeal airway in place, at a rate of _____ ventilations per minute.
   (a) 8
   (b) 10
   (c) 12
   (d) 20–24
   (e) 50–60

38. Which of the following statements regarding assembling and preparing the equipment needed for orotracheal intubation is false?

   (a) The selected ET tube's cuff should be inflated and tested for leaks.

   (b) The syringe for air-injection should remain attached to the ET tube cuff inflation valve during intubation.

   (c) A securing device must be within easy reach.

   (d) A functional suction unit must be within easy reach, with a rigid tip suction catheter attached and ready for use.

   (e) A functional suction unit must be within easy reach, with a French (ET tube) suction catheter attached and ready for use.

39. To achieve optimal airway alignment, the correct positioning of the patient's head is vitally important to successful orotracheal intubation. When trauma is not suspected, the patient should be positioned with his

   (a) head and neck in a neutral position, with someone manually maintaining in-line stabilization.

   (b) neck flexed and chin lifted (the "sniffing" position).

   (c) head tilted back and chin lifted.

   (d) Answers (a) or (b).

   (e) Answers (b) or (c).

40. When a trauma patient requires orotracheal intubation, the patient should be positioned with his

   (a) head and neck in a neutral position, with someone manually maintaining in-line stabilization.

   (b) neck flexed and chin lifted.

   (c) head tilted back and chin lifted.

   (d) Answers (a) or (b).

   (e) Answers (b) or (c).

41. When beginning orotracheal intubation, the _____ should be held in the left hand, and the _____ should be held in the right hand.

   (a) suction catheter / laryngoscope

   (b) ET tube / laryngoscope

   (c) laryngoscope / ET tube

   (d) suction catheter / ET tube

   (e) Answers (b) or (c); right-handed and left-handed providers will use opposite techniques.

42. When using the laryngoscope to visualize the glottic opening, the EMT should
   (a) lift the patient's mandible up and away from the patient.
   (b) use a sweeping motion to lift the tongue up and to the left.
   (c) gently use the teeth as a fulcrum for the laryngoscope handle to achieve the best visualization possible.
   (d) Answers (a) and (b).
   (e) Answers (a) or (c), and answer (b), depending upon personal preference.

43. Application of *Sellick's maneuver* during attempts at orotracheal intubation may be helpful. Which of the following statements regarding Sellick's maneuver is false?
   (a) Sellick's maneuver consists of another rescuer using his thumb and index finger to apply direct pressure to the patient's anterior neck, at the cricoid cartilage level.
   (b) Sellick's maneuver consists of the intubating rescuer using the laryngoscope to apply direct pressure to the patient's cricoid cartilage.
   (c) Sellick's maneuver may help to compress the esophagus, thus reducing the risk of vomiting during intubation.
   (d) Sellick's maneuver may help to bring the glottic opening into better view.
   (e) If used, Sellick's maneuver should be continued until the patient is intubated.

44. Which of the following statements regarding visualization of the glottic opening is true?
   (a) The best confirmation of correct ET tube placement is when the ET tube is actually visualized entering the glottic opening.
   (b) Introduction of the ET tube into the oropharynx will always obscure glottic opening visualization; simply hold the laryngoscope steady and blindly advance the ET tube.
   (c) Visualization of the ET tube entering the glottic opening is preferred. However, if the glottic opening cannot be visualized, do not delay intubation. Simply make as many attempts as necessary to pass the ET tube into the trachea (this is often called "blind intubation").
   (d) Answers (b) and (c) are true.
   (e) None of the above answers is true.

45. Do not remove the laryngoscope until after the ET tube's cuff
   (a) has gone through the glottic opening and just past the vocal cords.
   (b) is halfway through the vocal cords.
   (c) has passed the vocal cords by at least 10 centimeters.
   (d) has passed the vocal cords and the tube's adapter is even with the patient's teeth.
   (e) has passed the vocal cords by at least 10 centimeters and the tube cannot be advanced any further.

46. After the tube has been placed, the EMT should
   (a) remove the stylet (if one was used).
   (b) inflate the ET tube's cuff.

    (c) have the bag-valve device attached to the ET tube.

    (d) Answers (a) and (c).

    (e) Answers (a), (b), and (c).

47.   The most accurate way to confirm the correct placement of the ET tube is to

    (a) auscultate for breath sounds over the epigastrium.

    (b) auscultate for breath sounds over the apex of the left lung.

    (c) auscultate for breath sounds over the apex of the right lung.

    (d) visualize the ET tube passing through the vocal cords of the glottic opening.

    (e) Any of the above (all are equally accurate methods of tube placement confirmation).

48.   When verifying correct placement of the ET tube with a stethoscope, the first place the EMT should listen is over the

    (a) epigastrium.

    (b) apex of the left lung.

    (c) apex of the right lung.

    (d) base of the left lung.

    (e) base of the right lung.

49.   After the first intubation attempt, if breath sounds are present and clear on the right, but diminished or absent on the left, the EMT should

    (a) immediately secure the ET tube, hyperventilate the patient, and continue hyperventilation until delivery to the emergency department. (The patient has an absent or collapsed left lung and requires sustained hyperventilation to survive.)

    (b) remove the ET tube and immediately reattempt orotracheal intubation with the same tube.

    (c) deflate the ET tube cuff and slowly withdraw it, without completely removing the tube, while periodically auscultating for improved breath sounds on the left.

    (d) remove the ET tube and immediately reattempt orotracheal intubation with a fresh tube.

    (e) remove the ET tube and discontinue any further attempts at orotracheal intubation.

50.   After intubation, if breath sounds are heard in the epigastrium, the EMT should immediately

    (a) secure the ET tube, hyperventilate the patient, and continue hyperventilation until the patient is delivered to the emergency department. (Both of the patient's lungs have collapsed, and sustained hyperventilation is required if the patient is to survive.)

    (b) deflate the ET tube cuff and completely remove the tube.

    (c) deflate the ET tube cuff and slowly withdraw it, without completely removing the tube, while auscultating for improved breath sounds in either of the lungs.

    (d) check the left lung for breath sounds, followed by checking the right lung for breath sounds.

    (e) remove the ET tube and discontinue any further attempts at orotracheal intubation.

51. Once the epigastrium is free of sounds and breath sounds have been heard over both the right and left lungs, the ET tube should be manually held in place while the patient is appropriately ventilated, and the EMT should

   (a) inflate the ET tube cuff with the appropriate amount of air.

   (b) secure the tube in place with tape or a tube-tie, noting the markers on the tube to record the distance that the tube has been inserted.

   (c) insert an oral airway into the patient's mouth to prevent the patient from obstructing the tube by biting down on it.

   (d) Answers (a) and (b).

   (e) Answers (a), (b), and (c).

52. Following successful orotracheal intubation, the EMT should proceed with normal patient care and transportation measures, remembering that

   (a) after an ET tube has been secured, time does not need to be wasted reassessing breath sounds.

   (b) the external ET tube depth measurement should be frequently checked, to be sure it shows no tube movement.

   (c) breath sounds must be frequently reassessed, especially following every major movement of the patient (such as moving the patient in or out of the ambulance).

   (d) Answers (a) and (b).

   (e) Answers (b) and (c).

53. Indications for orotracheal intubation of pediatric patients include all of the following, except when

   (a) prolonged artificial ventilation will be required.

   (b) adequate artificial ventilation cannot be achieved by other means.

   (c) the pediatric patient is in cardiac arrest.

   (d) the pediatric patient is in respiratory arrest.

   (e) oropharyngeal airway insertion causes the unconscious pediatric patient to cough or sputter.

54. The average size of pediatric ET tubes required by full-term newborns and small infants is _____ millimeters in diameter.

   (a) 1.0

   (b) 2.0

   (c) 3.0 to 3.5

   (d) 4.0

   (e) 5.0 to 6.0

55. The mathematical formula for selecting the best ET tube size for a pediatric patient is as follows: the patient's _____ plus 16, divided by 4, indicates the ET tube size number.

    (a) age

    (b) weight

    (c) height

    (d) Answers (a) or (b).

    (e) Answers (b) or (c).

56. Another means of selecting the best ET tube size for the pediatric patient is to select a tube with a diameter that is the same size as the patient's

    (a) thumb.

    (b) small finger.

    (c) nostril opening.

    (d) Answers (a) or (c).

    (e) Answers (b) or (c).

57. Probably the best (and fastest) method of selecting an ET tube size for intubating the pediatric patient is to

    (a) consult a pediatric information guide that provides age- and weight-related identification of equipment appropriate for use with pediatric patients.

    (b) use a pediatric patient measuring device (such as the Broselow™ tape) to determine the equipment appropriate for use with pediatric patients.

    (c) call the Medical Director and describe the patient's height and weight, requesting official identification of the appropriately sized equipment for each individual pediatric patient.

    (d) Answers (a) or (b).

    (e) None of the above. (There is no "short cut" to knowing the correct size.)

58. Which of the following statements regarding use of ET intubation tubes with or without inflatable cuffs is true?

    (a) Children 8 years old and younger should not be intubated with a cuffed ET tube.

    (b) Uncuffed ET tubes are only used for infant intubation.

    (c) All patients older than 2 years should be intubated with a cuffed ET tube.

    (d) All patients older than 3 years should be intubated with a cuffed ET tube.

    (e) All patients older than 5 years should be intubated with a cuffed ET tube.

59. Which of the following statements regarding laryngoscope blades and orotracheal intubation of pediatric patients is true?

    (a) The EMT should have pediatric sizes of both curved and straight blades.

    (b) The smallest available straight blade is preferred for intubation of infants and small children.

    (c) The smallest available curved blade is preferred for intubation of infants and small children.

    (d) Answers (a) and (b) are true.

    (e) Answers (a) and (c) are true.

60. Which of the following statements regarding considerations related to orotracheal intubation procedure for pediatric patients is false?

    (a) The procedure for pediatric orotracheal intubation is basically the same as for adult orotracheal intubation.

    (b) The artificial ventilation rate that should be performed before and after intubation is faster for children than for adults.

    (c) As in adult patients, orotracheal intubation may stimulate rapid heart rates in pediatric patients. However, pediatric patients have much healthier hearts and are not adversely affected by intubation-related heart rate alterations.

    (d) Just as in adults, if trauma is suspected, the pediatric patient's head and neck must be manually stabilized in a neutral, in-line position during intubation.

    (e) If a pediatric patient's heart rate begins to slow during intubation efforts, immediately remove the laryngoscope blade and the ET tube and hyperventilate the patient.

61. To achieve optimal airway alignment, the correct positioning of the pediatric patient's head is vitally important to successful orotracheal intubation. When trauma is not suspected, the pediatric patient should be positioned with his

    (a) head and neck manually maintained in a neutral position, with in-line stabilization continued until after intubation, when his head is mechanically secured.

    (b) torso elevated by folded towels or a blanket.

    (c) head and neck manually maintained in a neutral position, with his chin lifted into a "sniffing" position.

    (d) Answers (a) and (b).

    (e) Answers (b) and (c).

62. If good visualization of the pediatric glottic opening is not well achieved by the previously mentioned head positioning, the EMT should

    (a) flex the patient's head and neck more forward.

    (b) flex the patient's head and neck more backward.

    (c) turn the patient's head slightly to the left side.

    (d) turn the patient's head slightly to the right side.

    (e) use additional folded towels (or the like) to further raise the patient's torso by one or more inches.

63.   In infants and small children, the best indicators of a correctly placed ET tube and adequately delivered ventilations are an improvement in skin color and when
    (a) breath sounds are heard on the left side of the patient's chest.
    (b) breath sounds are heard on the right side of the patient's chest.
    (c) epigastric sounds are heard (children are "belly" breathers).
    (d) both sides of the chest gently rise and fall with each ventilation.
    (e) the abdomen rises with each ventilation (children are "belly" breathers).

64.   If the ET tube is properly placed (you saw it go through the glottic opening and there are no gastric sounds on ventilation), but the child's chest does not expand adequately with ventilation, the problem is probably an ET tube that is
    (a) blocked by secretions. Suction the tube. If suctioning fails, the tube should be removed and replaced with a fresh tube, after hyperventilation.
    (b) too small for the patient, and air is escaping around the tube at the glottic opening. The tube should be removed and replaced with a larger tube, after hyperventilation.
    (c) too large for the patient. The cricoid cartilage is pinching off the tube, and air is not reaching the lungs. The tube should be removed and replaced with a smaller tube, after hyperventilation.
    (d) Answers (a) or (b).
    (e) Answers (a) or (c).

65.   Indications for adult or pediatric "deep suctioning" of the lower airway (suctioning through the ET tube) include
    (a) when moist, bubbling noises are heard while auscultating the patient's chest during ventilation, indicating that excessive secretions are present in the lower airway.
    (b) when secretions are visible, bubbling up into the ET tube.
    (c) when poor or decreasing compliance (chest excursion) is noticed after ventilating the patient for a period of time.
    (d) Answers (a) and (b).
    (e) Answers (a), (b), and (c).

66.   Using a sterile technique to perform deep suctioning of the lower airway
    (a) is an unrealistic expectation for prehospital emergency care performance. "Clean" suctioning is the best that can be achieved in the field.
    (b) is unnecessary because the suction catheter will be inside the ET tube, and will not contact patient tissues.
    (c) is very important because it is an invasive form of suctioning. A contaminated suction catheter would introduce dangerous pathogens to the highly vulnerable lung tissue of the patient.
    (d) will require too much time to accomplish and would threaten the patient's life by increasing hypoxia from the continued secretion interference. A "clean" suctioning technique is acceptable.
    (e) is only done in school and for testing situations. In "real life," only a fool would bother with sterile techniques in the prehospital emergency care environment.

67. Before inserting a soft (French) suction catheter into the ET tube for deep suctioning, the EMT should

   (a) estimate the length of catheter to be inserted by measuring from the patient's lips, to his ear, to his nipple line (an approximation of the distance from the top of the ET tube to the carina).

   (b) preoxygenate the patient by hyperventilating with a high concentration of oxygen.

   (c) deflate the ET tube's cuff to allow for residual ventilation during ET suction.

   (d) Answers (a) and (b).

   (e) Answers (a), (b), and (c).

68. The suction catheter should be advanced

   (a) until resistance is met or the desired, premeasured, length of catheter is inserted (as far as the carina).

   (b) until 33 centimeters of catheter has been inserted (the length of an average, adult ET tube). If it were advanced any further, the nonsterile catheter would have contact with patient tissues and contaminate the patient.

   (c) as far as it can be inserted (well past the carina). In this way, actual intralung-suctioning is accomplished (hence the name "deep suctioning").

   (d) only until its tip can no longer be visualized in the exposed ET tube (some systems will advance it an additional 3 centimeters, but no more than that).

   (e) Any of the above lengths (every system is different).

69. Suction should be engaged

   (a) while inserting the catheter, to assist in the passage of the catheter down into the ET tube. Discontinue suctioning once the desired level of catheter advancement has been reached. Withdraw the tube without suctioning.

   (b) once the desired level of catheter advancement has been reached. Suction while remaining at that level. Withdraw the tube without suctioning.

   (c) only after the desired level of catheter advancement has been reached. Suction while withdrawing the catheter, twisting the catheter back and -forth as you withdraw.

   (d) Answers (a) or (b).

   (e) Answers (a), (b), or (c).

70. The patient may be deep-suctioned for a maximum of _____ at a time. Hyperventilation of the patient must be repeated before suctioning again.

   (a) 5 seconds

   (b) 15 seconds

   (c) 20 seconds

   (d) 30 seconds

   (e) 1 minute

71.   Complications of deep suctioning via the ET tube include all of the following, except

    (a) oxygen deprivation (hypoxia) and cardiac arrhythmias.

    (b) stimulation of the patient's cough reflex (when the carina is reached).

    (c) damage to the airway's lining (mucosa).

    (d) spasm of the vocal cords.

    (e) bronchospasm (if the catheter advances past the carina).

72.   The purpose of prehospital pediatric nasogastric tube (NG tube) insertion is to

    (a) confirm the placement of an ET tube.

    (b) administer glucose to an unresponsive diabetic patient before transportation to the emergency department.

    (c) reduce gastric distention caused by air having accumulated in the stomach and proximal bowel.

    (d) Answers (a) and (b).

    (e) Answers (a), (b), and (c).

73.   Which of the following is an indication for prehospital insertion of a nasogastric tube in the pediatric patient?

    (a) Inability to ventilate the infant or child due to gastric distention (which often occurs in infants and children from bag-valve-mask ventilations prior to orotracheal intubation).

    (b) An unconscious infant or child with gastric distention.

    (c) An infant or child with an altered level of consciousness from head trauma (head injuries are often accompanied by profuse vomiting).

    (d) Answers (a) and (b).

    (e) Answers (a), (b), and (c).

74.   Which of the following statements regarding complications of pediatric nasogastric tube insertion is true?

    (a) The NG tube may accidentally enter the trachea, especially if the patient has not been intubated with an ET tube.

    (b) Passing of the NG tube may cause nasal trauma, with severe bleeding, or may stimulate vomiting.

    (c) Although it is a rare occurrence, if the patient has major facial or head trauma, the NG tube may pass into the cranium through a basilar skull fracture. (This is why insertion of a nasogastric tube is contraindicated in patients with major facial or head trauma. Consider insertion of an *oro*gastric tube, instead.)

    (d) Answers (a), (b), and (c) are true.

    (e) None of the above is true. Nasogastric tube insertion is not accompanied by any kind of serious complications when the procedure is performed correctly.

75. Which of the following statements regarding NG tube insertion preparation is false?

(a) Measure the NG tube from the tip of the patient's nose, around the ear, to below the xiphoid process to determine the maximum length of insertion.

(b) Measure the NG tube from the tip of the patient's nose, down to the xiphoid process to determine the minimum length of insertion.

(c) Use an 8 French for newborns and infants, or a 10 French for toddlers and preschoolers.

(d) Use a 12 French for school-aged children, or a 14 to 16 French for adolescents.

(e) Lubricate the distal end of the NG tube with a water-soluble lubricant prior to insertion.

The answer key for Test Section Ten is on page 366.

11

ALS-Assist Skills (An Elective Section)

AUTHOR'S NOTE: Each group of questions in this section is headed by the group's subject title. In this way, subjects unrelated to an EMT's local requirements may be skipped.

Subjects:

- Assisting with Endotracheal Intubation
- Assisting with ECG Application and Use
- Assisting with IV Therapy

Test Section Eleven consists of 40 questions and, if the entire section is used, is allotted 40 minutes for completion.

ASSISTING WITH ENDOTRACHEAL INTUBATION

1.   Prior to any intubation attempt, the patient should be hyperventilated with 100% oxygen, at a rate of _____ ventilations per minute.
        (a) 8
        (b) 10
        (c) 12
        (d) 20–24
        (e) 50–60

2.   Which of the following statements regarding bag-valve-mask (BVM) ventilation prior to intubation is true?
        (a) One-person operation of the BVM is the least effective method of delivering ventilations. But, because the patient will soon be intubated, one-person BVM operation is sufficient prior to intubation.
        (b) The BVM must be operated by two EMTs. It is important that the best possible ventilations be delivered to the patient prior to discontinuing ventilation for intubation performance.
        (c) An oral airway must be inserted to achieve optimal BVM ventilations.
        (d) Answers (a) and (c) are true.
        (e) Answers (b) and (c) are true.

3.   To achieve optimal airway alignment, the correct positioning of the patient's head is vitally important for successful orotracheal intubation. When trauma is not suspected, the patient should be positioned with his
        (a) head and neck in a neutral position, with someone manually maintaining in-line stabilization.
        (b) neck flexed and chin lifted.
        (c) head tilted back and chin lifted.
        (d) Answers (a) or (b).
        (e) Answers (b) or (c).

4.   When a trauma patient requires orotracheal intubation, the patient should be positioned with his
        (a) head and neck in a neutral position, with someone manually maintaining in-line stabilization.
        (b) neck flexed and chin lifted.
        (c) head tilted back and chin lifted.
        (d) Answers (a) or (b).
        (e) Answers (b) or (c).

5. Application of *Sellick's maneuver* during orotracheal intubation may be helpful to the person intubating. Which of the following statements regarding the performance of Sellick's maneuver is false?

    (a) Sellick's maneuver consists of the assisting EMT using his thumb and index finger to apply direct pressure to the patient's anterior neck, at the cricoid cartilage level.

    (b) Sellick's maneuver consists of the intubating rescuer using the laryngoscope to apply direct, upward, pressure to the patient's cricoid cartilage. An assisting EMT may be asked to stabilize the patient's cricoid cartilage during this maneuver, by gently placing the palm of his hand on the patient's anterior neck and depressing the neck approximately 1 to 2 inches.

    (c) Sellick's maneuver may help to compress the esophagus, thus reducing the risk of vomiting during intubation.

    (d) Sellick's maneuver may help to bring the glottic opening into better view.

    (e) If used, Sellick's maneuver should be continued until the patient is intubated.

6. If the intubating person asks the assisting EMT to listen for tube placement confirmation, the EMT should first auscultate

    (a) over the epigastrium, to check for noises indicating that air is entering the stomach.

    (b) for breath sounds over the apex of the left lung.

    (c) for breath sounds over the base of the left lung.

    (d) for breath sounds over the base of the right lung.

    (e) for breath sounds over the apex of the right lung.

7. Which of the following statements regarding ventilation of an intubated patient is true?

    (a) While ventilating via an endotracheal (ET) tube as it is being secured to the patient, pay strict attention to keeping the ET tube from moving. Once secured, the ET tube requires no further special attention.

    (b) ET tube ventilation requires strict observation of the centimeter marks along the side of the ET tube. Note the centimeter number at the level of the patient's teeth and ensure that the tube stays at that level.

    (c) Even after the ET tube has been secured to the patient, strict attention must be paid to prevent the ET tube from moving, especially if you must disconnect the bag-valve-mask (for defibrillation or the like).

    (d) Answers (a) and (b) are true.

    (e) Answers (b) and (c) are true.

8.   While ventilating the intubated patient, if the ET tube appears to sink lower into the patient's airway, you should

   (a)   pull it back up and resume ventilation of the patient. Do not interrupt ventilations or the activities of others.

   (b)   leave it where it is; there is no need for concern. The ET tube has a cuff at its distal end, which will hold the tube's opening in the correct place, even though the exposed section of the tube appears shorter. Do not interrupt ventilations or the activities of others.

   (c)   immediately notify the person who performed the intubation. Returning the tube to its correct placement level will require deflation of the tube's cuff and careful withdrawal, while one EMT is ventilating the patient, and another EMT is auscultating the patient's chest.

   (d)   immediately pull the ET tube completely out of the patient's airway and return to bag-valve-mask ventilation. Then notify the person who performed the intubation.

   (e)   Answers (a) or (d), depending on your local protocol.

9.   Considering the anatomy of the human body, an ET tube that appears to sink lower into the patient's airway is most likely entering the patient's

   (a)   left mainstem bronchus.

   (b)   right mainstem bronchus.

   (c)   stomach.

   (d)   esophagus.

   (e)   mediastinum.

10.   While ventilating the intubated patient, if the ET tube appears to begin sliding out of the patient's airway (or you suddenly notice there is more of the tube visible), you should

   (a)   push it back in and resume ventilation of the patient. Do not interrupt ventilations or the activities of others.

   (b)   leave it where it is; there is no need for concern. The ET tube has a cuff at its distal end, which will hold the tube's opening in the correct place, even though the exposed section of the tube appears longer. Do not interrupt ventilations or the activities of others.

   (c)   immediately notify the person who performed the intubation. Checking the tube's placement will require one EMT to auscultate the epigastric area and chest, while another EMT ventilates the patient. If the tube has come out of the trachea or entered the patient's esophagus, it will have to be removed or the patient could die.

   (d)   immediately pull the ET tube completely out of the patient's airway and return to bag-valve-mask ventilation. Then notify the person who performed the intubation.

   (e)   Answers (a) or (d), depending on your local protocol.

11.   When ventilating an intubated patient who has her own respiratory effort, you
       should
       (a) time your ventilations to coincide with the patient's natural inhalations, as
            long as the patient is breathing at an appropriate rate.
       (b) assist the patient to attain a more rapid respiratory rate if she is breathing too
            slowly (or requires hyperventilation). Do this by ventilating with the patient's
            own inhalations, and gently interposing extra ventilations between them.
       (c) continue to observe that the tube placement level does not change, and
            monitor that the patient continues to breathe on her own. A breathing patient
            does not need to be artificially ventilated. Simply hold the bag-valve device
            steady, supporting its weight.
       (d) Answers (a) or (b).
       (e) None of the above. This is a trick question. A patient who is intubated will not
            have her own respiratory effort.

12.   When ventilating an intubated patient, if you notice an increase in the resistance of
       the patient's lungs (if the bag-valve device becomes more difficult to squeeze), it
       may be a sign that
       (a) the patient is waking up. As long as the patient is restrained, disregard the
            increased resistance and squeeze more forcefully to continue ventilations.
       (b) the lungs are being obstructed by something. This is a serious development.
            Immediately notify the intubating EMT.
       (c) the esophagus needs to be decompressed. Notify the intubating EMT only if
            she/he is not busy with other activities (gastric distention in an intubated
            patient is not an immediate concern).
       (d) Answers (a) or (c).
       (e) None of the above. Increased lung resistance is a natural side effect of
            endotracheal ventilation and should be disregarded. Squeeze more forcefully
            to continue ventilations, without interrupting the other provider's activities.

13.   When ventilating an intubated patient, if you notice any change in the resistance of
       the patient's lungs (if the bag-valve device becomes more difficult *or* less difficult to
       squeeze), it may be a sign that
       (a) the patient is about to vomit. Immediately discontinue ventilations and gather
            the suctioning equipment.
       (b) the esophagus needs to be decompressed. Notify the intubating EMT only if
            she/he is not busy with other activities (gastric distention in an intubated
            patient is not an immediate concern).
       (c) the ET tube has slipped out of the trachea or has entered the esophagus. This
            could be a fatal development. Immediately notify the intubating EMT.
       (d) Answers (a) or (b).
       (e) None of the above. Changes in lung resistance (whether increased or
            decreased) are natural side effects of endotracheal ventilation and should be
            disregarded. Continue ventilations without interrupting the other provider's
            activities.

14. When ventilating an intubated cardiac arrest patient who is about to be defibrillated, you should

  (a) continue ventilations without worry. The rubber bag of the bag-valve device is designed to "ground" you and protect you from electrical shock. It is vitally important that a cardiac arrest patient's ventilations not be interrupted, for any reason.

  (b) immediately drop the bag-valve device and get away from the patient. Do not disconnect it from the secured ET tube, because doing so would delay your return to ventilating after the defibrillation.

  (c) remind the defibrillating EMT to deflate the tube's cuff and remove the ET tube before defibrillation.

  (d) carefully disconnect the bag-valve device from the ET tube and then hold the ET tube in place. Make sure that you are not in contact with the patient's lips or body during defibrillation. The plastic ET tube is designed to "ground" you and protect you from electrical shock.

  (e) carefully disconnect the bag-valve device from the ET tube and then move away from the patient.

15. While ventilating an intubated patient, you also need to observe the patient for signs of level of consciousness (LOC) changes. If the patient begins to move, in any manner, you should

  (a) immediately notify the person you are assisting. She/he will want to prevent the patient from attempting to remove the ET tube by administering a sedative via the IV.

  (b) immediately notify the person you are assisting. If the patient's hands are free, they will need to immediately be restrained.

  (c) stop ventilations and observe for a return of the patient's respiratory effort. If the patient has resumed breathing, discontinue ventilations and simply support the weight of the bag-valve device until the ET tube can be removed and a nonrebreather mask applied.

  (d) Answers (a) and (b).

  (e) Answers (a) and (c).

16. While ventilating an intubated patient who has an oropharyngeal airway inserted as a "bite block," if you notice the patient beginning to gag or chew or cough, you should

  (a) partially withdraw the oral airway, removing its tip from the posterior oropharynx, but keeping a portion of the airway between the patient's teeth to continue to act as a bite block. Then, continue ventilations as you notify the person you're assisting of the patient's LOC change.

  (b) hold the oral airway in place (fully inserted), but stop ventilations and observe for a return of the patient's respiratory effort. If the patient has resumed breathing, discontinue ventilations and simply continue holding the airway in place, while supporting the weight of the bag-valve device.

    (c) hold the oral airway in place (fully inserted) and continue ventilations. It may be helpful to tape the airway in place so that the patient cannot dislodge it from the posterior oropharynx.

    (d) remove the oral airway completely, before it stimulates the patient to vomit.

    (e) None of the above. Oral airways are not inserted after a patient is intubated, for any reason (ET tubes are hard enough to be their own "bite block").

17. Which of the following statements regarding assisting with medication delivery via the ET tube is true?

    (a) Only paramedics may administer medications via the ET tube. If asked to assist with this in any manner, the EMT should respectfully (but firmly) decline.

    (b) After the medication is injected down the ET tube, the assisting EMT may be asked to hyperventilate the patient. This will increase the rate of medication absorption.

    (c) After the medication is injected down the ET tube, the assisting EMT should wait for at least 15 seconds before resuming ventilation (to give the medication opportunity to be absorbed). When resumed, ventilations should be very slow to continue allowing the medication to be absorbed.

    (d) Any of the above, depending on local protocols.

    (e) None of the above. Medication does not get injected into the airway!

ASSISTING WITH ECG APPLICATION AND USE

18. The electrocardiogram (ECG) provides graphic information about the

    (a) electrical activity of the heart.

    (b) electrical activity of the brain.

    (c) force and effectiveness of cardiac contraction.

    (d) Answers (a) and (c).

    (e) Answers (a), (b), and (c).

19. EMTs who wish to assist with ECG application and use should learn all of the following, except

    (a) how to turn the machine on and off.

    (b) how to record an ECG strip.

    (c) how to defibrillate a patient using transcranial ECG paddle placement.

    (d) how to change the ECG batteries.

    (e) how to change the ECG paper.

20. Types of electrodes (patches or pads) used for the prehospital ECG include
   (a) small electrodes for monitoring only and large electrodes that can deliver an electrical shock (defibrillate) as well as monitor.
   (b) large electrodes for monitoring only and small electrodes that can deliver an electrical shock (defibrillate) as well as monitor.
   (c) dry (unlubricated) electrodes for monitoring only and prelubricated electrodes that can deliver an electrical shock (defibrillate) as well as monitor.
   (d) Answers (a) or (b), depending upon the brand of the electrode.
   (e) Answers (a), (b), or (c), depending upon the brand of the electrode.

21. Which of the following statements regarding application of ECG electrodes is false?
   (a) The best quality of ECG monitoring is achieved by electrodes placed on dry, bare skin.
   (b) It may be necessary to shave off the patient's hair in the areas where the electrodes will be placed.
   (c) If the patient has very oily skin, it may be necessary to wash the areas where the electrodes will be placed.
   (d) If the patient continues to be very sweaty (after initially wiping the skin dry), consider applying an antiperspirant to the areas where the electrodes will be placed.
   (e) In an emergency, speed is more important than ensuring that electrodes are placed on bare skin. If the electrodes begin to lift off the patient after application to a hairy site, taping over the electrode will hold it in place and allow it to function adequately.

22. Monitoring electrode placement may differ from system to system. The most common placement site for the electrode attached to the white (negative) ECG cable is
   (a) on the right arm or beneath the right clavicle.
   (b) on the left arm or beneath the left clavicle.
   (c) on the right leg or at the lowest corner of the right chest.
   (d) on the left leg or at the lowest corner of the left chest.
   (e) Answers (c) or (d).

23. The most common placement site for the electrode attached to the red (positive) ECG cable is
   (a) on the right arm or beneath the right clavicle.
   (b) on the left arm or beneath the left clavicle.
   (c) on the right leg or at the lowest corner of the right chest.
   (d) on the left leg or at the lowest corner of the left chest.
   (e) Answers (c) or (d).

24. The most common placement site for the electrode attached to the black or green (grounding) ECG cable is
   (a) on the right arm or beneath the right clavicle.
   (b) on the left arm or beneath the left clavicle.

    (c) on the right leg or at the lowest corner of the right chest.

    (d) on the left leg or at the lowest corner of the left chest.

    (e) Answers (c) or (d).

ASSISTING WITH IV THERAPY

25.   The abbreviation *IV* stands for the medical term

    (a) intervascular.

    (b) injection-venous.

    (c) inner-venous.

    (d) into-vessel.

    (e) intravenous.

26.   There are three basic types of IV fluids commonly administered in the prehospital environment. Which of the following statements regarding IV fluid consisting of dextrose 5% in sterile water (D_5W) is false?

    (a) D_5W is a "sugar water" solution that is usually supplied in small quantities (50, 250, and 500 cc bags or bottles).

    (b) D_5W may be used for pediatric patients or adult patients.

    (c) D_5W is only used for patients who do not need "volume replacement."

    (d) Because D_5W is rapidly absorbed by the patient's tissues, it is impossible to "overload" any patient with D_5W, and the EMT need not be concerned about monitoring the fluid flow rate.

    (e) Because D_5W is rapidly absorbed by the patient's tissues, it should not be used for trauma patients or dehydrated medical patients.

27.   Which of the following statements regarding Normal Saline (NS) or Lactated Ringer (LR) IV fluid solutions is false?

    (a) Because NS and LR are most often used as "volume replacement" fluids, they are usually supplied in large (1,000 cc) bags.

    (b) NS and LR are the only IV fluids that should ever be used for diabetics, whether they are trauma patients or medical emergency patients.

    (c) NS and LR are more versatile IV fluids than D_5W, because they may be used for trauma patients or medical emergency patients.

    (d) If NS or LR is used for a patient who does not need "volume" replacement, the infusion rate must be strictly controlled and frequently monitored to prevent fluid overload.

    (e) Some medications cannot be administered through an IV of LR, and IV administration of NS is dangerous for some patients. If both NS and LR are available, be very sure that you correctly select the specific fluid requested by the paramedic you are assisting.

28. There are two basic types of IV fluid administration sets (administration tubing). The primary difference between these sets is the number of drops required to deliver 1 cc (cubic centimeter) or mL (milliliter) of fluid. The IV tubing type that delivers 1 cc with every 60 drops is called the
- (a) mini drip (or micro drip) administration set.
- (b) little drop administration set.
- (c) infant drip (or pedi drip) administration set.
- (d) small drip administration set.
- (e) Answers (b) or (c).

29. The IV tubing type that delivers 1 cc with every 10 or 15 drops is called the
- (a) macro drip (or maxi drip) administration set.
- (b) big drop administration set.
- (c) adult drip administration set.
- (d) large drip administration set.
- (e) Answers (b) or (c).

30. The biggest difference in the physical appearance of these two IV tubing types consists of the different drip rate monitoring chamber configurations. The drip chamber of the IV administration set that delivers _____ drops per 1cc/ml contains a special, tiny metal barrel, from which the drops emerge.
- (a) 10
- (b) 15
- (c) 60
- (d) Answers (a) or (b).
- (e) Answers (b) or (c).

31. Which of the following statements regarding an IV extension tubing set is false?
- (a) Attaching an extension set can make it easier to disrobe the patient without disturbing the IV site.
- (b) IV extension tubing comes in two sizes: a 60 drop/1cc size, and a 10 or 15 drop/1cc size.
- (c) Attaching an extension set can make it easier to carry or move a patient without disturbing the IV site.
- (d) Extension tubing is rarely used with a 10 or 15 drop/1cc administration set, because the extra length may slow the rate of administration.
- (e) If used, extension tubing must be attached to the main tubing and well flushed prior to being connected to the IV catheter.

32. When assisting with IV therapy, non-IV-certified EMT-B responsibilities may include all of the following, except
- (a) inspecting the IV fluid to make sure it is clear and free of contaminants.
- (b) squeezing the IV fluid bag to check for any leaks.

(c) IV needle insertion under the direct supervision of a paramedic.

(d) correctly identifying the requested IV fluid and administration set.

(e) maintaining connection site sterility during assembly.

33. Before connecting the administration set to the IV fluid container, the EMT must

(a) assemble the tubing's flow regulator.

(b) attach a flow regulator to the tubing.

(c) disconnect the flow regulator from the tubing.

(d) close the tubing's flow regulator.

(e) open the tubing's flow regulator.

34. Which of the following statements regarding IV assembly sterility factors is true?

(a) Although it would be best to keep the attaching parts sterile, speed of assembly is more important than sterility in the prehospital emergency setting.

(b) After removal of the tubing spike's protective cover, if the spike contacts an unsterile surface, cleanse it with an alcohol wipe and proceed with assembly.

(c) Antibiotics will be administered at the hospital and will correct any infection caused by nonsterile IV-assembly techniques.

(d) All of the above are true.

(e) None of the above is true.

35. The administration set's drip chamber should be

(a) free of fluid (to avoid obstruction of drip rate visualization).

(b) completely filled with fluid to prevent air from entering the IV tubing.

(c) filled only about one-third-full of fluid (leaving two-thirds of the chamber filled with air).

(d) completely filled with fluid only for the 60 drops/1 cc administration set.

(e) completely filled with fluid only for the 10 or 15 drops/1 cc administration sets.

36. Which of the following statements regarding "flushing" air from the IV tubing is true?

(a) The cap at the patient-connection-end of the tubing must be removed and discarded in order to flush air from any kind of IV tubing.

(b) All of the air bubbles (large and small) must be flushed from the IV tubing.

(c) Expelling excessive IV fluid will alter the patient's fluid "intake" record. Only the largest air bubbles must be flushed from the tubing. Small (2 to 3 cc) air bubbles will not endanger the patient because they will be absorbed by the patient's body tissues.

(d) Answers (a) and (b) are true.

(e) Answers (a) and (c) are true.

37.   When the drips stop dripping in the drip chamber, it means that the IV fluid is no longer flowing through the tubing (into the patient). Which of the following is not a potential cause for the drips to stop dripping?
   (a) A closed flow regulator or a closed tubing clamp.
   (b) IV tubing that has become kinked or folded.
   (c) IV tubing that has become caught under the patient's body or a piece of equipment.
   (d) IV tubing that has become disconnected from the patient's IV catheter.
   (e) The constricting band used to engorge the vein for IV catheter insertion has been left on the patient.

38.   If the IV fluid stops flowing through the patient's IV catheter,
   (a) a blood clot may have formed inside the catheter, rendering the IV site useless.
   (b) the EMT should pull the catheter slightly out of the patient (1 or 2 centimeters), and forcefully squeeze the bag to get the IV running again.
   (c) the EMT should inject 30 to 50 cc of air through the medication administration port, to clear the IV of debris, and get it running again.
   (d) Answers (b) or (c).
   (e) Answers (a), (b), or (c).

39.   A "runaway IV"
   (a) is an IV that is flowing too fast (faster than what the patient's condition requires).
   (b) is when the IV needle or catheter has punctured the vein, and fluid is flowing into the tissues around the IV site instead of into the vein.
   (c) may cause a fluid overload that can create serious problems for the patient.
   (d) Answers (a) and (c).
   (e) Answers (a), (b), and (c).

40.   An "infiltrated IV"
   (a) is an IV that is flowing too fast (faster than what the patient's condition requires).
   (b) is when the IV needle or catheter has punctured the vein, and fluid is flowing into the tissues around the IV site instead of into the vein.
   (c) may cause a fluid overload that can create serious problems for the patient.
   (d) Answers (a) and (c).
   (e) Answers (b) and (c).

The answer key for Test Section Eleven is on page 369.

Appendix
Contents

DIRECTIONS FOR COPYING THE MASTER BLANK ANSWER SHEETS

To use this Self-Test text, photocopy the "Blank Answer Sheet" forms we have created and included in this text. (We have provided two copies of each.) The first page of our Blank Answer Sheet form provides answer sets for questions 1 through 120. The second page provides another 120 answer sets (questions 121 through 240), for a total of 240 answer sets if both pages are copied. But, only 4 of the 11 Test Sections go over 120 questions. So, you don't need to make 11 copies of the second Blank Answer Sheet.

To make a *full set* of Blank Answer Sheets (to use all 11 Test Sections):

- Make 11 photocopies of a Blank Answer Sheet page 1.
- Make 4 photocopies of a Blank Answer Sheet page 2 (for Test Sections One, Four, Five, and Nine).

EMT-B National Standards Self Test, 3ʳᵈ Edition

BLANK ANSWER SHEET Page 1 for Test Section _____.

#		#		#	
1. ⓐ ⓑ ⓒ ⓓ ⓔ		25. ⓐ ⓑ ⓒ ⓓ ⓔ		49. ⓐ ⓑ ⓒ ⓓ ⓔ	
2. ⓐ ⓑ ⓒ ⓓ ⓔ		26. ⓐ ⓑ ⓒ ⓓ ⓔ		50. ⓐ ⓑ ⓒ ⓓ ⓔ	
3. ⓐ ⓑ ⓒ ⓓ ⓔ		27. ⓐ ⓑ ⓒ ⓓ ⓔ		51. ⓐ ⓑ ⓒ ⓓ ⓔ	
4. ⓐ ⓑ ⓒ ⓓ ⓔ		28. ⓐ ⓑ ⓒ ⓓ ⓔ		52. ⓐ ⓑ ⓒ ⓓ ⓔ	
5. ⓐ ⓑ ⓒ ⓓ ⓔ		29. ⓐ ⓑ ⓒ ⓓ ⓔ		53. ⓐ ⓑ ⓒ ⓓ ⓔ	
6. ⓐ ⓑ ⓒ ⓓ ⓔ		30. ⓐ ⓑ ⓒ ⓓ ⓔ		54. ⓐ ⓑ ⓒ ⓓ ⓔ	
7. ⓐ ⓑ ⓒ ⓓ ⓔ		31. ⓐ ⓑ ⓒ ⓓ ⓔ		55. ⓐ ⓑ ⓒ ⓓ ⓔ	
8. ⓐ ⓑ ⓒ ⓓ ⓔ		32. ⓐ ⓑ ⓒ ⓓ ⓔ		56. ⓐ ⓑ ⓒ ⓓ ⓔ	
9. ⓐ ⓑ ⓒ ⓓ ⓔ		33. ⓐ ⓑ ⓒ ⓓ ⓔ		57. ⓐ ⓑ ⓒ ⓓ ⓔ	
10. ⓐ ⓑ ⓒ ⓓ ⓔ		34. ⓐ ⓑ ⓒ ⓓ ⓔ		58. ⓐ ⓑ ⓒ ⓓ ⓔ	
11. ⓐ ⓑ ⓒ ⓓ ⓔ		35. ⓐ ⓑ ⓒ ⓓ ⓔ		59. ⓐ ⓑ ⓒ ⓓ ⓔ	
12. ⓐ ⓑ ⓒ ⓓ ⓔ		36. ⓐ ⓑ ⓒ ⓓ ⓔ		60. ⓐ ⓑ ⓒ ⓓ ⓔ	
13. ⓐ ⓑ ⓒ ⓓ ⓔ		37. ⓐ ⓑ ⓒ ⓓ ⓔ		61. ⓐ ⓑ ⓒ ⓓ ⓔ	
14. ⓐ ⓑ ⓒ ⓓ ⓔ		38. ⓐ ⓑ ⓒ ⓓ ⓔ		62. ⓐ ⓑ ⓒ ⓓ ⓔ	
15. ⓐ ⓑ ⓒ ⓓ ⓔ		39. ⓐ ⓑ ⓒ ⓓ ⓔ		63. ⓐ ⓑ ⓒ ⓓ ⓔ	
16. ⓐ ⓑ ⓒ ⓓ ⓔ		40. ⓐ ⓑ ⓒ ⓓ ⓔ		64. ⓐ ⓑ ⓒ ⓓ ⓔ	
17. ⓐ ⓑ ⓒ ⓓ ⓔ		41. ⓐ ⓑ ⓒ ⓓ ⓔ		65. ⓐ ⓑ ⓒ ⓓ ⓔ	
18. ⓐ ⓑ ⓒ ⓓ ⓔ		42. ⓐ ⓑ ⓒ ⓓ ⓔ		66. ⓐ ⓑ ⓒ ⓓ ⓔ	
19. ⓐ ⓑ ⓒ ⓓ ⓔ		43. ⓐ ⓑ ⓒ ⓓ ⓔ		67. ⓐ ⓑ ⓒ ⓓ ⓔ	
20. ⓐ ⓑ ⓒ ⓓ ⓔ		44. ⓐ ⓑ ⓒ ⓓ ⓔ		68. ⓐ ⓑ ⓒ ⓓ ⓔ	
21. ⓐ ⓑ ⓒ ⓓ ⓔ		45. ⓐ ⓑ ⓒ ⓓ ⓔ		69. ⓐ ⓑ ⓒ ⓓ ⓔ	
22. ⓐ ⓑ ⓒ ⓓ ⓔ		46. ⓐ ⓑ ⓒ ⓓ ⓔ		70. ⓐ ⓑ ⓒ ⓓ ⓔ	
23. ⓐ ⓑ ⓒ ⓓ ⓔ		47. ⓐ ⓑ ⓒ ⓓ ⓔ		71. ⓐ ⓑ ⓒ ⓓ ⓔ	
24. ⓐ ⓑ ⓒ ⓓ ⓔ		48. ⓐ ⓑ ⓒ ⓓ ⓔ		72. ⓐ ⓑ ⓒ ⓓ ⓔ	

#		#	
73. ⓐ ⓑ ⓒ ⓓ ⓔ		97. ⓐ ⓑ ⓒ ⓓ ⓔ	
74. ⓐ ⓑ ⓒ ⓓ ⓔ		98. ⓐ ⓑ ⓒ ⓓ ⓔ	
75. ⓐ ⓑ ⓒ ⓓ ⓔ		99. ⓐ ⓑ ⓒ ⓓ ⓔ	
76. ⓐ ⓑ ⓒ ⓓ ⓔ		100. ⓐ ⓑ ⓒ ⓓ ⓔ	
77. ⓐ ⓑ ⓒ ⓓ ⓔ		101. ⓐ ⓑ ⓒ ⓓ ⓔ	
78. ⓐ ⓑ ⓒ ⓓ ⓔ		102. ⓐ ⓑ ⓒ ⓓ ⓔ	
79. ⓐ ⓑ ⓒ ⓓ ⓔ		103. ⓐ ⓑ ⓒ ⓓ ⓔ	
80. ⓐ ⓑ ⓒ ⓓ ⓔ		104. ⓐ ⓑ ⓒ ⓓ ⓔ	
81. ⓐ ⓑ ⓒ ⓓ ⓔ		105. ⓐ ⓑ ⓒ ⓓ ⓔ	
82. ⓐ ⓑ ⓒ ⓓ ⓔ		106. ⓐ ⓑ ⓒ ⓓ ⓔ	
83. ⓐ ⓑ ⓒ ⓓ ⓔ		107. ⓐ ⓑ ⓒ ⓓ ⓔ	
84. ⓐ ⓑ ⓒ ⓓ ⓔ		108. ⓐ ⓑ ⓒ ⓓ ⓔ	
85. ⓐ ⓑ ⓒ ⓓ ⓔ		109. ⓐ ⓑ ⓒ ⓓ ⓔ	
86. ⓐ ⓑ ⓒ ⓓ ⓔ		110. ⓐ ⓑ ⓒ ⓓ ⓔ	
87. ⓐ ⓑ ⓒ ⓓ ⓔ		111. ⓐ ⓑ ⓒ ⓓ ⓔ	
88. ⓐ ⓑ ⓒ ⓓ ⓔ		112. ⓐ ⓑ ⓒ ⓓ ⓔ	
89. ⓐ ⓑ ⓒ ⓓ ⓔ		113. ⓐ ⓑ ⓒ ⓓ ⓔ	
90. ⓐ ⓑ ⓒ ⓓ ⓔ		114. ⓐ ⓑ ⓒ ⓓ ⓔ	
91. ⓐ ⓑ ⓒ ⓓ ⓔ		115. ⓐ ⓑ ⓒ ⓓ ⓔ	
92. ⓐ ⓑ ⓒ ⓓ ⓔ		116. ⓐ ⓑ ⓒ ⓓ ⓔ	
93. ⓐ ⓑ ⓒ ⓓ ⓔ		117. ⓐ ⓑ ⓒ ⓓ ⓔ	
94. ⓐ ⓑ ⓒ ⓓ ⓔ		118. ⓐ ⓑ ⓒ ⓓ ⓔ	
95. ⓐ ⓑ ⓒ ⓓ ⓔ		119. ⓐ ⓑ ⓒ ⓓ ⓔ	
96. ⓐ ⓑ ⓒ ⓓ ⓔ		120. ⓐ ⓑ ⓒ ⓓ ⓔ	

EMT-B National Standards Self Test, 3rd Edition

BLANK ANSWER SHEET Page 2 for Test Section _____

121. (a) (b) (c) (d) (e)
122. (a) (b) (c) (d) (e)
123. (a) (b) (c) (d) (e)
124. (a) (b) (c) (d) (e)
125. (a) (b) (c) (d) (e)
126. (a) (b) (c) (d) (e)
127. (a) (b) (c) (d) (e)
128. (a) (b) (c) (d) (e)
129. (a) (b) (c) (d) (e)
130. (a) (b) (c) (d) (e)
131. (a) (b) (c) (d) (e)
132. (a) (b) (c) (d) (e)
133. (a) (b) (c) (d) (e)
134. (a) (b) (c) (d) (e)
135. (a) (b) (c) (d) (e)
136. (a) (b) (c) (d) (e)
137. (a) (b) (c) (d) (e)
138. (a) (b) (c) (d) (e)
139. (a) (b) (c) (d) (e)
140. (a) (b) (c) (d) (e)
141. (a) (b) (c) (d) (e)
142. (a) (b) (c) (d) (e)
143. (a) (b) (c) (d) (e)
144. (a) (b) (c) (d) (e)

145. (a) (b) (c) (d) (e)
146. (a) (b) (c) (d) (e)
147. (a) (b) (c) (d) (e)
148. (a) (b) (c) (d) (e)
149. (a) (b) (c) (d) (e)
150. (a) (b) (c) (d) (e)
151. (a) (b) (c) (d) (e)
152. (a) (b) (c) (d) (e)
153. (a) (b) (c) (d) (e)
154. (a) (b) (c) (d) (e)
155. (a) (b) (c) (d) (e)
156. (a) (b) (c) (d) (e)
157. (a) (b) (c) (d) (e)
158. (a) (b) (c) (d) (e)
159. (a) (b) (c) (d) (e)
160. (a) (b) (c) (d) (e)
161. (a) (b) (c) (d) (e)
162. (a) (b) (c) (d) (e)
163. (a) (b) (c) (d) (e)
164. (a) (b) (c) (d) (e)
165. (a) (b) (c) (d) (e)
166. (a) (b) (c) (d) (e)
167. (a) (b) (c) (d) (e)
168. (a) (b) (c) (d) (e)

169. (a) (b) (c) (d) (e)
170. (a) (b) (c) (d) (e)
171. (a) (b) (c) (d) (e)
172. (a) (b) (c) (d) (e)
173. (a) (b) (c) (d) (e)
174. (a) (b) (c) (d) (e)
175. (a) (b) (c) (d) (e)
176. (a) (b) (c) (d) (e)
177. (a) (b) (c) (d) (e)
178. (a) (b) (c) (d) (e)
179. (a) (b) (c) (d) (e)
180. (a) (b) (c) (d) (e)
181. a (b) (c) (d) (e)
182. (a) (b) (c) (d) (e)
183. (a) (b) (c) (d) (e)
184. (a) (b) (c) (d) (e)
185. (a) (b) (c) (d) (e)
186. (a) (b) (c) (d) (e)
187. (a) (b) (c) (d) (e)
188. (a) (b) (c) (d) (e)
189. (a) (b) (c) (d) (e)
190. (a) (b) (c) (d) (e)
191. (a) (b) (c) (d) (e)
192. (a) (b) (c) (d) (e)

193. (a) (b) (c) (d) (e)
194. (a) (b) (c) (d) (e)
195. (a) (b) (c) (d) (e)
196. (a) (b) (c) (d) (e)
197. (a) (b) (c) (d) (e)
198. (a) (b) (c) (d) (e)
199. (a) (b) (c) (d) (e)
200. (a) (b) (c) (d) (e)
201. (a) (b) (c) (d) (e)
202. (a) (b) (c) (d) (e)
203. (a) (b) (c) (d) (e)
204. (a) (b) (c) (d) (e)
205. (a) (b) (c) (d) (e)
206. (a) (b) (c) (d) (e)
207. (a) (b) (c) (d) (e)
208. (a) (b) (c) (d) (e)
209. (a) (b) (c) (d) (e)
210. (a) (b) (c) (d) (e)
211. (a) (b) (c) (d) (e)
212. (a) (b) (c) (d) (e)
213. (a) (b) (c) (d) (e)
214. (a) (b) (c) (d) (e)
215. (a) (b) (c) (d) (e)
216. (a) (b) (c) (d) (e)

217. (a) (b) (c) (d) (e)
218. (a) (b) (c) (d) (e)
219. (a) (b) (c) (d) (e)
220. (a) (b) (c) (d) (e)
221. (a) (b) (c) (d) (e)
222. (a) (b) (c) (d) (e)
223. (a) (b) (c) (d) (e)
224. (a) (b) (c) (d) (e)
225. (a) (b) (c) (d) (e)
226. (a) (b) (c) (d) (e)
227. (a) (b) (c) (d) (e)
228. (a) (b) (c) (d) (e)
229. (a) (b) (c) (d) (e)
230. (a) (b) (c) (d) (e)
231. (a) (b) (c) (d) (e)
232. (a) (b) (c) (d) (e)
233. (a) (b) (c) (d) (e)
234. (a) (b) (c) (d) (e)
235. (a) (b) (c) (d) (e)
236. (a) (b) (c) (d) (e)
237. (a) (b) (c) (d) (e)
238. (a) (b) (c) (d) (e)
239. (a) (b) (c) (d) (e)
240. (a) (b) (c) (d) (e)

EMT-B National Standards Self Test, 3rd Edition
BLANK ANSWER SHEET Page 1 for Test Section _____.

1. (a) (b) (c) (d) (e)
2. (a) (b) (c) (d) (e)
3. (a) (b) (c) (d) (e)
4. (a) (b) (c) (d) (e)
5. (a) (b) (c) (d) (e)
6. (a) (b) (c) (d) (e)
7. (a) (b) (c) (d) (e)
8. (a) (b) (c) (d) (e)
9. (a) (b) (c) (d) (e)
10. (a) (b) (c) (d) (e)
11. (a) (b) (c) (d) (e)
12. (a) (b) (c) (d) (e)
13. (a) (b) (c) (d) (e)
14. (a) (b) (c) (d) (e)
15. (a) (b) (c) (d) (e)
16. (a) (b) (c) (d) (e)
17. (a) (b) (c) (d) (e)
18. (a) (b) (c) (d) (e)
19. (a) (b) (c) (d) (e)
20. (a) (b) (c) (d) (e)
21. (a) (b) (c) (d) (e)
22. (a) (b) (c) (d) (e)
23. (a) (b) (c) (d) (e)
24. (a) (b) (c) (d) (e)

25. (a) (b) (c) (d) (e)
26. (a) (b) (c) (d) (e)
27. (a) (b) (c) (d) (e)
28. (a) (b) (c) (d) (e)
29. (a) (b) (c) (d) (e)
30. (a) (b) (c) (d) (e)
31. (a) (b) (c) (d) (e)
32. (a) (b) (c) (d) (e)
33. (a) (b) (c) (d) (e)
34. (a) (b) (c) (d) (e)
35. (a) (b) (c) (d) (e)
36. (a) (b) (c) (d) (e)
37. (a) (b) (c) (d) (e)
38. (a) (b) (c) (d) (e)
39. (a) (b) (c) (d) (e)
40. (a) (b) (c) (d) (e)
41. (a) (b) (c) (d) (e)
42. (a) (b) (c) (d) (e)
43. (a) (b) (c) (d) (e)
44. (a) (b) (c) (d) (e)
45. (a) (b) (c) (d) (e)
46. (a) (b) (c) (d) (e)
47. (a) (b) (c) (d) (e)
48. (a) (b) (c) (d) (e)

49. (a) (b) (c) (d) (e)
50. (a) (b) (c) (d) (e)
51. (a) (b) (c) (d) (e)
52. (a) (b) (c) (d) (e)
53. (a) (b) (c) (d) (e)
54. (a) (b) (c) (d) (e)
55. (a) (b) (c) (d) (e)
56. (a) (b) (c) (d) (e)
57. (a) (b) (c) (d) (e)
58. (a) (b) (c) (d) (e)
59. (a) (b) (c) (d) (e)
60. (a) (b) (c) (d) (e)
61. (a) (b) (c) (d) (e)
62. (a) (b) (c) (d) (e)
63. (a) (b) (c) (d) (e)
64. (a) (b) (c) (d) (e)
65. (a) (b) (c) (d) (e)
66. (a) (b) (c) (d) (e)
67. (a) (b) (c) (d) (e)
68. (a) (b) (c) (d) (e)
69. (a) (b) (c) (d) (e)
70. (a) (b) (c) (d) (e)
71. (a) (b) (c) (d) (e)
72. (a) (b) (c) (d) (e)

73. (a) (b) (c) (d) (e)
74. (a) (b) (c) (d) (e)
75. (a) (b) (c) (d) (e)
76. (a) (b) (c) (d) (e)
77. (a) (b) (c) (d) (e)
78. (a) (b) (c) (d) (e)
79. (a) (b) (c) (d) (e)
80. (a) (b) (c) (d) (e)
81. (a) (b) (c) (d) (e)
82. (a) (b) (c) (d) (e)
83. (a) (b) (c) (d) (e)
84. (a) (b) (c) (d) (e)
85. (a) (b) (c) (d) (e)
86. (a) (b) (c) (d) (e)
87. (a) (b) (c) (d) (e)
88. (a) (b) (c) (d) (e)
89. (a) (b) (c) (d) (e)
90. (a) (b) (c) (d) (e)
91. (a) (b) (c) (d) (e)
92. (a) (b) (c) (d) (e)
93. (a) (b) (c) (d) (e)
94. (a) (b) (c) (d) (e)
95. (a) (b) (c) (d) (e)
96. (a) (b) (c) (d) (e)

97. (a) (b) (c) (d) (e)
98. (a) (b) (c) (d) (e)
99. (a) (b) (c) (d) (e)
100. (a) (b) (c) (d) (e)
101. (a) (b) (c) (d) (e)
102. (a) (b) (c) (d) (e)
103. (a) (b) (c) (d) (e)
104. (a) (b) (c) (d) (e)
105. (a) (b) (c) (d) (e)
106. (a) (b) (c) (d) (e)
107. (a) (b) (c) (d) (e)
108. (a) (b) (c) (d) (e)
109. (a) (b) (c) (d) (e)
110. (a) (b) (c) (d) (e)
111. (a) (b) (c) (d) (e)
112. (a) (b) (c) (d) (e)
113. (a) (b) (c) (d) (e)
114. (a) (b) (c) (d) (e)
115. (a) (b) (c) (d) (e)
116. (a) (b) (c) (d) (e)
117. (a) (b) (c) (d) (e)
118. (a) (b) (c) (d) (e)
119. (a) (b) (c) (d) (e)
120. (a) (b) (c) (d) (e)